Optimization in Drug Discovery

METHODS IN PHARMACOLOGY AND TOXICOLOGY

Y. James Kang, Series Editor

Optimization in Drug Discovery: In Vitro Methods, edited by **Zhengyin Yan** *and* **Gary W. Caldwell**, *2004*

Cardiac Drug Development Guide, edited by **Michael K. Pugsley**, *2003*

Apoptosis Methods in Pharmacology and Toxicology: Approaches to Measurement and Quantification, edited by **Myrtle A. Davis**, *2002*

Ion Channel Localization: Methods and Protocols, edited by **Anatoli N. Lopatin** *and* **Colin G. Nichols**, *2001*

Preface

Recent analyses of drug attrition rates reveal that a significant number of drug candidates fail in the later stage of clinical development owing to absorption, distribution, metabolism, elimination (ADME), and toxicity issues. Lead optimization in drug discovery, a process attempting to uncover and correct these defects of drug candidates, is highly beneficial in lowering the cost and time to develop therapeutic drugs by reducing drug candidate failures in development.

At present, parallel synthesis combining with high-throughput screening has made it easier to generate highly potent compounds (i.e., hits). However, to be a potential drug, a hit must have drug-like characteristics in addition to potency, which include optimal physicochemical properties, reasonable pharmacokinetic parameters, and good safety profiles. Therefore, research tools must be available in drug discovery to rapidly screen for compounds with favorable drug-like properties, and thus adequate resources can be directed to projects with high potential. *Optimization in Drug Discovery: In Vitro Methods* is a compilation of detailed experimental protocols necessary for setting up a variety of assays important in compound evaluation. A total of 25 chapters, contributed by many experts in their research areas, cover a wide spectrum of subjects including physicochemical properties, absorption, plasma binding, metabolism, drug interactions, and toxicity.

A good pharmacokinetic profile has long been recognized as an important drug-like characteristic. Pharmacokinetic parameters are affected by many properties of drug molecules such as physicochemical nature, absorption, metabolic stability, and so on. Physicochemical properties influence the transfer of a drug across cell membranes, and thus affect absorption and distribution of the drug. Chapter 1 provides experimental methods measuring pK_a solubility and lipophilicity, the most fundamental physicochemical properties of a drug candidate. These parameters are vital for preparing an optimal drug formulation. A good absorption profile is another important requirement for drug effectiveness. Drug absorption is primarily governed by a passive transport mechanism, and many drug transporters play a very important role in absorption and disposition. Several chapters address different issues on this aspect. The Caco-2 model described in Chapter 2 is most commonly used to investigate drug absorption mechanism. Parallel artificial membrane permeability (PAMPA) is a rapid screening approach for the earliest ADME primary screening of research compounds. Chapter 3 covers a wide background about PAMPA and also experimental procedures to perform the assay. The perfused rat intestinal model outlined in Chapter 4 has long been considered the definitive or "gold standard" for evaluation of drug absorption. Because CNS drugs need to penetrate the blood–brain barrier, the brain microvessel endothelial cell model has recently been proposed (Chapter 5) to screen compounds targeting CNS diseases. Because of important roles played by the transporter P-glycoprotein (MDR1) in absorption and resistance in anticancer chemotherapy, an enzymatic activity-based method is described in Chapter 6 for rapidly screening MDR1 substrates; the following chapter outlines a different approach to investigate the involvement of drug transporters using oocytes injected with cRNAs (Chapter 7).

Plasma protein binding may also have significant effects on a wide variety of phenomena such as pharmacokinetics, drug–drug interaction potential, or interindividual variability. Chapters 8 and 9 present several different methods evaluating plasma protein binding, which include equilibrium dialysis, ultrafiltration and isothermal titration calorimetry. It is obvious that each approach has unique advantages.

Optimal metabolic stability is essential for a drug to have lasting pharmacological effects on the action site. With respect to optimizing pharmacokinetic parameters such as bioavailability and clearance, the metabolic stability of drug candidates can be determined from in vitro incubations with either hepatocytes or microsomes as described in Chapter 10. As stated, each metabolism system has clear advantages and bears different objectives. Characterization of major metabolites in drug discovery has unique objectives: (1) identifying potent metabolites with better "drug-like" properties; (2) understanding the metabolism fate of drug candidates; and (3) using metabolism information to guide new synthesis and generate more stable compounds. Chapter 11 outlines methods for identifying oxidative metabolites using microsomes or S9 fractions. Glucuronidation catalyzed by UDP-glucuronosyltransferases (UGTs) represents another important drug metabolism pathway. Chapter 12 describes a general approach identifying UGTs responsible for metabolizing a given drug candidate.

For safety reasons, drug–drug interaction has been of increasing concern in drug discovery. Most drug interactions involve alternations in the metabolic pathways within the cytochrome P450 (CYP) system. Induction of CYP expressions by a given drug could lead to lower efficacy of the drug and coadministered agents. CYP induction can be evaluated using human hepatocytes as described in Chapter 13. Inhibition of CYPs is currently recognized as the major mechanism for drug–drug interactions observed in clinic. CYP inhibition can be assessed in different in vitro systems. Chapter 14 describes a high throughput approach screening for 13 individual CYPs by using fluorescent substrates and cDNA-expressed enzymes, and Chapter 15 presents a traditional method assessing the inhibition of those major CYPs in human liver microsomes. Each system has its own advantages and limitations, and the decision to use a particular approach depends on the goal of the drug evaluation. CYP inhibition can be further classified into reversible and irreversible, and understanding the inhibition mechanism is critical for compound selection in drug discovery. A systemic approach is given in Chapter 16 to identify mechanism-based CYP inhibitors. Drug interaction related to the phase II reaction of glucuronidation is not covered in this book.

Toxicity is a major cause of drug candidate failures in both clinical development and after market launch. One aspect of toxicity results from the interaction of a drug or its metabolites with either nucleic acids or specific proteins important in normal cellular function. The interaction of xenobiotics with DNAs potentially results in DNA damage or covalent modifications, leading to genotoxicity. As assessment of genotoxicity remains an important aspect in drug discovery and development, several chapters are devoted to genotoxicity assessment. In Chapter 17, detection of DNA adducts is described using ^{32}P-postlabeling combining with PAGE or HPLC radioactive analysis; analysis of CYP-mediated covalent DNA adducts is presented in Chapter 18. Two methods detecting DNA damage at the level of individual eukaryotes induced by xenobiotics are provided, including a traditional Comet assay (Chapter 19) and a rapid cell-based reporter system (Chapter 20). Although the Ames test has long been used to detect mutagens and possible carcinogens, an improved version assay given in Chapter 21 significantly reduces background resulting from contamination in S9 fractions. Also, a modified mouse lymphoma assay (MLA) is outlined in Chapter 22, because this assay has been recommended as one of core toxicology tests.

Toxicity caused by interaction of a drug or its metabolites with cellular proteins is more difficult to detect, simply because both targeting proteins and interaction mechanism (covalent or noncovalent) are largely unknown at the drug discovery stage. Because of the complexity of this aspect, this book only treats several topics of more general interest. As QT prolongation caused by interaction of drug molecules with HERG channels remains to be a common concern in drug discovery, a high throughput in vitro assay is devised in Chapter 23 to screen compounds for interaction with HERG. Recently, it has been recognized that covalent modification of cellular proteins by reactive drug metabolites is potentially associated with idiosyncratic toxicity. Reactive metabolites generated by CYPs can be trapped by the addition of glutathione to in vitro incubations and structurally characterized using mass spectrometry (Chapter 24). Another well-known class of reactive metabolites is acyl glucuronides formed by the Phase II conjugation. Acyl glucuronides are electrophilic intermediates that are unstable and can interact with amino acid residues to form covalent protein adducts. The last chapter presents a new in vitro assay assessing the reactivity of acyl glucuronides (Chapter 25).

Each chapter contains introduction, materials, methods, and notes sections. The introduction contains important background information. The materials section lists all the equipment and reagents necessary to carry out the assay, while step-by-step protocols are outlined in the methods section. Finally, information dealing with common and unexpected experimental problems is detailed in the notes section.

We want to express our tremendous gratitude to all contributors who were so receptive to contributing chapters to this book. Without their time and energy, this book would not have been possible.

Zhengyin Yan
Gary W. Caldwell

Contents

Preface .... *v*

Contributors .... *xiii*

1 pK_a, Solubility, and Lipophilicity: *Assessing Physicochemical Properties of Lead Compounds*
Yushen Guo and Hong Shen *1*

2 Use of Caco-2 Cell Monolayers to Study Drug Absorption and Metabolism
Ming Hu, Jie Ling, Huimin Lin, and Jun Chen *19*

3 Absorption Screening Using the PAMPA Approach
Jeffrey A. Ruell and Alex Avdeef *37*

4 *In Situ* Single-Pass Perfused Rat Intestinal Model for Absorption and Metabolism
Eun Ju Jeong, Yan Liu, Huimin Lin, and Ming Hu *65*

5 In Vitro Permeation Study With Bovine Brain Microvessel Endothelial Cells
Seong-Hee Park, Sung-Hack Lee, Yaming Su, and Patrick J. Sinko *77*

6 An Enzymatic Microplate Assay for Testing P-Glycoprotein Substrates and Inhibitors
S. Orlowski, J. Nugier, and Eric Ezan *89*

7 Evaluation of Drug–Transporter Interactions Using In Vitro Cell Models
Yaming Su and Patrick J. Sinko *103*

8 Plasma Protein-Binding Methods in Drug Discovery
Lucinda H. Cohen *111*

9 Isothermal Titration Calorimetry Characterization of Drug-Binding Energetics to Blood Proteins
Gary W. Caldwell and Zhengyin Yan *123*

10 Metabolic Stability Assessed by Liver Microsomes and Hepatocytes
David C. Ackley, Kevin T. Rockich, and Timothy R. Baker *151*

11 In Vitro Drug Metabolite Profiling Using Hepatic S9 and Human Liver Microsomes
Wu-Nan Wu and Linda A. McKown ***163***

12 In Vitro Identification of UDP-Glucuronosyltransferases Involved in Drug Metabolism
Michael H. Court ***185***

13 In Vitro CYP Induction in Human Hepatocytes
Daniel R. Mudra and Andrew Parkinson ***203***

14 High-Throughput Screening of Human Cytochrome P450 Inhibitors Using Fluorometric Substrates: *Methodology for 25 Enzyme/Substrate Pairs*
David M. Stresser ***215***

15 Evaluation of Cytochrome P450 Inhibition in Human Liver Microsomes
Zhengyin Yan and Gary W. Caldwell ***231***

16 Identification of CYP Mechanism-Based Inhibitors
Amin A. Nomeir, Jairam R. Palamanda, and Leonard Favreau ***245***

17 Detection of DNA Adducts by ^{32}P-Postlabeling Analysis
Naomi Suzuki, Padmaja M. Prabhu, and Shinya Shibutani ***263***

18 Covalent DNA Adduct Formation Mediated by Cytochrome P450
Marie Stiborová ***279***

19 Application of In Vitro Comet Assay for Genotoxicity Testing
Bojana Žegura and Metka Filipič ***301***

20 Assessing DNA Damage Using a Reporter Gene System
Xuming Jia and Wei Xiao ***315***

21 Improvement of the Ames Test Using Human Liver S9 Preparation
Atsushi Hakura, Satoshi Suzuki, and Tetsuo Satoh ***325***

22 Screening for Chemical Mutagens Using the Mouse Lymphoma Assay
Tao Chen and Martha M. Moore ***337***

23 A High-Throughput Binding Assay for HERG
Keith Finlayson and John Sharkey ***353***

24 In Vitro Drug Metabolism: *Thiol Conjugation*
Wei Tang and Randy R. Miller ***369***

25 In Vitro Screening Assay of the Reactivity of Acyl Glucuronides
Sébastien Bolze ***385***

Index ***405***

Contributors

DAVID C. ACKLEY • *Drug Safety Assessment-Disposition, Procter and Gamble Pharmaceuticals, Mason, OH*

ALEX AVDEEF • *pION INC., Woburn, MA*

TIMOTHY R. BAKER • *Research Analytical, Procter and Gamble Pharmaceuticals, Mason, OH*

SÉBASTIEN BOLZE • *DMPK Department, MerckSanté, Lyon, France*

GARY W. CALDWELL • *Drug Discovery, Johnson & Johnson Pharmaceutical Research & Development, LLC, Spring House, PA*

TAO CHEN • *Division of Genetic and Reproductive Toxicology, National Center for Toxicological Research, US Food and Drug Administration, Jefferson, AR*

JUN CHEN • *Department of Pharmaceutical Sciences, College of Pharmacy, Washington State University, Pullman, WA*

LUCINDA H. COHEN • *Dynamics & Metabolism, Department of Pharmacokinetics, Bioanalytical Research, Pfizer Global Research and Development, Pfizer, Ann Arbor, MI*

MICHAEL H. COURT • *Comparative and Molecular Pharmacogenetics Laboratory, Department of Pharmacology and Experimental Therapeutics, Tufts University School of Medicine, Boston, MA*

ERIC EZAN • *CEA/Direction des Sciences du Vivant-Saclay, Gif-sur-Yvette, France*

LEONARD FAVREAU • *Exploratory Drug Metabolism, Department of Drug Metabolism and Pharmacokinetics, Schering-Plough Research Institute, Kenilworth, NJ*

METKA FILIPIČ • *Department of Genetic Toxicology and Cancer Biology, National Institute of Biology, Ljubljana, Slovenia*

KEITH FINLAYSON • *Fujisawa Institute of Neuroscience, Division of Neuroscience, University of Edinburgh, Edinburgh, United Kingdom*

YUSHEN GUO • *Pharmaceutical Sciences, Aventis Pharmaceuticals Inc., Bridgewater, NJ*

ATSUSHI HAKURA • *Drug Safety Research Laboratories, Eisai Co. Ltd., Kawashima, Hashima, Gifu, Japan*

MING HU • *Department of Pharmaceutical Sciences, College of Pharmacy, Washington State University, Pullman, WA*

EUN JU JEONG • *Department of Pharmaceutical Sciences, College of Pharmacy, Washington State University, Pullman, WA*

XUMING JIA • *Department of Microbiology and Immunology, University of Saskatchewan, Saskatoon, Canada*

SUNG-HACK LEE • *Department of Pharmaceutics, Ernest Mario School of Pharmacy, Rutgers, The State University of New Jersey, Piscataway, NJ*

HUIMIN LIN • *Department of Pharmaceutical Sciences, College of Pharmacy, Washington State University, Pullman, WA*

YAN LIU • *Department of Pharmaceutical Sciences, College of Pharmacy, Washington State University, Pullman, WA*

LINDA A. MCKOWN • *Division of Preclinical Drug Evaluation, Johnson & Johnson Pharmaceutical Research & Development, LLC., Spring House, PA*

RANDY R. MILLER • *Department of Drug Metabolism, Merck Research Laboratories, Rahway, NJ*

MARTHA M. MOORE • *Division of Genetic and Reproductive Toxicology, National Center for Toxicological Research, US Food and Drug Administration, Jefferson, AR*

DANIEL R. MUDRA • *Department of Pharmaceutical Chemistry, University of Kansas, Lawrence, KS*

AMIN A. NOMEIR • *Exploratory Drug Metabolism, Department of Drug Metabolism and Pharmacokinetics, Schering-Plough Research Institute, Kenilworth, NJ*

J. NUGIER • *CEA/Direction des Sciences du Vivant-Saclay, Gif-sur-Yvette, France*

S. ORLOWSKI • *CEA/Direction des Sciences du Vivant-Saclay, Gif-sur-Yvette, France*

JAIRAM R. PALAMANDA • *Exploratory Drug Metabolism, Department of Drug Metabolism and Pharmacokinetics, Schering-Plough Research Institute, Kenilworth, NJ*

SEONG-HEE PARK • *Department of Pharmaceutics, Ernest Mario School of Pharmacy, Rutgers, The State University of New Jersey, Piscataway, NJ*

ANDREW PARKINSON • *XenoTech, LLC, Lenexa, KS*

PADMAJA M. PRABHU • *Laboratory of Chemical Biology, Department of Pharmacological Sciences, State University of New York at Stony Brook, Stony Brook, NY*

KEVIN T. ROCKICH • *Drug Safety Assessment-Disposition, Procter and Gamble Pharmaceuticals, Mason, OH*

Jeffrey A. Ruell • *pION INC, Woburn, MA*

Tetsuo Satoh • *HAB Biomedical Research Institute, Hiratsuka, Shiroi, Chiba, Japan*

Sébastien Bolze • *Department of Drug Metabolism and Pharmacokinetics, MerckSanté, Lyon, France*

John Sharkey • *Fujisawa Institute of Neuroscience, Division of Neuroscience, University of Edinburgh, Edinburgh, United Kingdom*

Hong Shen • *Structural and Physical Chemistry, Aventis Pharmaceuticals Inc., Bridgewater, NJ*

Shinya Shibutani • *Laboratory of Chemical Biology, Department of Pharmacological Sciences, State University of New York at Stony Brook, Stony Brook, NY*

Patrick J. Sinko • *Department of Pharmaceutics, Ernest Mario School of Pharmacy, Rutgers, The State University of New Jersey, Piscataway, NJ*

Marie Stiborová • *Department of Biochemistry, Faculty of Natural Sciences, Charles University, Prague, Czech Republic*

David M. Stresser • *BD Biosciences, Discovery Labware Inc., Woburn, MA*

Yaming Su • *Department of Pharmaceutics, Ernest Mario School of Pharmacy, Rutgers, The State University of New Jersey, Piscataway, NJ*

Satoshi Suzuki • *HAB Biomedical Research Institute, Hiratsuka, Shiroi, Chiba, Japan*

Naomi Suzuki • *Laboratory of Chemical Biology, Department of Pharmacological Sciences, State University of New York at Stony Brook, Stony Brook, NY*

Wei Tang • *Department of Drug Metabolism, Merck Research Laboratories, Rahway, NJ*

Wu-Nan Wu • *Division of Preclinical Drug Evaluation, Johnson & Johnson Pharmaceutical Research & Development, LLC, Spring House, PA*

Wei Xiao • *Department of Microbiology and Immunology, University of Saskatchewan, Saskatoon, Canada*

Zhengyin Yan • *Drug Discovery, Johnson & Johnson Pharmaceutical Reseařch & Development, LLC, Spring House, PA*

Bojana Zegura • *Department of Genetic Toxicology and Cancer Biology, National Institute of Biology, Ljubljana, Slovenia*

1

pK_a, Solubility, and Lipophilicity

Assessing Physicochemical Properties of Lead Compounds

Yushen Guo and Hong Shen

Summary

In the drug discovery process, the lead candidates must have proper physicochemical properties, in addition to affinity and potency, in order to have a better chance of success in development. Many pharmacologically active compounds fail to become drugs because of poor bioavailability, unacceptable pharmacokinetics, or unexpected safety problems, which sometimes are related to inappropriate physicochemical characteristics. As a result, physicochemical parameters have been incorporated into drug discovery programs, along with other properties, to rank the lead compounds and filter out unsuitable compounds. The pK_a, solubility, and lipophilicity are among the most fundamental physicochemical properties of a drug candidate, and their measurements are essential for both *in silico* and in vitro evaluation of drug-like properties. In this chapter, the authors present some widely used methods for measuring these three parameters . Because of space limitations, only one method is discussed in detail for each parameter, using chlophedianol as an example. The GLpKa method was used for measuring pK_a. The solubility in buffer solutions was measured with liquid chromatography–mass spectrometry (LC-MS) on a 96-well plate setting. Finally, a microscale shake-flask method was used to measure partition coefficients of chlophedianol between 1-octanol and buffer solutions.

Key Words: Drug discovery; physicochemical properties; pK_a; solubility; lipophilicity; chlophedianol.

From: *Methods in Pharmacology and Toxicology*
Optimization in Drug Discovery: In Vitro Methods
Edited by: Z. Yan and G. W. Caldwell © Humana Press Inc., Totowa, NJ

1. Introduction

With increasing pressure to accelerate drug discovery and development while reducing costs, it is critical for pharmaceutical companies to make the lead optimization process more efficient. Many efforts have been undertaken to determine potential drug leads' absorption, distribution, metabolism, excretion, and toxicological (ADMET) properties and developability early, based on *in silico* and high-throughput in vitro approaches ***(1–3)***. With a major shift to early attrition of poor drug candidates, it is important to have a fast and reliable evaluation of critical parameters to make informed decisions. During the lead optimization process, the goal is to quickly find drug candidates with high in vitro activity and selectivity, suitable physicochemical characteristics, acceptable pharmacokinetics, and minimal toxicity. Among all these desired properties, proper physicochemical characteristics were often overlooked in the past, and their negative effects were then discovered late in the development stage, with an adverse impact on clinical success and overall costs. The pK_a, solubility, and lipophilicity are among the basic and important physicochemical properties of a new drug candidate. They are also the fundamental parameters for assessing ADMET properties of drug candidates ***(1,4)***, whose deficiencies account for 50–60% of compound failures during development. Any reduced confidence in the results of these physicochemical properties will cast doubts on the predictions based on them. Their early assessments during the discovery stage also provide critical information that can help better interpret screening results and design new molecules ***(5)***. Drug-like properties should be optimized in parallel to pharmacological activity against the target. Although poor physicochemical properties should not be the only reason to reject a promising lead compound with great in vitro receptor affinity and selectivity, the challenges and risks are much greater when the compound is developed at a later stage. The increasing popularity of the *in silico* estimation of pK_a, solubility, and lipophilicity by no means will totally replace the experimental measurements. The use of *in silico* methods and high-throughput assays is important at the lead generation stage, when planning for library synthesis or when only a limited amount of material is available. But in-depth assessment of lead candidates should be done at lead optimization or the early development stage. High-quality experimental data using reliable methods are especially valuable for any new class of compounds. The results should be routinely incorporated into *in silico* prediction methods to enhance the predictability. In recent years, the importance of physicochemical properties in designing bioavailable drugs has been widely recognized ***(6–8)***, and increased efforts have been spent on assessing the drug "developability" based on calculated and measured physicochemical parameters ***(9,10)***. Some integrated processes for measuring the physicochemical properties of drug candidates have been implemented into drug discovery research in a number of pharmaceutical companies *(11,12)*. The task of making a comprehensive review of all the methods is nearly impossible in this chapter. Instead, we will use chlophedianol, an antitussive drug *(13)*, as a model compound to illustrate the experimental procedures on one of the commonly used methods for each parameter.

2. Materials

All the chemicals, except where specified, were analytical grade and purchased from Fisher Scientific, Inc. (Pittsburgh, PA). The model compound, chlophedianol HCl, was purchased from Sigma (St. Louis, MO). Special materials and instruments required for each method are listed below.

2.1. pK_a

1. GLpKa instrument (Sirius, UK). A semi-microelectrode with Ag/AgCl double junction was used for the pH measurement. The system also contains a thermostated autosampler tray with a capacity of 50 titration vials. Once set up, the system will carry out the experiments fully automated.
2. Solvents: distilled or deionized high-performance liquid chromatography (HPLC)–grade water.
3. Solutions: 0.15 *M* KCl (as the matrix for titrations), 0.5 *M* KOH (as base), 0.5 *M* HCl (as acid), and 0.5% Triton X-100 solution (as wash solution).
4. Potassium hydrogen phthalate (KHP): used to standardize the KOH titrant.
5. Tris(hydroxymethyl)-methylamine (TRIS): used to standardize the HCl titrant.
6. Argon: as inert gas (~200 cc/min) to protect samples from absorbing atmospheric CO_2, especially in the basic pH region.

2.2. Solubility

1. An LC-MS system with the following components: an Agilent 1100 HPLC system with photodiode array (PDA) and Finnigan TSQ 700 mass spectrometer detectors, a Gilson 215 autosampler, and an extra loading pump (Perkin-Elmer LC 200). A two-position 10-port electronic-actuated LabPRO™ switching valve from Rheodyne (Rohnert Park, CA) was used to facilitate column switching (**Fig. 1**).
2. HPLC mobile phase: A: 0.1% formic acid and 5% acetonitrile in water; B: 0.1% formic acid and 5% water in acetonitrile (all in v/v ratio).
3. Autosampler rinsing solution: 1:1 ratio of methanol and water with 1% formic acid (for better rinsing results).
4. Loading solution: the same as mobile phase A.
5. Test samples supplied as solid or in a plate format as a stock solution in dimethylsulfoxide (DMSO).

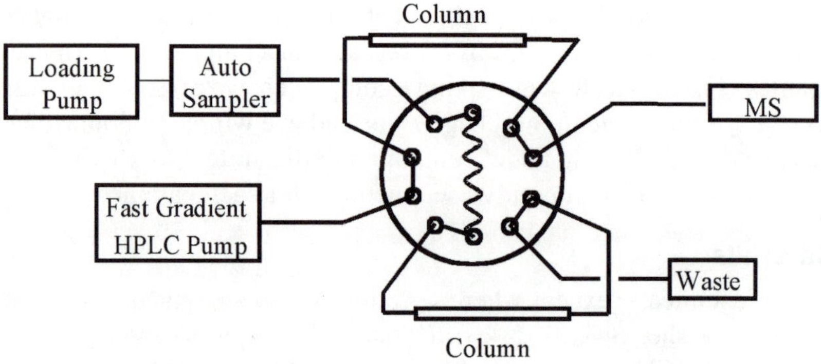

Fig. 1. An instrument setup for a high-throughput LC/MS assay.

2.3. Lipophilicity

1. Buffer solutions at pH ~2.0, 5.0, 6.5, 7.4, 8.0, 9.6, and 11.5 (50 m*M*). All buffer solutions were phosphate buffers, except the one at pH 5.0, which was an acetate buffer. The ionic strength of all buffer solutions was adjusted to 154 m*M* (isotonic of 0.9% saline) using NaCl, except the phosphate buffer at pH 11.5, which had an ionic strength of about 250 m*M*, and no NaCl was added (*see* **Subheading 4.3., Note 1**).
2. 1-Octanol (99+%) HPLC grade (Aldrich, Milwaukee, WI), was used without further purification (*see* **Subheading 4.3., Note 1**).
3. HPLC system: an Agilent 1100 HPLC system with a Zobax SB-C18 column (3.5 μm, 3.0 × 150 mm) was used for quantification. The mobile phase used was a mixture of acetonitrile and 0.3% trifluoroacetic acid (TFA) water solution in a 40/60 (v/v) ratio. The flow rate was 0.45 mL/min, the injection volume was 50 μL, and the column temperature was 25°C. The UV detector wavelength was set at 210 and 260 nm (*see* **Subheading 4.3., Note 2**).

3. Methods

3.1. pK_a

The pK_a of the ionization group of a molecule determines the ratio of the neutral form to the ionized form at a given pH (*see* **Subheading 4.1., Note 1**). It greatly affects the solubility and lipophilicity of a drug molecule, which are closely related to its bioavailability ***(14)***. The pK_a is also an important parameter for chemical development when the selected drug molecule needs to be converted to a suitable salt form to achieve better solubility and/or stability. During salt selection screening of a basic drug compound, the acid used should have a pK_a at least two units lower. In the traditional potentiometric titration method, the pK_a of a compound is obtained by titrating its aqueous solution with a standard HCl or NaOH solution *(15)*. GLpKa (Sirius), a commercially available instrument, has been widely used in both discovery and development settings because of its relatively high throughput (up to 30 compounds per day) and minimum sample requirement. For compounds with low aqueous solubility, multiple titrations are performed in the presence of a water-miscible cosolvent (i.e., methanol, DMSO), and the results are extrapolated to a zero cosolvent content using the Yasuda-Shedlovsky method *(16)*. Other methods, such as capillary electrophoresis (CE) and spectral gradient analysis (SGA), have been reviewed recently *(12)*. The method described below outlines the general pK_a measurement procedures of a typical compound using the GLpKa instrument (*see* **Subheading 4.1., Note 2**).

1. Install water and titrant solutions. Check the solvent dispensers, syringes, pH electrode, stirrer, temperature probe, and Argon line to ensure the proper working condition. Before the GLpKa system can be used in determining sample pK_a, several fundamental coefficients must be assessed. First, a blank titration is performed to standardize the electrode. Second, an acid/base standard (KHP or TRIS) is used to determine the true concentration of the prepared base (KOH) or acid (HCl).
2. Once these factors are known and refined, the pK_a of a given sample can be assessed. Typically, several milligrams of the test compound are dissolved in a titration vial with 10 to 20 mL of 0.15 *M* KCl solution (typical sample concentration of 0.25–0.5 m*M*). The standard titrant solution of an acid or base is then automatically added into the solution to adjust it to the desired starting pH (*see* **Subheading 4.1., Note 3**).
3. Once the desired pH is reached, the titration will start with the addition of the titration solution while the solution pH is monitored continuously. Typical titration range is within pH 1.8 to 12.2 to cover the range from one to two units below the lowest expected pK_a to one or two pH units above the highest expected pK_a.
4. A difference curve (Bjerrum plot) is obtained by subtracting the blank titration curve from the sample titration curve. The pK_a value can then be obtained by automated fitting of the experimental data points with refinement of the difference plot. In the chlophedianol example, the solution was first titrated to pH 3.0 using a standard HCl solution and then to pH 11.0 using a standard KOH solution. The pK_a of chlophedianol was determined as 9.13 ± 0.02 based on triple titrations.
5. To determine the pK_a of a water-insoluble compound, cosolvents can be used to ensure that the compound dissolves in the titration media throughout the tested pH range. In this approach, the apparent dissociation constants (p_sK_a) at three or more cosolvent ratios are determined. The true pK_a is obtained by extrapolating the Yasuda-Shedlovsky plot (*see* **Subheading 4.1., Note 4**). By this approach (**Fig. 2**), the pK_a of chlophedianol was determined to be 8.91 ($R^2 = 0.998$) when DMSO was used as a cosolvent at three concentrations (7%, 16%, and 25%, w/w).

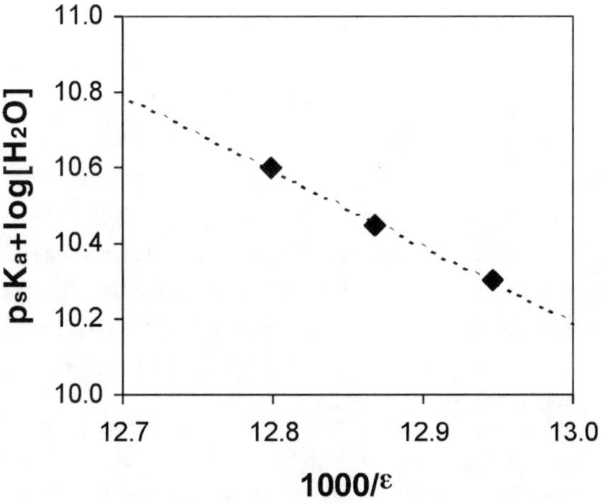

Fig. 2. The Yasuda-Shedlovsky plot of chlophedianol in DMSO-water mixtures at 25°C and an ionic strength of 0.15 *M*.

From the pK_a value, the percentage of ionization of chlophedianol at a particular pH can be calculated using **Eq. 1**.

$$\% \text{ ionized} = \frac{100}{1 + 10^{(pH - pk_a)}} \tag{1}$$

Figure 3 provides a complete visual profile for the distribution of both neutral (B) and ionized (BH^+) species at different pH. Notice that the pK_a value is equal to the pH at which a compound is 50% ionized.

3.2. Solubility

The intrinsic solubility (S_o) is defined as the solubility of the native neutral form of a compound (free base or acid), which is a characteristic value for a defined solid form at a given temperature and pressure. In practice, it corresponds to the measured solubility at a pH about two units below the pK_a of an acidic compound or about two units above the pK_a of a basic compound. The apparent solubility (S) is the total solubility of both ionized form(s) and the neutral form at a defined pH (*see* **Subheading 4.2.**, **Note 1**). Drug candidates with low aqueous solubility can cause erroneous results during different biochemical and functional assays, with increased risk of false hits or leads. Low solubility is often associated with high plasma protein binding, slow tissue distribution, and drug-drug interactions. Extra time and resources are required to develop a poorly soluble drug candidate. The lowest acceptable solubility limit of a drug candidate is related to its permeability and pharmacological

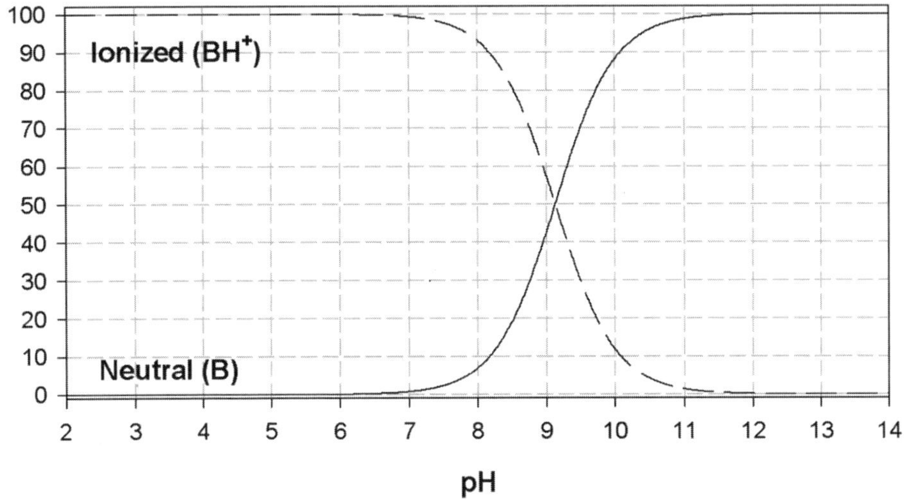

Fig. 3. Percentages of chlophedianol species as a function of pH.

potency *(6)*. Sometimes, high solubility may be able to overcome low permeability if the compound's potency is moderate to high *(9)*. In early drug discovery studies, a large number of pharmaceutical compounds are assessed, with only a limited amount of material available either in a DMSO solution or as an amorphous solid. The consideration of such solubility determination is somewhat different from that during the development stage. Here the apparent solubility information at pH 7.4 is usually combined with other data of the compound, such as potency and early ADMET characteristics, to rank the lead compounds. A number of high-throughput methods have been developed and widely used in pharmaceutical companies to measure the "kinetic solubility" of drug compounds *(9,17,18)*. Among those methods, the potentiometric titration and the nephelometric assay gain popularity for the fast determination of drug solubility in a discovery setting. Although these methods have a clear advantage of higher throughput, the solubility range is limited by the sensitivity of the detection methods and the concentration of the stock DMSO solution. The result obtained is also less reliable for designing in vivo animal toxicity and drug metabolism and pharmacokinetics (DMPK) studies, in which solubilization of the drug substance in proper media is often required to prepare liquid formulations at various concentrations.

The method described below can be used to measure compound solubility in either an aqueous buffer solutions or mixtures of cosolvents with relatively high-throughput capability while maintaining adequate accuracy of the results.

Either solid samples or DMSO stock solutions can be used. Solubility from solid samples provides important information on early IV formulations, with pH adjustment and cosolvent being two of the most used methods to solubilize low-solubility drug compounds. Chlophedianol is used as an example to illustrate the application of this generic LC/MS-based solubility determination protocol. In this method, sample was mixed with buffer solutions. The supernatant of the saturated solution was then quantified by the LC/MS method.

1. A standard solution (50 µ*M*) is prepared by diluting 1.5 µL of DMSO stock solution (10 m*M*) into 300 µL of mixture of mobile phases A and B (A/B = 70/30, v/v) in a Costar 96-well plate (Corning) (*see* **Subheading 4.2.**, **Note 2**). The typical up limit for saturated solutions prepared from DMSO stock solutions is 100 µ*M* (with 1% DMSO content). This range is determined based on the requirement of the early ADMET assay and other screenings (*see* **Subheading 4.2.**, **Note 3**).
2. About 4.0 µL of a DMSO stock solution (10 m*M*) is transferred into a deep well plate (Costar 0.5-mL general assay plate, well volume ~650 µL) and diluted with 396 µL phosphate buffer solution (pH 7.4).
3. The sample plate is sonicated in a water bath for 15 min and allowed to equilibrate at room temperature for 30 min thereafter (*see* **Subheading 4.2.**, **Note 4**). The mixture is then centrifuged at 4000 rpm for 10 min, and about 250 µL of supernatant is transferred into a clean plate (as a saturated sample solution).
4. The concentration of this saturated solution (solubility) is analyzed by the LC/MS system along with the standard solution (*see* **Subheading 4.2.**, **Note 5**).
5. For compounds with higher solubility (>100 µ*M*), as in the case of chlophedianol, the above procedure is modified to determine solubility directly from solid samples. Excess solid sample is allocated to plate wells, and different buffer solutions are then added. The plate is sonicated briefly and then agitated for up to 24 h, followed by the same centrifugation to separate supernatant from precipitates. The standard solutions were prepared directly from accurately weighted solid samples, and the LC/MS procedures are the same as described above from DMSO solutions.

The solubility-pH profile of chlophedianol was obtained based on solubility measurements of the solid sample in different buffer solutions (**Fig. 4**), which showed that the maximum solubility could be obtained around pH 5.0. Similarly, the solubility profile based on the amount of cosolvent (i.e., propylene glycol, PEG-400) could also be obtained. These profiles provide important information for liquid formulations during early toxicology and DMPK studies while high drug concentrations are often required.

3.3. Lipophilicity

Partition coefficient (P) and distribution coefficient (D) values between two immiscible solvent phases (1-octanol/water) are commonly used to express the

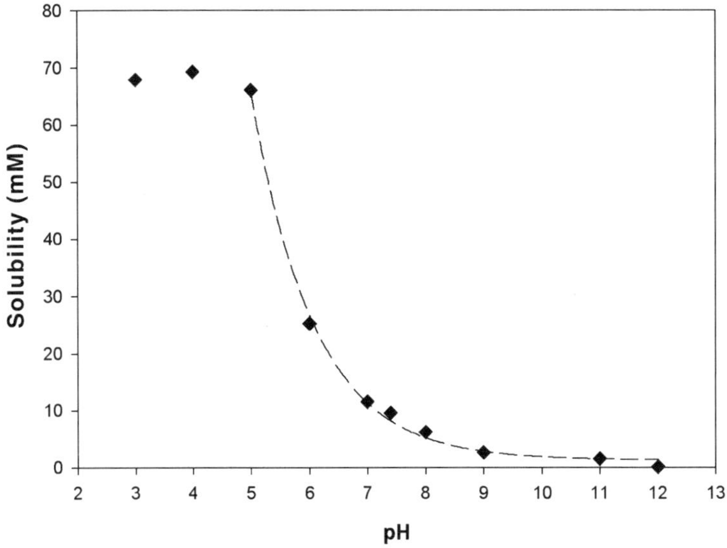

Fig. 4. Solubility-pH profile of chlophedianol.

lipophilicity (or hydrophobicity) of organic molecules. The term *logP* is related to the logarithm of the equilibrium concentration ratio of a single species (i.e., un-ionized neutral species of a molecule), which, in practice, can be measured at a pH about two units below the pK_a of an acid molecule or about two units above the pK_a of a basic compound. logD is related to all species (neutral and charged) of a molecule, which is sometimes also referred to as an apparent or observed partition coefficient. In a drug discovery setting, the logD at pH 7.4 ($logD_{7.4}$) is widely used to give an indication of the lipophilicity of a drug molecule at the pH of blood plasma. The lipophilicity profile as a function of pH is usually measured during a drug development study to correlate with the changing pH environment of the GI tract. For a drug candidate, its lipophilicity is closely related to its ADMET properties ***(19–21)***. A drug molecule should have proper lipophilicity to transverse the biological membranes of the GI tract as well as targeted organelles. Compounds with increasing lipophilicity generally show increased permeability, plasma protein binding and volume of distribution, and decreased renal extraction ***(22)***. Drugs with an extremely low lipophilicity value are not easily absorbed through passive transport, whereas drugs with a very high lipophilicity value may get trapped inside membranes after absorption. Compounds of high lipophilicity may also have other problems such as poor aqueous solubility, which leads to challenges for formulation development. A drug-like molecule generally should not have a logP more than 5 ("Rule of Five") *(9)*. Various approaches to measure logP values different lipophilicity descriptors have been reviewed *(23)*. In recent years, a number of indirect methods have been developed to measure logP in a drug discovery environment *(11,24,25)*. Among those, the reverse-phase HPLC method has long been recognized as a potential high-throughput indirect method for lipophilicity determination *(24)*. In this method, the gradient retention times were converted to chromatographic hydrophobicity indices (CHI). This method could be used for a high-throughput lipophilicity screen of combinatorial libraries based on experimental lipophilicity data of a few structurally related reference compounds. Other advantages include easy automation, a minimum sample requirement (<1 μg), being compatible with DMSO solutions and impurities, and easy to use for MS identity confirmation. A detailed discussion of this method is beyond the scope of this chapter. It should be realized that the conventional shake-flask method and its modified versions are still among the most widely used techniques because of their simplicity, cost-effectiveness, and proven reliability. In this section, we present experimental procedures of the microscale shake-flask method to measure the lipophilicity of chlophendianol.

In the microscale shake-flask method, the drug material is first dissolved in the more soluble phase, and a small volume of this solution is equilibrated with another phase. After centrifugation, the two phases are separated and analyzed using HPLC. Although each phase can be injected directly by setting the autosampler needle position, in most cases, only drug concentration in one phase (mostly the phase with the lower concentration and larger volume) is measured. The concentration in the other phase is calculated by subtracting the amount of compound in the measured phase from the total amount of compound used, assuming no significant drug substance loss. The following procedures outline the lipophilicity measurement of a typical compound. This method could also be used in a high-throughput setting by adapting 96-well plate technology and modern laboratory automation.

1. Transfer an appropriate amount (100–400 μL) of the drug solution (0.25–0.50 mg/mL) in 1-octanol (presaturated with water) into a 2-mL HPLC vial along with 1000 μL buffer solution (presaturated with 1-octanol). The concentration of the initial solution depends on the approximate logD estimation and the dynamic range of the detector. Generally, the concentration should be kept to the lower range as allowed by the detection limit (*see* **Subheading 4.3., Note 3**).
2. The vials are agitated for 2 h using a shaking mixer (*see* **Subheading 4.3., Note 4**).
3. After centrifuging for 25 min at 3300 rpm (1380*g*), the drug content in the lower aqueous layer is analyzed by HPLC. Occasionally, sample from the upper 1-octanol phase is also analyzed to confirm the mass balance (*see* **Subheading 4.3., Note 5**).

Distribution coefficients of an acid or base compound at a particular pH are related to the pK_a and partition coefficient of both the neutral (P) and the ionized species (P_i) by **Eqs. 2a** and **2b**, respectively. When the solubility of the ionized species in 1-octanol is insignificant, **Eqs. 2a** and **2b** can be simplified and still provide an estimate in the pH range of physiologic interest with enough accuracy *(26)*.

$$D_{\mathrm{pH(acid)}} = \frac{P}{1 + K_a/[\mathrm{H}^+]} + \frac{P_i}{1 + [\mathrm{H}^+]/K_a} \tag{2a}$$

$$D_{\mathrm{pH(base)}} = \frac{P}{1 + [\mathrm{H}^+]/K_a} + \frac{P_i}{1 + K_a/[\mathrm{H}^+]} \tag{2b}$$

The mean experimental logD values of chlophendianol were plotted as a function of pH, which were fitted to **Eq. 2b** using SigmaPlot2002 (Windows Version 8.0, SPSS, Inc.) (**Fig. 5**). The partition coefficients of the neutral (log$P$) and the ionized form (logP_i) were estimated to be 2.76 and 0.14, respectively (*see* **Subheading 4.3.**, **Note 6**).

At the drug discovery stage, the lead candidates are frequently available in DMSO solutions. The log$P$ of DMSO is about –1.35 (calculated), so most of the DMSO is in the aqueous phase. It is interesting to investigate the effect of DMSO on experimental results, although theoretically the volume of DMSO should be kept to the minimum. The log$D$ of chlophedianol in the presence of different amount of DMSO at different pH was studied to simulate the use of the DMSO solution (**Fig. 6**). The volume of 1-octanol and buffer was kept at 200 μL and 1000 μL, respectively. **Figure 5** clearly shows that there was no significant effect from the presence of DMSO in the studied pH range. In addition, the effect of DMSO with different 1-octanol/water ratios was also studied. The log$D_{7.4}$ values at different DMSO contents (0 to 40 μL) were measured under various 1-octanol/water ratios (100–400 μL/1000 μL). The average log$D_{7.4}$ is 1.79 (RSD = 1.49%, n = 9), and there is no significant effect from DMSO content and relative amounts of 1-octanol and water.

4. Notes

4.1. pK_a

1. pK_a values are usually temperature and ionic-strength dependent. The standard practice is to measure pK_a at 25°C in a constant ionic-strength medium of 0.15 *M* KCl. Data from some simple acids and bases showed that the temperature coefficients are mostly negative and usually not greater than about –0.03 log units/°C *(27)*.
2. D-PAS (Dip Probe Absorption Spectroscopy), an accessory of the existing GLpKa instrument, is available from Sirius. In this method, the change of the UV absorption spectrum of the compound with chromophore(s) close to the ionizable

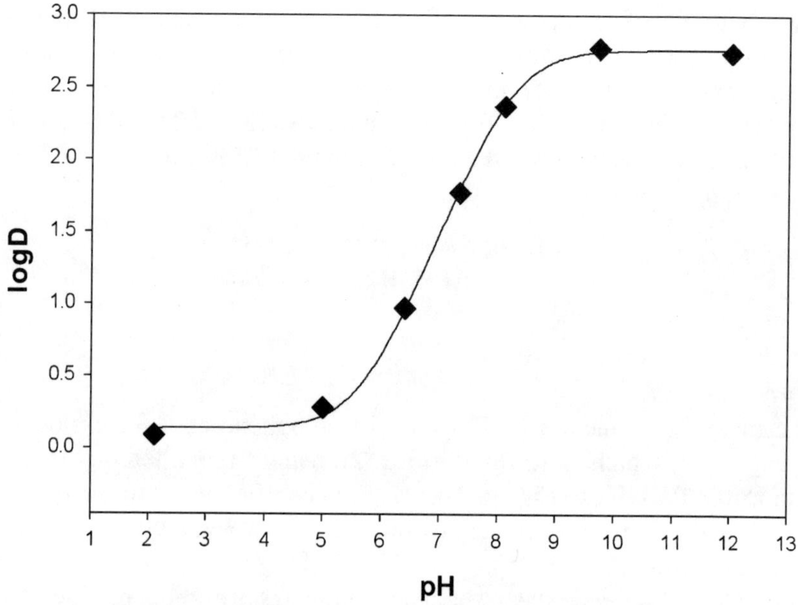

Fig. 5. Lipophilicity (log*D*-pH) profile of chlophedianol.

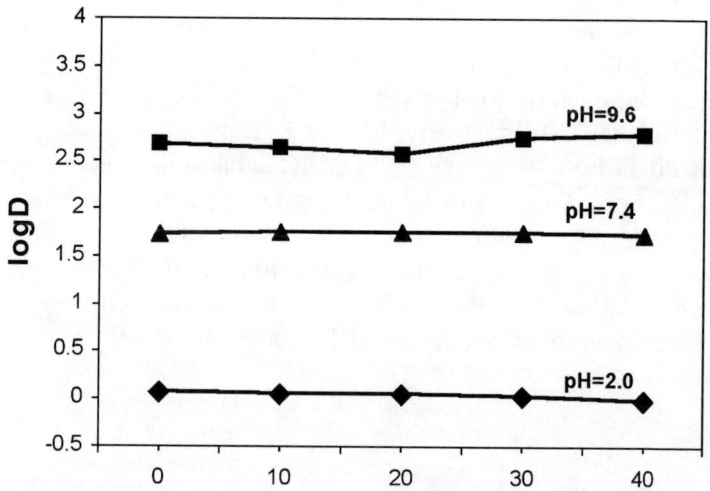

Fig. 6. Effect of DMSO content on log*D* values at different pH.

group is measured during the pH titration when the charge state of the compound changes. The D-PAS addition enables the sample concentration to be about two orders of magnitude lower than that of pH-metric titration because of the increased sensitivity of UV detection as well as the data-processing algorithm.

3. The starting titration point is usually chosen from where the solubility is the highest to ensure that the compound is totally soluble at the beginning of the experiment. With this setting, the pK_a of certain compounds can still be determined even if it precipitates near the end of the titration. During the refinement process, the data can be "clipped" to include only the valid data points that are not affected by the precipitation. A turbidity probe could be installed in the electrode holder of GLpKa to detect the appearance of precipitate during titration when mirrored vials are used. The probe is calibrated using $BaSO_4$ suspensions.
4. The Yasuda-Shedlovsky extrapolation is expressed as **Eq. 3**, where p_sK_a is the apparent dissociation constants measured in the presence of cosolvents, $[H_2O]$ represents the molar water concentration (equal to 55.5 for pure water), and ε denotes the dielectric constant of the mixture.

$$p_sK_a + \log[H_2O] = A/e + B \quad (3)$$

When using cosolvent/water mixtures with ε values greater than 50, the linear extrapolation to the pure aqueous system ($[H_2O] = 55.5$, $\varepsilon = 78.3$) can be used to predict aqueous pK_a with relatively high accuracy ***(16)***. Several cosolvent systems (methanol, 1,4-dioxane, ethanol, ethylene glycol, DMSO, DMF, tetrahydrofuran [THF], and acetonitrile) have been studied with GLpKa and incorporated into the software. Methanol is the most widely used because it has a wide extrapolation range (0–75%) and is also less affected by carbon dioxide and pH-metric errors ***(27)***.

4.2. Solubility

1. Theoretically, by knowing the pK_a and the intrinsic solubility (S_o) of a basic compound, the apparent solubility (S) at a different pH can be estimated from the following equation:

$$S = S_o\,(1 + 10^{pka-pH}) \quad (4)$$

2. A diluted solution prepared from the same stock solution will serve as a single-point standard. For compounds that have extremely low solubility, even in an acidified 30% methanol solution, a further diluted standard solution with more methanol content will be used. Because solution derived from the common stock solution is used, the accuracy of the determined solubility results will also be affected by the initial concentration accuracy of the stock solutions.
3. The solubility of a given compound can be influenced by the presence of DMSO. Because most of the pharmaceutical compounds in early stage are stored as DMSO stock solution, the compound solutions used in other screening tests are also derived from the same stock solution, and the presence of a certain percent-

age of DMSO is inevitable. The kinetic solubility determined from the DMSO solution is related more to early in vitro biological assays, whereas the thermodynamic solubility from well-defined solid material is more meaningful to later development.

4. Different sonication time settings (5, 10, 15, 30, and 60 min) were compared. The sonication both enhanced mixing and accelerated reaching equilibrium after a solid compound or a stock solution was mixed with buffer solutions. It was observed that 15 to 30 min of sonication was adequate, whereas prolonged sonication could generate excessive heat and affect the temperature of the solution.
5. A fast gradient is generally used to achieve high-sample throughput for the LC/MS system. A typical gradient runs linearly from 100% mobile phase A to 100% mobile phase B in 1 min. The mobile phase B remains for another 30 sec before the system steps back to 100% mobile phase A. The overall runtime is around 1.5 min. The two-column setup with column switching eliminates the equilibrating time needed after gradient elution. While one column is undergoing fast gradient separation, the other column is equilibrated with sample loading buffer and prepared for next sample. The added benefit of using a mass spectrometer as the detector is that any coeluting or degradation products can be identified. The system can handle roughly 200 samples in an overnight run. The data collected from the LC/MS system will be analyzed automatically by a series of macros in the Excel sheet.

4.3. Lipophilicity

1. Both 1-octanol and buffer stock solutions were presaturated by adding a few drops of their counterpart. The solutions were shaken briefly and required to sit for at least 48 h before use. The solubility of water in 1-octanol is about 3.1% (v/v), whereas the solubility of 1-octanol in water is about 0.08% (v/v) ***(28,29)***.
2. The range and accuracy of the shake-flask method are affected by the analytical methods (commonly UV). Based on the UV absorption of the test compound, the concentration dynamic range could be increased by about two magnitudes when a dual-wavelength UV detector is used. More sensitive detection methods such as mass spectroscopy should be used when measuring extremely high lipophilic or hydrophilic compounds. The accuracy of the method may also be affected by other factors, including the precision of the phase volume ratio, the purity of the solvents and solutes, and the efficiency of breaking down the microemulsions with centrifuge.
3. Generally, the solute concentration should be kept to the minimum, without sacrificing detection, to avoid possible compound aggregation. Multiple samples with different water to 1-octanol ratios should be tested.
4. About 2 h of agitation using a mechanic mixer is generally enough for reaching equilibration based on our experience and literature reports. The vials, which have 1/4 to 1/3 void space, should be in the horizontal position during mixing to increase the efficiency. Extensive and vigorous shaking is not necessary and could

cause increasing temperature and microemulsion. Microdroplets or emulsions may form easily, especially for drugs with surfactant activity. Centrifugation at 3000 rpm for 20 min is necessary to thoroughly separate the two phases.

5. The experimental temperature should be close to 25°C if possible. It was reported that the temperature dependence of logP is on the order of ±0.01 log unit/degree for some small organic compounds ***(30)***.
6. The shake-flask method is applicable for measuring log*D* in the range of about –2 to 4. A "slow-stirring" method has been widely used in environmental studies for highly hydrophobic compounds with log*P* > 5 ***(31,32)***. In this method, the exchange of the test compound between the two phases is mediated by stirring to minimize the effect of possible microemulsion. The drawback of this method is the requirement of longer equilibration time (days).

5. Conclusion

The measurement of pK_a, solubility, and lipophilicity should become an integral part of the pharmaceutical profiling of the lead compounds. Meanwhile, some information related to other properties such as the chemical stability (i.e., hydrolysis, oxidation) of the test compounds in solution should be monitored. This will ensure proper sample handling during measurements and also provide possible explanations of any erratic results. The drug material used should be of the highest purity available to ensure reliable results. Impurity and process-related polymorph changes can have significant effects on the solubility and bioavailability of a drug substance. Further tests using later purer batches may be necessary to confirm the results. Impurity and process-related polymorph changes can have significant effects on the solubility and bioavailability of a drug substance. It should also be realized that pK_a, solubility, and lipophilicity are only the starting point of a more comprehensive physicochemical characterization for any selected drug candidate ***(33)***, which should be done during the course of the development phase.

References

1. Smith, D. A., Jones, B. C., and Walker, D. K. (1996) Design of drugs involving the concepts and theories of drug metabolism and pharmacokinetics. *Med. Res. Rev.* **16,** 243–266.
2. Tarbit, M. H. and Berman, J. (1998) High-throughput approaches for evaluating absorption, distribution, metabolism, and excretion properties of lead compounds. *Curr. Opin. Chem. Biol.* **2,** 411–416.
3. Stenberg, P., Norinder, U., Luthman, K., and Artursson, P. (2001) Experimental and computational screening models for the prediction of intestinal drug absorption. *J. Med. Chem.* **44,** 1927–1937.
4. Lin, J. H. and Lu, A. Y. H. (1997) Role of pharmacokinetics and metabolism in drug discovery and development. *Pharmacol. Rev.* **49,** 403–449.

5. Hamilton, H. W., Steinbaugh, B. A., Stewart, B. H., Chan, O. H., Schmid, H. L., Schroeder, R., et al. (1995) Evaluation of physicochemical parameters important to the oral bioavailability of peptide-like compounds: implications for the synthesis of rennin inhibitors. *J. Med. Chem.* **38,** 1446–1455.
6. Curatolo, W. (1998) Physical chemical properties of oral drug candidates in the discovery and exploratory development settings. *Pharm. Sci. Tech. Today* **1,** 387–393.
7. Krämer, S. D. (1999) Absorption prediction from physicochemical parameters. *Pharm. Sci. Tech. Today* **2,** 373–380.
8. Avdeef, A. (2001) Physicochemical profiling (solubility, permeability and charge state). *Current Topics in Med. Chem.* **1,** 277–351.
9. Lipinski, C. A., Lombardo, F., Dominy, B. W., and Feeney, P. J. (1997) Experimental and computational approaches to estimate solubility and permeability in drug discovery and development settings. *Adv. Drug Deliv. Rev.* **23,** 3–25.
10. Venkatesh, S. and Lipper, R. A. (2000) Role of development scientist in compound lead selection and optimization. *J. Pharm. Sci.* **89,** 145–154.
11. Kibbey, C. E., Poole, S. K., Robinson, B., Jackson, J. D., and Durham, D. (2001) An integrated process for measuring the physicochemical properties of drug candidates in a preclinical discovery environment. *J. Pharm. Sci.* **90,** 1164–1175.
12. Kerns, E. H. (2001) High throughput physicochemical profiling for drug discovery. *J. Pharm. Sci.* **90,** 1838–1858.
13. Budavari, S., O'Neil, M. J., Smith, A., Heckelman, P. E., and Kinnerary, J. F., eds. (1996) *The Merck Index*, 12th ed., Merck & Co., Inc., Whitehouse Station, NJ.
14. Chan, O. H. and Stewart, B. H. (1996) Physicochemical and drug-delivery considerations for oral drug bioavailability. *Drug Discov. Today* **1,** 461–473.
15. Albert, A. and Serjeant, E. P. (1984) *The Determination of Ionization Constants*, Chapman & Hall, London.
16. Avdeef, A., Box, K. J., Comer, J. E. A., Gilges, M., Hadley, M., Hibbert, C., et al. (1999) pH-metric logP 11. pK_a determination of water-insoluble drugs in organic solvent-water mixtures. *J. Pharm. Biomed. Anal.* **20,** 631–641.
17. Quarterman, C. P., Bonham, N. M., and Irwin, A. K. (1998) Improving the odds-high throughput techniques in new drug selection. *Eur. Pharm. Rev.* **18,** 27–32.
18. Bevan, C. D. and Lloyd, R. S. (2000) A high-throughput screening method for the determination of aqueous drug solubility using laser nephelometry in microtiter plates. *Anal. Chem.* **72,** 1781–1787.
19. Pliska, V., Testa, B., and van de Waterbeemd, H., eds. (1996) *Lipophilicity in Drug Action and Toxicology*. VCH Publishers, Weinheim, Germany.
20. Walter, W. P., Murcko, A., and Murcko, M. A. (1999) Recognizing molecules with drug-like properties. *Curr. Opin. Chem. Biol.* **3,** 384–387.
21. Lobell, M., Molnár L., and Keserü, G. M. (2003) Recent advances in the prediction of blood-brain partitioning from molecular structure. *J. Pharm. Sci.* **92,** 360–370.
22. Van de Waterbeemd, H., Smith, D. A., Beaumont, K., and Walker, D. K. (2001)

Property-based design: optimization of drug absorption and pharmacokinetics. *J. Med. Chem.* **44,** 1313–1333.
23. Caron, G., Reymond, F., Carrupt, P., Girault, H., and Testa, B. (1999) Combined molecular lipophilicity descriptors and their role in understanding intramolecular effects. *Pharm. Sci. Tech. Today* **2,** 327–335.
24. Valko, K., Bevan, C., and Reynolds, D. (1997) Chromatographic hydrophobicity index by fast-gradient RP-HPLC: a high-throughput alternative to logP/logD. *Anal. Chem.* **69,** 2022–2029.
25. Lombardo, F., Shalaeva, M. Y., Tupper, K. A., Gao, F., and Abraham, M. H. (2000) ElogPoct: a tool for lipophilicity determination in drug discovery. *J. Med. Chem.* **43,** 2922–2928.
26. Scott, D. C. and Clymer J. W. (2002) Estimation of distribution coefficients from the partition coefficient and pK_a. *Pharm. Tech.* **26,** 30–40.
27. Sirius Analytical Instruments Ltd. (1993) *Applications and Theory Guide to pH-Metric pKa and logP Determination*, East Sussex, UK, pp. 62–63.
28. Leahy, D. E., Taylor, P. J., and Wait, A. R. (1989) Model solvent systems for QSAR: I. Propylene glycol dipelargonate (PGDP). A new standard solvent for use in partition coefficient determination. *Quant. Struct.-Act. Relat.* **8,** 17–31.
29. Margolis, S. A. and Levenson, M. (2000) Centification by the Karl Fischer method of the water content in SRM 2890, water saturated 1-octanol, and the analysis of associated interlaboratory bias in the measurement process. *J. Anal. Chem.* **367,** 1–7.
30. Leo, A., Hansch, C., and Elkins, D. (1971) Partition coefficients and their uses. *Chem. Rev.* **71,** 525–616.
31. Brooke, D. N., Dobbs, A. J., and Williams, N. (1986) Octanol:water partition coefficients (P): measurement, estimation, and interpretation, particularly for chemical with P>10e5. *Ecotoxicol. Environ. Saf.* **11,** 251–260.
32. Fisk, A. T., Rosenberg, B., Cymbalisty, C. D., Stern, G. A., and Muir, D. C. G. (1999) Octanol/water partition coefficients of toxaphene congeners determined by the "slow-stirring" method. *Chemosphere* **39,** 2549–2562.
33. Streng, W. H. (1997) Physical chemical characterization of drug substances. *Drug Discov. Today* **2,** 415–426.

2

Use of Caco-2 Cell Monolayers to Study Drug Absorption and Metabolism

Ming Hu, Jie Ling, Huimin Lin, and Jun Chen

Summary

The Caco-2 cell culture model is used to determine the absorption potentials of drug candidates and the transport and metabolism mechanisms of drugs and dietary chemicals. The Food and Drug Administration (FDA) recognized the model system as useful in classifying a compound's absorption characteristics in the Biopharmaceutics Classification System. In addition to its usefulness as an absorption model, the Caco-2 cells are useful for studying the metabolism of drugs. More recently, they have been used to determine the efflux mechanisms of phase II conjugates of drugs and natural products. However, Caco-2 cells do not always express appropriate amounts of transporters or enzymes, which may introduce bias in the determination of their transport via a carrier-mediated process or their metabolism via a particular pathway. Additional genetic manipulation of the Caco-2 cells will be needed to further advance the utility of this model in the drug development process and to ultimately establish this model as the "gold standard" for studying intestinal disposition of drugs.

Key Words: Caco-2; absorption screening; transporter; metabolism; efflux; transepithelial transport; Biopharmaceutics Classification System.

1. Introduction

The Caco-2 cell culture model is a well-recognized and commonly used cell culture model of the human intestine. It is used in many pharmaceutical companies to screen drug candidates for their absorption potential as a part of the absorption, distribution, metabolism, and excretion (ADME) package. It is also used in academic and industrial laboratories to determine the mechanisms of intestinal absorption and, less frequently, metabolism. It is one of the two mod-

From: *Methods in Pharmacology and Toxicology*
Optimization in Drug Discovery: In Vitro Methods
Edited by: Z. Yan and G. W. Caldwell © Humana Press Inc., Totowa, NJ

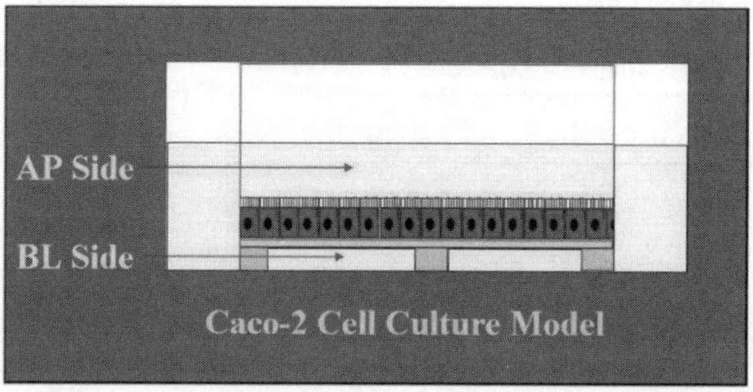

Fig. 1. A schematic representation of the Caco-2 cell monolayer grown onto a collagen-coated porous polycarbonate membrane. The apical (AP) and basolateral (BL) sides of the cell monolayers are easily accessible, making it an ideal model to study both absorption and excretion.

els recognized by FDA to perform absorption studies so that a drug or drug candidate can be classified according to the Biopharmaceutics Classification System. The special feature of this model is that both the apical and basolateral sides of the intestinal epithelium are easily accessible, which makes this an excellent model for studying drug excretion or efflux. Another advantage of this model system is that it only needs small quantities of compounds (~1 mg) to perform transport experiments, critical for its function as a support tool for drug discovery. The model was originally developed in late 1980s at Dr. Ronald T. Borchardt's laboratories in the Department of Pharmaceutical Chemistry, School of Pharmacy, University of Kansas (Lawrence, KS) *(1)* and at Ciba-Geigy in England *(2)*. This is the first cellular model of intestinal absorption widely adapted by pharmaceutical industries and academic laboratories. This model is by far the best-characterized cellular model for intestinal transport and is also an excellent model for epithelial transport in general. Another useful model of epithelial transport is the Madin Darby canine kidney (MDCK) cells *(3)*. The Caco-2 cells are human colon adenocarcinoma cells that differentiate spontaneously when they reach confluence on a porous polymer membrane. They form tight monolayers after about 3 wk in culture and have a useful window of 3 to 5 d. Typical transepithelial electrical resistance of mature Caco-2 cell monolayers is 420 ohm cm^2 or above. **Figure 1** shows a schematic representation of the Caco-2 cell monolayer.

The primary use of the Caco-2 model is to study the drug's absorption potential. This is based on various published correlation data that have shown excellent correlation between permeability in the Caco-2 model and percent absorption in humans (for review, *see* **refs. *3*** and ***4***). The correlation data represent the scientific evidence that the Caco-2 model works and are commonly

Table 1
Permeability of Model Compounds in Caco-2 TC7 Cell Monolayers

Compound	Permeability (10^{-6} cm/s)	% Absorption in humans	Reference
Mannitol	1.7	16	–
Guanabenz	6.23	79	–
Propranolol	11.3	90	–
Linopirdine	17.1	100	–
Amlodipine	21.6	85	–
Simvastatin	25.7	85	–
Testosterone	33	100	–
Genistein	36.6	100	–
Warfarin	44.2	98	–
Sulpiride*	0.038	30	*5*
Nadolol*	0.09	35	*6*
Atenolol*	0.28	50	*7*
Sulfasalazine*	0.34	13	*8*
AG337*	4.1	82	*9*
Ciprofloxacin*	2.14	70	*10*
Phenylalanine*	6.55	100	*11*
Cephalexin*	8.72	90	*12,13*

Note: Compounds with the asterisk indicate the involvement of a transporter (either for uptake or for efflux), which could make their permeabilities deviate from the established correlation. The experiments were performed using mature Caco-2 TC7 cell monolayers in a 37°C environmental shaker running at 50 rpm.

used as to validate the model system when it is implemented at a particular research site. It is necessary to validate the Caco-2 model using in-house data because the cells tend to evolve or undergo "phenotypical drift" as they adapt to local growth conditions and passages *(3)*. Published correlation appears to work well within a lab, and combinations of several sets of correlation data from several laboratories have shown very little correlation and are a poor tool for validating the model system *(3,4)*. Therefore, validation work should be performed in house, and cell passages should be kept at a relatively narrow range. In our own laboratories, we keep the passage numbers at 10 passages, using one split (1:10) per week. **Table 1** contains a list of model compounds with their permeability in the Caco-2 TC7 monolayers and percent absorption in humans. For compounds that are absorbed via passive diffusion, absorption is correlated with permeability. In contrast, for compounds whose transport involved a carrier-mediated process, the permeabilities are usually smaller than what they ought to be, perhaps as the result of the underexpression of uptake carriers, such as amino acids and peptide carriers, or the overexpression of efflux carriers, such as P-glycoprotein.

Another important use of the cell culture model was to determine transport mechanisms of drugs. There are two main areas of research: absorption mechanisms and efflux mechanisms. Earlier reports concentrated on the characterization of various nutrient transporters, including amino acids, peptides, fatty acids, nucleobases, nucleotides, sugars, and others (for review, *see* **refs. *4*** and ***14***). More recently, efflux transporters such as P-glycoprotein, the multidrug-resistance related protein (MRP) family of efflux transporters, and other excretion pathways have been characterized ***(3)***. It can be said that the Caco-2 model system is the most characterized intestinal model system. A MedLine search using the word combination *Caco-2 intestinal* generated nearly 2000 hits in April 2003.

Another use of the Caco-2 model system is to determine the intestinal metabolism of drugs ***(15)***, nutrients ***(16)***, and herbal supplements ***(17)***. A unique feature of the Caco-2 cell culture model is that it allows the determination of transport characteristics of metabolites ***(17,18)***, which is facilitated by the fact that both the apical and basolateral membranes of the Caco-2 cell monolayers are easily accessible. Compared to commonly used animal models, such as the perfused rat intestinal model, isolated segments of rat intestine, and isolated sheets of intestinal epithelium, the Caco-2 cells are the only model of human intestinal cells. The Caco-2 model is easy to manipulate and can be grown via an automated process. Compared to other epithelial models of absorption, such as MDCK cell monolayers, the Caco-2 model is much better characterized as an absorption model because major absorption pathways and transport carriers have been carefully studied. However, culturing Caco-2 cells could be more time-consuming than culturing other epithelial cells (e.g., MDCK), and therefore the model may be more expensive to use. Although the Caco-2 cell culture model is an excellent model of human intestinal absorption, there are several significant concerns with its use. For example, there is no mucus covering the Caco-2 cell monolayer, and many enzymes and transporters are not expressed at the levels comparable to the human intestine. Several groups of investigators have attempted to develop a hybrid cell culture model that has mucus. These investigators have cocultured Caco-2 cells and intestinal cell variants such as HT29-MTX cells ***(19,20)***. These cells produce cell monolayers with mucus of different viscosity and thicknesses. They may be more useful for intestinal toxicity studies, but reports of their use as a transport model have not been forthcoming because cells of the same type tend to form a colony of pure cells, possibly altering the uniformity of the cell monolayers. We and other research groups have tried to correct for the lack of CYP3A4 expression by either introducing human CYP3A4 into the cells ***(21)*** or inducing its expression using 1-α-2,5-dihydroxyvitamin D3 *(22)* because the expression level of cytochrome CYP3A4 in Caco-2 cells was much less than normal *(21)*. The expression level of CYP3A4 in the Caco-2 cells via the introduction of a CYP3A4 gene was comparable to what was seen in the human intestine. However, the expression decreased as a function of time, with a half-life of about 3 wk *(23)*. Addition of a DNA methylation inhibitor 2'-deoxyazacytidine increased the half-life of the decay to about 6 wk *(23)*. The level of expression of CYP3A4 with vitamin D3 treatment was much higher than the wild-type cells but was substantially less than the intestinal CYP3A4 expression *(22)*, making the system an excellent tool to study CYP3A4 regulation and functions, but it is less capable of predicting human intestinal metabolism via CYP3A4. To further remediate the apparent lack of CYP3A4 activities, we incorporated the expressed CYP3A4 plus the nicotinamide adenosine dinucleotide phosphate (NADPH) regenerating system into the BL side to better measure the effect of first-pass metabolism. We used a series of calcium channel inhibitors that are mainly metabolized by CYP3A4 and determined their transcellular permeabilities in the absence or presence of the expressed CYP3A4 system at the BL side. The results indicated that permeabilities in the presence of the BL CYP3A4 system correlated better with bioavailability than permeabilities in the absence of the BL CYP3A4 system, especially when Caco-2 TC7 cells were used (**Table 2**). Further improvement of this approach will be necessary because isoforms other than CYP3A4 were involved in the metabolism of some of the calcium channel inhibitors.

In summary, the Caco-2 cell culture model system is an excellent model for determining the absorption potential of drug candidates, elucidating the absorption mechanisms of drugs, and delineating the excretion mechanisms of drugs and their metabolites. The major strength and limitations of the model system are well documented, which improves their usefulness. Further improvement of this model system is difficult to achieve due to the fact that these cells are resistant to genetic manipulation.

2. Materials

2.1. Chemicals, Reagents, and Supplies

1. Feeding media (Dulbecco's modified Eagle's medium [DMEM]): DME media (Hyclone, cat. no. SH30003.04 or equivalent) with 10% fetal bovine serum (FBS) (Hyclone or equivalent), supplemented with 25 m*M* HEPES (Sigma) and 25 m*M* glucose adjusted to pH 7.4 (*see* **Note 1**).
2. Cell Inserts (Nunc, cat. no. 137435, polycarbonate membrane, 3.0 or 0.4 μm), with an absorption surface area of about 4.2 cm^2 (*see* **Note 2**).
3. Six-well cell culture cluster and assorted disposable supplies of serological pipets (Corning).

Table 2
Bidirectional Transcellular Transport of Model Compounds in the Presence or Absence of CYP3A4 Microsomes Using Wild-Type Caco-2 and Caco-2 TC7 Cells

P (10^{-5} cm/s)	Amlodipine	Nifedipine	Nitrendipine	Nimodipine
Wild-type Caco-2 cells				
AP-BL				
w/o E*	1.51 ± 0.06	5.74 ± 0.17	4.79 ± 0.3	3.59 ± 0.07
w/E*	3.01 ± 0.25	1.18 ± 0.09	1.6 ± 0.18	1.24 ± 0.02
BL-AP				
w/o E*	1.19 ± 0.08	5.81 ± 0.54	4.49 ± 0.01	4.03 ± 0.03
Ratio of BL-AP/AP-BL				
w/o E*	0.79	1.012	0.937	1.123
Caco-2 TC7 cells				
AP-BL				
w/o E*	2.66 ± 0.33	4.89 ± 0.27	3.33 ± 0.12	2.12 ± 0.15
w/ E**	ND	1.84 ± 0.09	ND	0.45 ± 0.04
BL-AP				
w/o E*	2.22 ± 0.15	5.06 ± 0.09	4.02 ± 0.17	3.33 ± 0.07
Ratio of BL-AP/AP-BL				
w/o E*	0.83	1.03	1.21	1.57
Bioavailability	64	45	22	6.6

Note: Transport experiments were performed in triplicate (average ± SD) using an initial donor concentration of 20 μ*M* at room temperature. The shaking speed is 50 rpm. w/o E, without expressed CYP3A4; w/ E, with 10 pmol/mL expressed CYP3A4 microsome on the basolateral side; ND, not determined.

4. Hemocytometer (Corning) or other instruments that can be used to determine cell numbers in a cell suspension.
5. Rat Tail Collagen, Type I (Collaborative Biomedical Product, Bedford, MA, cat. no. 40326) dissolved in 0.5% (v/v) acetic acid and sterile filtered in the biological safety cabinet.
6. Trypsin (10X solution).
7. D-PBS without Ca^{++}/Mg^{++}(Sigma), but with 0.2% (w/v) ethylenediaminetetraacetic acid (EDTA) (Sigma).

2.2. Equipment

1. Low-speed centrifuge (5000 rpm): sufficient to spin down the cells (e.g., Beckman).
2. Biological safety cabinet (Type II): working surface leveled with a bulb leveler (e.g., NuAire).

3. CO_2 incubator: shelves all leveled with a bulb level (e.g., Forma Scientific).
4. Inverted microscope: ×200 top magnification (e.g., Olympus).

3. Methods

3.1. Coating and Preparing Culture Inserts for Seeding

The whole process must be performed in the biological safety cabinet using aseptic procedures.

1. Dilute rat tail collagen 1:9 with 0.5% acetic acid (10X dilution).
2. Coat each insert with 200 μL of diluted collagen solution.
3. Tilt the insert so that the entire surface is covered with the collagen solution.
4. Remove the excess collagen solution.
5. Air-dry the coated collagen overnight with lit slightly/partially opened.
6. After the inserts are dry, use UV irradiation for 30 to 45 min to further sterilize the inserts (*see* **Note 3**).
7. Put 2 mL of DMEM on the top and bottom side of the insert, and leave the wetted inserts inside the incubator overnight.

3.2. Seeding Cells Onto an Insert

The whole process must be performed in the biological safety cabinet using aseptic procedures.

1. Get the Caco-2 cells from a flask of a suitable size. The cells should have reached at least 95% confluence but have not been overgrown (<2 d past confluence).
2. Aspirate the media out.
3. Put an appropriate volume (12 mL for T75 flask) of phosphate-buffered saline (PBS) in the flask and wash at least once. Add the PBS again into the flask and let the flask sit in a 37°C incubator for 3 to 5 min or slightly longer (*see* **Note 4**).
4. Aspirate the PBS off.
5. Put 3 mL of trypsin (1–5X solution diluted in D-PBS with EDTA) on the cell monolayer to ensure that the whole surface is covered with the trypsin solution. Aspirate out the excess amount and leave the T75 in the incubator (cap loosened) for 5 to 10 min, depending on the cells. Observe every 2 to 3 min and tap the T-flask. When the incubation time is long enough, the cells will form sand-like domes when tapped. If this loosening of the cells does not happen, continue to incubate the cells in trypsin. If after 10 min, the loosening still does not happen, the concentration of trypsin is too low. Another flask of untreated cells will be needed to repeat the treatment using higher (2–5X) trypsin concentrations until suitable cell clumps are made (*see* **Note 5**).
6. Add 10 mL of DMEM into the T75 flask, break cells further by rigorously pipetting (use 5- or 10-mL pipets) the cell suspensions up and down in the pipet. Make sure that the cell suspension hits the bottom of the flask as hard as possible when peptizing the suspension into the flask (achieved by putting the mouth of the pipet near the bottleneck).

7. Put the cell suspension into a sterile centrifuge tube (15 mL). Centrifuge at 3000 rpm for 5 to 10 min to pellet the cells. Aspirate the top media, and add new DMEM. Resuspend the cells in the media and break up the cell clumps gently with pipet.
8. Use a sterile pipet to take a sample (100–200 μL) of cell suspension.
9. Load the cell suspension sample in a hemocytometer (nonsterile procedure).
10. Count the cells (nonsterile procedure).
11. Dilute the cell suspension appropriately such that each 2 mL of diluted suspension will contain 400,000 cells, 90% or more of which should be singular cells (*see* **Note 6**).
12. Take out the wetted inserts precoated with collagen and aspirate out the media from both sides.
13. Add 2 mL of cell suspension to the top and 2 mL of DMEM on the bottom.
14. Gently shake the 6-well cell culture cluster (avoid circular shaking).
15. Put the cell culture cluster into the incubator, which must be leveled.
16. Change the media after 1 d (*see* **Note 7**).
17. Change the media every other day afterward.
18. Always feed the cells 24 h prior to experiments unless you want to investigate the effect of not fasting the cells or fasting the cells for a long time. Properly seeded and grown, the cells will mature in 19 d and can be used from 19 to 22 d. A longer interval (e.g., 18 or 23 d) may be acceptable depending on the cells and the purposes of the studies.

3.3. Transport Experiments

3.3.1. Reagents and Supplies

1. Hank's balanced salt solution, pH 7.4 (Sigma Chemical Company, powder form), supplemented with 25 m*M* glucose and 25 m*M* HEPES (pH >6.0) or 2-(*N*-morpholino) ethanesulfonic acid (MES) (pH <6.0) (HBSS).
2. Millicell-ERS with electrodes (for measuring transepithelial electrical resistance [TEER]) (Millipore Corp.)
3. Drug solution containing the compound(s) of interest (should be near or equal to iso-osmotic).
4. Shaking incubator (e.g., New Brunswick).
5. Pipets (e.g., Pipetman).
6. Mature Caco-2 cell monolayers that have been fed a day before (*see* **Note 8**).

3.3.2. Experiment

All components should be as clean as possible, although the aseptic procedure is not required unless the experiments will last for more than 6 h.

1. Aspirate the media out.
2. Wash the cell monolayers three times with HBSS. Add 2.5 mL of HBSS to the outside and 2 mL to the inside of the insert.

3. Measure the TEER values using Millicell-ERS. We found that the difference between the blank and the cell monolayers should be at least 100 ohm/4.2 cm^2, or 420 ohm/cm^2, for the monolayer to be useful and give relatively consistent results (*see* **Note 9**).
4. Incubate the cells with HBSS at 37°C for 1 h to allow the cells to release all the materials it may have taken up during incubation with the growth media.
5. Aspirate HBSS out and load the drug either to the apical or basolateral side.
6. Take three to four samples afterward at appropriate time intervals, but the whole sampling period is usually not longer than 4 h. For the rapid transported compound, the sampling interval is 15 min, and for the slowly transported compound, the sampling interval is 1 h (*see* **Note 10**).
7. Analyze the sample with high-performance liquid chromatography (HPLC) or other methods (*see* **Note 11**).
8. Caco-2 cells associated with the monolayer may be broken up via a freeze-and-thaw cycle (3×) or by sonication at 100 Wfor up to 30 min. Fresh cell lysate may be used to study the cellular metabolism and enzyme activities by incorporating the necessary coenzymes.
9. Amounts in the cytosolic domain (not tightly associated with membrane) are determined after the supernatant is withdrawn following centrifuge at 16,000*g* for 15 min. Amounts of drugs associated with membrane are determined using methanol to further extract the drugs from the pellets.

3.4. Data Analysis

The rate of transport is often obtained from the amount transported vs the time curve using linear regression. In general, the amount of transport increases linearly with time (pseudo-zero order) so long as the sink conditions are not violated (i.e., the concentration in the donor chamber is sufficiently high to replenish what is being transported out of the cellular domain). To facilitate comparison, permeability of a compound is often calculated using the following equation:

$$P = \frac{V}{SC}\frac{dC}{dt} = \frac{dM}{dt}\frac{1}{SC}$$

where V is the volume of the receiver in units of milliliters or cm^3 (typical volume is 2.5 mL), S is the surface area of the cell monolayer in units of cm^3 (typical surface area is 4.2 cm^2), C is the initial concentration in μ*M*, and is the rate of concentration change on the receiver side in units of μ*M*/min or μ*M*/s. We used $\frac{dM}{dt}$ as the rate of drug transport in units of nmol/min (or B in **Figs. 2** and **3**). The rate of drug transport is obtained by linear regression analysis of amounts transported vs the time plot (*see* the plot in **Fig. 2**). It is also worthwhile to calculate percent recovery using the following equation:

$$\% \text{ Recovery} = \frac{M_r + M_d + M_c}{M_L} \times 100\%$$

Date of Experiment: dd/mm/yy
Cell Info: type, passage, days in culture
180 ul injection in HPLC

Drug A Transport
Apical to Basolateral

A-B,pH6.5-pH6.5

C(μM): 50

Standard Curve

μM	Drug A Peak Area
0.78125	112.8
1.5625	222.6
3.125	409.5
6.25	787.1
12.5	1516.9
25	3034.7
50	5899.0

slope = 118.93
intercept= 0
r^2 0.9995

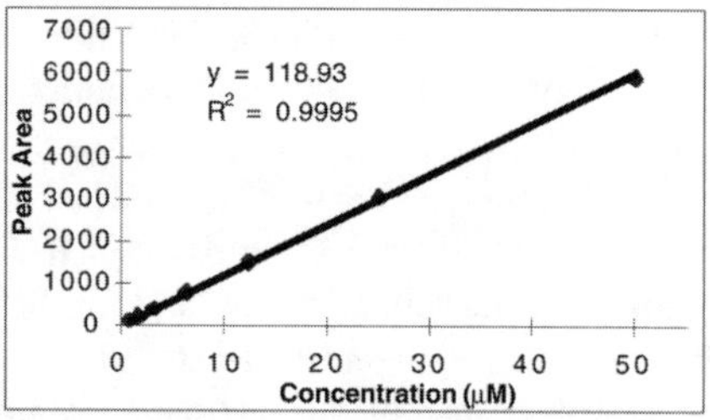

Receiver (ml) 2.5
sample (ml) 0.5 final (ml) 0.5

	receiver	area	con (μM)	actual(μM)	cum(μM)	nmol
A	60	462.7	3.89	3.89	3.89	9.7
	120	846	7.11	7.11	7.89	19.7
	180	1377.6	11.58	11.58	13.78	34.5
	240	1512.3	12.72	12.72	17.23	43.1
B	60	461.7	3.88	3.88	3.88	9.7
	120	1010.1	8.49	8.49	9.27	23.2
	180	1440	12.11	12.11	14.58	36.5
	240	1636.4	13.76	13.76	18.66	46.6
C	60	550.2	4.63	4.63	4.63	11.6
	120	1007.2	8.47	8.47	9.39	23.5
	180	1600.9	13.46	13.46	16.08	40.2
	240	1926.2	16.20	16.20	21.51	53.8

TEER Measurement: ohms 4.2 cm²			
BLANk	154	153	164
1	358	357	356
2	353	356	360
3	364	363	360

TEER Values (ohms cm²)			
BLANk	0	0	0
1	844	840	836
2	823	836	853
3	869	865	853

Transport

Time (min)	nmol	nmol	nmol	Average	SD
60	9.73	9.71	11.57	10.33	1.07
120	19.73	23.17	23.49	22.13	2.08
180	34.46	36.46	40.20	37.04	2.91
240	43.08	46.64	53.77	47.83	5.44
rateB(nmol)	0.1913	0.2068	0.2389	0.2123	0.0242
A(nmol)	-1.95	-2.03	-3.58	-2.52	0.92
R	0.9952	0.9980	0.9981	0.9971	0.0016
P (cm/sec)	1.50E-5	1.75E-5	1.73E-5	1.66E-5	1.39E-6

Fig. 2. Sample worksheet. The column headed by "con (μ*M*)" represents the measured concentration of drug A in a sample based on the slope of regression curve. The column headed by "actual (μ*M*)" represents the actual concentration after correcting for any dilution/concentration of samples prior to injection into HPLC. The column headed by "cum (μ*M*)" represents the cumulative concentration of drug A after correcting for amounts of drug A taken out in the sampling process. The column headed by "nmol" represents amounts of drug A transported after multiplying the cumulative concentration with the receiver volume (2.5 mL).

where M_x, M_d, and M_c are amounts of the drug recovered from the receiver side, donor side, and cell monolayer at the end of the experiment, respectively, and M_L is the amount of drug loaded to the donor side at time zero.

Plot

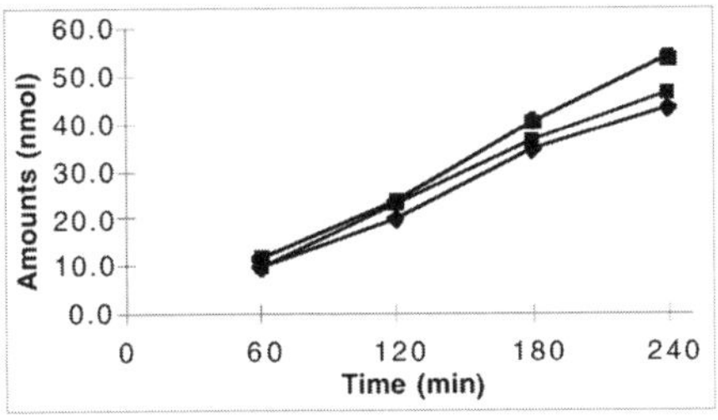

Cellular Uptake

in the cell(Buffer)	dilute(ml)		0.5 ml	Buffer		
	area	con(uM)	nmol	average/sd	Total average/sd	
1	397.2	3.34	1.7	1.78	2.66	2.88
2	406	3.41	1.7	0.15	2.71	0.33534
3	464.9	3.91	2.0		3.26	

in the cell(MeOH/Buff	dilute(ml)		0.5 ml	Methanol/Buffer
	area	con(uM)	nmol	average/sd
1	235.7	1.98	1.0	1.10
2	238.3	2.00	1.0	0.18
3	311.5	2.62	1.3	

Experimental Recovery

Donor				Recovery%
A				A
Begin	5974.8	50.24	125.6	95.94
End	3545.8	29.81	74.5	
Difference			51.1	
B				B
Begin	5541.9	46.60	116.5	105.98
End	3517.4	29.58	73.9	
Difference			42.6	
C				C
Begin	6453.3	54.26	135.7	104.32
End	4037.5	33.95	84.9	
Difference			50.8	

Fig. 2. (*continued*).

When a drug is metabolized during transport, it is often possible to measure amounts of metabolites on both the apical and basolateral sides of the cell monolayers as a function of time. Therefore, it is possible to calculate the rate of metabolite efflux using the same equation. **Figure 2** presents the worksheets that we normally use to perform various calculations. Information in the shaded area must be updated for each set of triplicate experiments. We usually use a standard curve that is forced to origin because the transport of some drugs could be slow initially, and a large intercept complicates the calculation of concentration, especially at early time points when transport could be slow.

3.5. Interpretation of Transport Results

When studying a new compound in some detail, the first experiment is to determine the transepithelial transport in the apical to basolateral and basolateral to apical directions. For compounds that are transported via passive diffusion, the directional rates of transport should be the same. For compounds that are taken up by an uptake transporter located in the apical membrane, the apical to basolateral transport rate should significantly exceed the basolateral to apical transport rate. For compounds that are excreted or effluxed by an apical transporter, the basolateral to apical transport rate could significantly exceed the apical to basolateral transport rate. In this first set of studies, it is also important to determine the percent recovery. If percent recovery is 85% or less, it is possible that the compound was metabolized during transport or that the compound sticks to the surface of the study apparatus, both of which will negatively bias the actual permeability or the rate of transport. If transport mechanisms need to be studied in greater detail because of the involvement of the transport carrier, it is often necessary to determine the effect of concentration, pH, and temperature on the transport. To determine the transporter responsible, specific chemical inhibitors are often used. Confirmation studies may also be conducted using special cell lines that overexpress a transporter of interest. Occasionally, the plot of amounts transported vs time will not be linear. There are several possible explanations for this observation. First, there is a lag time before the amount of transport vs time will become linear (**Fig. 3A**), which usually means that the compound needs some time to accumulate inside cells, substantial binding of the compound (>10%) to cellular membrane occurs, or both. This is also common if one determines the amount of metabolite formed as a function of time. Second, the rate of transport decreases as a function of time (**Fig. 3B**), which usually results from the loss of too much compound from the donor side due to rapid transport, rapid metabolism, or both. Occasionally, the loss of donor concentration could be the result of rapid binding to the cellular membrane or precipitation of drug molecules from a supersaturated solution. Third, the rate of transport increases as a function of time (**Fig. 3C**), and this could be a sign that cell junctions are compromised or metabolism is approaching saturation. It may be necessary to employ additional marker compounds (e.g., ^{14}C-mannitol) that are predominantly transported via the paracellular pathway to determine if tight junctions are compromised. Compromised cellular junctions are often a sign of cellular toxicity, which will bias the permeability results.

4. Notes

1. It is prudent to buy a large batch of serum for proposed experiments if there is a possibility that the object of the study will change when there is a slight variation

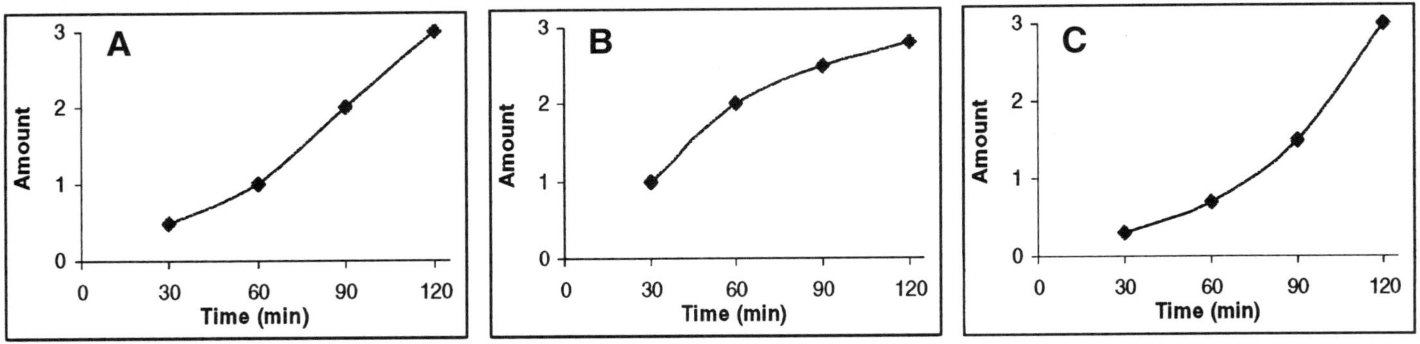

Fig. 3. Plots of the amount transported vs time curves. The time and amounts used in these plots are arbitrary.

in serum constituents. We normally do not change suppliers for serum. Other components of the DMEM could possibly be changed, but frequent change should be avoided.

2. Other suppliers may be used, but frequent change of suppliers is not recommended. We have used two suppliers in 13 yr, and we only switched because the first supplier stopped making the product. There are many types of polymer membrane available from the supplier for culture insert. We recommend polycarbonate because it is less likely to have drug adsorption.
3. We recommend coating using rat tail collagen to improve the homogeneity and uniformity of the Caco-2 cell monolayer. This step is not necessary to grow Caco-2 cell monolayers.
4. The purpose of this procedure is to allow the extraction of C_a^{++}/M_g^{++} from the intracellular space via chelation with EDTA. A small numbers of cells (<5%) may slough off during the incubation process, but cells should not come off as a sheet. If the cells are sloughed off as a sheet, the cells are probably overgrown (i.e., they are grown for too many days past confluence).
5. Trypsin dislodges the cells from the flask and from each other. Excessive treatment of cells with trypsin can damage cells and causes certain cells to die, creating selective pressure that allows cells with the ability to withstand the trypsin treatment to dominate, which can gradually change the composition of cell populations as a function of time.
6. Alternatively, cells could be centrifuged again after counting so we can freeze them for later use. This is necessary because cells will change over time, and we want to start from the same point every 10 passages. The freezing of cells are achieved by (1) preparing a cell suspension of 10 to 20×10^6 cells/mL containing 50% FBS in DMEM, (2) mixing 0.5 mL of the cell suspension with an equal volume of 20% DMSO (sterile cell culture grade), and (3) freezing the cells in a –20°C freezer for 3 h and at –80°C for 24 h and then transferring them to liquid nitrogen for permanent storage (which can be viable for years).
7. This is important because dead cells should be eliminated to allow normal growth.
8. Time of the last feeding to the experiments should be carefully controlled because it may affect the transport and metabolism of a compound, especially if the transport is mediated by a nutrient carrier.
9. You need to establish a threshold value in the laboratory where the validation is being established using known compounds. The value around 400 ohm per cm^2 is commonly used, but different values have been used before. It is not useful to make monolayers that are particularly tight because too tight cell monolayers are not necessarily good. Indeed, some people argue that the Caco-2 cell monolayer is already too tight as it is.
10. Unless the drug molecule is transported by a carrier-mediated process (uptake or efflux) in the Caco-2 cells, any compound without measurable transport (usually less than 1% absorption in 4 h) is unlikely to be absorbed (<5%) in humans via passive diffusion.

11. It may be necessary to preserve the samples by acidifying them or adding methanol at sufficient quantities to prevent bacteria growth. We also commonly add interval standard before samples are centrifuged.
12. It is often necessary to prepare the samples against chemical and microbiological instability. These samples have bacteria that can consume your chemical at room temperature (most autosamplers) in less than a day. We commonly acidify the samples to pH 2.0 or less. Sometimes, antioxidants are added too.

5. Preliminary Studies

Preliminary studies must first be conducted to determine the chemical stability of the test compound in buffers of various pHs. The best buffer is the one that has been incubated with cell monolayers for some time (1–24 h depending on what is being studied). Stability of the test compounds may be enhanced through the use of the stabilizing agent (e.g., acidification of the samples). Stability studies should also be performed using freshly prepared cell lysate if possible to determine if the compounds are metabolically stable. One can study the stability at a different pH or at pH 7.4. Spiking concentrated solution into the homogenate is acceptable for the starting solution. One should harvest the enterocytes if possible.

6. Preparation To Be Done the Day Before or Earlier

Stock solutions of the compound of interest need to be prepared, along with the labeling of containers. A typical experiment with two plates of six wells each could potentially generate more than 120 samples, and it is critical to track these samples so they are not lost or mislabeled.

References

1. Hidalgo, I. J., Raub, T. J., and Borchardt, R. T. (1989) Characterization of the human colon carcinoma cell line (Caco-2) as a model system for intestinal epithelial permeability. *Gastroenterology* **96,** 736–749.
2. Dix, C. J., Hassan, I. F., Obray, H. Y., Shah, R., and Wilson, G. (1990) The transport of vitamin B12 through polarized monolayers of Caco-2 cells. *Gastroenterology* **98(5, Pt. 1),** 1272–1279.
3. Hidalgo, I. J. (2001) Assessing the absorption of new pharmaceuticals. *Curr. Top. Med. Chem.* **1,** 385–401.
4. Artursson, P., Palm, K., and Luthman, K. (2001) Caco-2 monolayers in experimental and theoretical predictions of drug transport. *Adv. Drug Deliv. Rev.* **46,** 27–43.
5. Watanabe, K., Sawano, T., Endo, T., Sakata, M., and Sato, J. (2002) Studies on intestinal absorption of sulpiride (2): transepithelial transport of sulpiride across the human intestinal cell line Caco-2. *Biol. Pharm. Bull.* **25,** 1345–1350.

6. Terao, T., Hisanaga, E., Sai, Y., Tamai, I., and Tsuji, A. (1996) Active secretion of drugs from the small intestinal epithelium in rats by P-glycoprotein functioning as an absorption barrier. *J. Pharm. Pharmacol.* **48,** 1083–1089.
7. Karlsson, J., Kuo, S. M., Ziemniak, J., and Artursson, P. (1993) Transport of celiprolol across human intestinal epithelial (Caco-2) cells: mediation of secretion by multiple transporters including P-glycoprotein. *Br. J. Pharmacol.* **110,** 1009–1016.
8. Liang, E., Proudfoot, J., and Yazdanian, M. (2000) Mechanisms of transport and structure-permeability relationship of sulfasalazine and its analogs in Caco-2 cell monolayers. *Pharm. Res.* **17,** 1168–1174.
9. Hu, M., Roland, K., Ge, L., Chen, L., Tyle, P., and Roy, S. (1998) Determination of absorption characteristics of AG337, a novel thymidylate synthase inhibitor, using a perfused rat intestinal model. *J. Pharm. Sci.* **87,** 886–890.
10. Ruiz-Garc'a, A., Lin, H., Plá-Delfina, J. M., and Hu, M. (2002) Kinetic characterization of secretory transport of a new ciprofloxacin derivative (CNV97100) across Caco-2 cell monolayers. *J. Pharm. Sci.* **91,** 2511–2519.
11. Hu, M. and Borchardt, R. T. (1992) Transport of a large neutral amino acid in a human intestinal epithelial cell line (Caco-2): uptake and efflux of phenylalanine. *Biochim. Biophys. Acta* **1135,** 233–244.
12. Hu, M., Zheng, L., Chen, J., Liu, L., Zhu, Y., Dantzig, A. H., et al. (1995) Mechanisms of transport of quinapril in Caco-2 cell monolayers: comparison with cephalexin. *Pharm. Res.* **12,** 1120–1125.
13. Hu, M., Zheng, L., Chen, J., Liu, L., Li, Y., Dantzig, A. H., et al. (1995) Peptide transporter function and prolidase activities in Caco-2 cells: a lack of coordinated expression. *J. Drug Target.* **3,** 291–300.
14. Artursson, P. and Borchardt, R. T. (1997) Intestinal drug absorption and metabolism in cell cultures: Caco-2 and beyond. *Pharm. Res.* **14,** 1655–1658.
15. Chikhale, P. J. and Borchardt, R. T. (1994) Metabolism of L-alpha-methyldopa in cultured human intestinal epithelial (Caco-2) cell monolayers: comparison with metabolism in vivo. *Drug Metab. Dispos.* **22,** 592–600.
16. Hu, M., Chen, J., Tran, D., Zhu, Y., and Leonardo, G. (1994) The Caco-2 cell monolayers as an intestinal metabolism model: metabolism of dipeptide Phe-Pro. *J. Drug Target* **2,** 79–89.
17. Hu, M., Chen, J., and Lin, H. (2003) Disposition of flavonoids via recycling: mechanistic studies of disposition of apigenin in the Caco-2 cell culture model. *J. Pharmacol. Exp. Ther.* **307,** 314–321.
18. Chen, J., Lin, H., and Hu, M. (2003) Metabolism of flavonoids via enteric recycling: role of intestinal disposition. *J. Pharmacol. Exp. Ther.* **304,** 1228–1235.
19. Pontier, C., Pachot, J., Botham, R., Lenfant, B., and Arnaud, P. (2001) HT29-MTX and Caco-2/TC7 monolayers as predictive models for human intestinal absorption: role of the mucus layer. *J. Pharm. Sci.* **90,** 1608–1619.
20. Walter, E., Janich, S., Roessler, B. J., Hilfinger, J. M., and Amidon, G. L. (1996) HT29-MTX/Caco-2 cocultures as an in vitro model for the intestinal epithelium:

in vitro–in vivo correlation with permeability data from rats and humans. *J. Pharm. Sci.* **85,** 1070–1076.

21. Crespi, C. L., Penman, B. W., and Hu, M. (1996) Development of Caco-2 cells expressing high levels of cDNA-derived cytochrome P4503A4. *Pharm. Res.* **13,** 1635–1641.
22. Schmiedlin-Ren, P., Thummel, K. E., Fisher, J. M., Paine, M. F., Lown, K. S., and Watkins, P. B. (1997) Expression of enzymatically active CYP3A4 by Caco-2 cells grown on extracellular matrix-coated permeable supports in the presence of 1-alpha,2,5-dihydroxyvitamin D3. *Mol. Pharmacol.* **51,** 741–754.
23. Hu, M., Li, Y., Penman, B. W., Huang, S. M., Thummel, K., and Crespi, C. L. (1999) Morphological and metabolic characterization of Caco-2 cells expressing high levels of cDNA-derived cytochrome P4503A4. *Pharm. Res.* **16,** 1352–1359.

3

Absorption Screening Using the PAMPA Approach

Jeffrey A. Ruell and Alex Avdeef

Summary

The parallel artificial membrane permeability assay (PAMPA), as a passive-permeability screen, is an excellent alternative to cellular models for the earliest absorption, distribution, metabolism, and excretion (ADME) primary screening of research compounds. PAMPA's popularity in the industry has risen rapidly. This chapter focuses on state-of-the-art PAMPA methods. Evidence will be cited demonstrating that as far as predicting passive permeability, PAMPA can outperform cellular models in speed, versatility, and especially cost, presenting a compelling and biologically relevant model of transport. The problem of low solubility of research compounds has been largely eliminated in the newest PAMPA variant, using a unique cosolvent method. This chapter also discusses how PAMPA has relevance in preformulation research. A detailed PAMPA protocol is presented, with step-by-step instructions for a popular version of the assay, using relatively inexpensive and readily obtainable components.

Key Words: Oral absorption; permeability; artificial membranes; PAMPA; in vitro–in vivo correlations; unstirred water layer; cosolvent method for low-solubility assay.

1. Introduction

At the 2002 Society for Biomolecular Screening meeting held in The Netherlands, Chris Lipinski *(1)* made some bold predictions about the future of permeability measurement. He indicated that Caco-2 screens will soon disappear, to be replaced by nonbiological assays, such as the parallel artificial membrane permeability assay (PAMPA), and single-mechanism assays. (An example of a single-mechanism assay may be P-glycoprotein-transfected MDCK cells.) He pointed out that for reasons of solubility, permeability screen-

From: *Methods in Pharmacology and Toxicology*
Optimization in Drug Discovery: In Vitro Methods
Edited by: Z. Yan and G. W. Caldwell © Humana Press Inc., Totowa, NJ

ing might be futile in some combinatorial libraries. That is, although the clinically relevant dose is typically 100 μ*M*, most of cellular-based permeability screening is done at 1 to 10 μ*M* or less, simply because a vast number of combinatorial compounds are not water soluble above 10 μ*M*. However, at these subclinical concentrations, another problem arises: many test compounds show up as substrates for efflux transporters and other active processes. Some of these transporters are low capacity and presumably can be saturated at clinical dosage levels. An often-cited example is that of verapamil: it is both a substrate for P-glycoprotein (P-gp) efflux and is 100% orally absorbed in humans. Therefore, this situation gives the medicinal chemist an overly pessimistic outlook about the fate of compounds that screen positive for biological activity against a particular target. The risk is of setting aside a possibly promising molecule—the dreaded condition of a "false negative."

Although many in the pharmaceutical industry may not entirely agree with Lipinski's outlook, his message spurs critical discussions. Most agree that cellular assays, such as Caco-2, are cumbersome and expensive to do and not practical to run on every molecule in a discovery library. It is also generally conceded that good interlaboratory reproducibility for Caco-2 measurement is hard to achieve because the expression of transporters seems to depend on growth conditions and other subtle factors that are not easily controlled. Most researchers agree that Caco-2 and similar cellular models are valuable and unique mechanistic probes, which are cost-effective as *secondary* permeability screens in lead optimization. In these later discovery settings, cellular models can be very effective for predicting efflux and other active transport processes, as well as intestinal barrier-based metabolism ***(2,3)***. Although active transport (especially efflux) can greatly affect blood-brain barrier penetration and plays a role in first-pass metabolism and clearance mechanisms, active transport is usually considered less of an obstacle to good oral absorption (as the above verapamil example demonstrates). That is, when oral absorption is poor for water-soluble molecules, often transcellular passive permeability is also poor. Screening for passive permeability, as a surrogate for oral absorption, may suffice in discovery applications ***(1)***. PAMPA, as a passive-permeability screen, is an excellent alternative to cellular models for the earliest absorption, distribution, metabolism, and excretion (ADME) *primary* screening of research compounds. PAMPA's popularity in the industry has risen rapidly. This chapter focuses on state-of-the-art PAMPA methods. Evidence will be cited demonstrating that as far as predicting *passive* permeability, PAMPA can outperform cellular models in speed, versatility, and especially cost, presenting a compelling and biologically relevant model of transport. The problem of solubility, mentioned by Lipinski above, has been largely eliminated in the newest PAMPA methods, as will be discussed. This chapter also discussed how PAMPA has relevance in preformulation research. In **Subheading 14.**, a detailed protocol will be presented, with step-by-step instructions for a popular version of the PAMPA assay, using relatively inexpensive and readily obtainable components.

2. The Rise of PAMPA

The acronym PAMPA, or parallel artificial membrane permeability assay, was coined by Manfred Kansy and coworkers at Hoffmann-La Roche in the widely read 1998 paper *(4)*. The Roche PAMPA method involves creating a filter-immobilized artificial membrane by infusing a lipophilic microfilter with 10% wt/vol egg lecithin dissolved in *n*-dodecane. The filter membrane is used to separate an aqueous solution containing a test molecule from an aqueous buffer initially free of the molecule. PAMPA enables the kinetics of transport by diffusion to be studied in this permeation cell. Microplate technology allows 96 permeation cells to be simultaneously formed, increasing the speed while lowering the cost. The fundamental basis of PAMPA has a longer history than is generally realized. In the early 1960s, Mueller et al. *(5)* described that when a droplet of phospholipid (2% wt/vol in *n*-decane) was deposited over a pinhole in a sheet of plastic suspended in water, a single bilayer membrane spontaneously formed over the hole. Because the membrane appears black under a microscope, the term *black lipid membrane* (BLM) was associated with this phenomenon. However, long before the BLM studies, mysterious "black spots" on the surface of soap films had been scrutinized by Robert Hooke and Isaac Newton in the 1600s and by Ben Franklin a hundred years later *(6)*. Mueller et al.'s report made it apparent that the in vitro-formed BLM has the same fundamental structure as natural biological membranes. BLMs were soon used to model the transport of molecules across biomembranes and, in many early instances, to further the design of biosensor probes *(6)*. Careful measurement of the permeability of weak acids across a single BLM was reported by Gutknecht and coworkers *(7–9)*, Antonenko et al. *(10)*, and Anderson and coworkers *(11–15)*. Performing these single-BLM experiments requires considerable skill and patience because the membranes are very delicate—as fragile as soap bubbles. Mountz and Tien *(16)* came up with the idea of using a microporous filter for the support of hundreds of thousands of BLMs to get more stable scaffold structures and increasing sensitivity. Perhaps this was the first single-well "PAMPA" experiment, done 20 yr before the Kansy report, long before parallel (microplate) assays were done. Later, Thompson et al. *(17)* apparently proved that when a polycarbonate filter was used (which has well-defined straight-through cylindrical holes), a single BLM formed in each pore. **Figure 1** shows

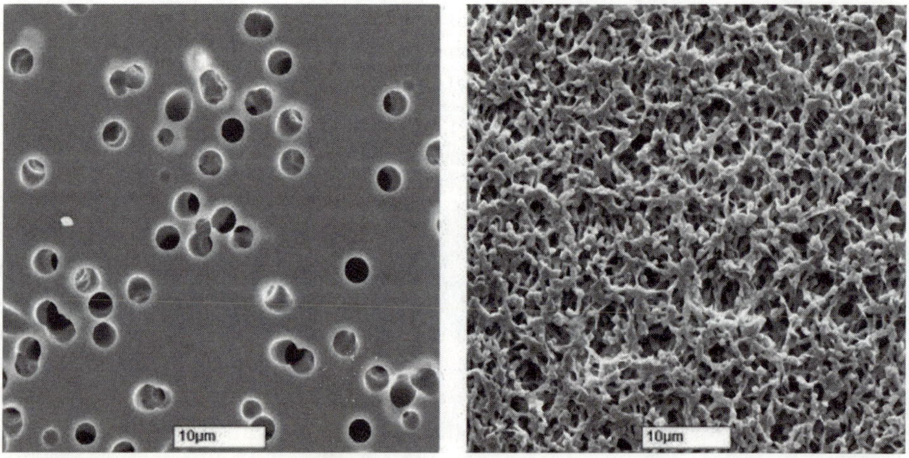

Fig. 1. Micrographs of two types of microporous filter material used in PAMPA: **(A)** polycarbonate (nominal porosity 0.2) and **(B)** IPVH (nominal porosity 0.7). Courtesy of Millipore Corporation.

the structures of polycarbonate filters used by Thompson and of IPVH filters used by Kansy. Cools and Janssen ***(18)*** impregnated filters with *n*-octanol and studied how ion-paired warfarin permeated membranes in high-pH solutions. Given how popular octanol-water partition coefficient measurement was in the 1980s (log D was used as a membrane permeation model), it is surprising that the more direct method of Cools and Janssen did not capture the collective imagination of the pharmaceutical industry at that time. One year before Kansy's report, Camenisch et al. ***(19)*** published a study in which an octanol-infused microfilter was used to characterize the permeability of drug molecules and compared the results to those obtained by Caco-2 assays. A large-volume "H-cell" was employed, where high-throughput measurement was not practical. Because of this, the method appeared not to have attracted much attention.

The rise of PAMPA following Kansy's report depended greatly on the state of pharmaceutical research in the mid-1990s. Combinatorial chemistry and fast robotics were rapidly producing novel compounds, by the hundreds of thousands. Fast, reliable, compound-sparing, and inexpensive assay methods had to be developed to keep up with the demand for higher throughput. The Roche PAMPA method came at just the right moment. In the 2-yr period after the first Kansy publication, several companies developed their own versions of the assay. During this period, a commercial instrument was launched by *p*ION INC. At the logP2000 Conference, organized by Prof. Bernard Testa

(Lausanne, March 2000), Kansy et al. ***(20)***, Avdeef ***(21)***, and Faller and Wohnsland ***(22)*** discussed the emerging PAMPA technology. Since then, several other PAMPA papers have appeared: Avdeef et al. ***(23)***, Wohnsland and Faller ***(24)***, Sugano et al. ***(25–28)***, Zhu et al. ***(29)***, Veber et al. ***(30)***, and Di et al. ***(31)***. The first international symposium on the topic was held in San Francisco in July 2002 (www.pampa2002.com), where nearly all researchers known to be involved with the new technique presented papers and posters. Several reviews with PAMPA coverage have been published, citing the literature between 1998 and 2003 ***(2,3,32–37)***, and a book by Avdeef ***(38)*** devotes a large portion to the topic of PAMPA. Since Kansy's first paper ***(4)***, terms such as *filter-immobilized artificial membranes* (*filter-IAM*) ***(23,32)*** and *BAMPA* ***(25,26)*** have appeared. At the PAMPA 2002 meeting, it was proposed, in the interest of easy tracking of the PAMPA literature, that the term *PAMPA* be adopted. This has been largely accepted by practitioners. But what does *PAMPA* actually stand for? Does the Mountz and Tien 1978 method ***(16)*** qualify as PAMPA? Kansy stressed the use of phospholipids infused into hydrophobic filters. Does the use of other lipids, such as simple hexadecane ***(22)***, constitute PAMPA measurements? Does the use of a single "H-cell" holding a Teflon filter infused with 1,9-decadiene ***(14)*** constitute a PAMPA measurement? A definition of PAMPA is needed, and we propose the following:

> PAMPA is a permeability assay that uses a microporous filter, infused with a lipid or a mixture of lipids, to separate two aqueous, pH-buffered solutions in a multiwell microplate sandwich. The buffers may contain additives, such as solubilizing agents in the donor compartment and agents simulating protein binding in the receiver and/or donor compartments. Gradient-pH and stirring may be used to improve in vitro–in vivo correlations.

The Caco-2 assay is excluded from this definition because the cells are not infused *into* the filter. BLM experiments ***(5–12)*** are also excluded from the definition because just a single pore is used. Liposome-based permeability assays, as developed by Anderson's group ***(13,15)***, are also excluded because filter support is not used. Single "H-cell" models ***(14,16,17,19)*** are excluded as well because *parallel* in the PAMPA acronym suggests high throughput, which was not of interest in the earlier single-well studies. Therefore, PAMPA is a distinct new variant of permeability assays, consisting of a number of parallel cells, each having a lipophilic permeation barrier, composed of an enormous number of lipid membranes held in a plane by a thin microfilter, separating two aqueous compartments. Its characteristic variants, such as Bio-Mimetic ***(25–28)***, HexaDecane Membrane ***(22,24)***, or Double-Sink™ ***(38,39)***, can be called BM-PAMPA, HDM-PAMPA, and DS-PAMPA, respectively.

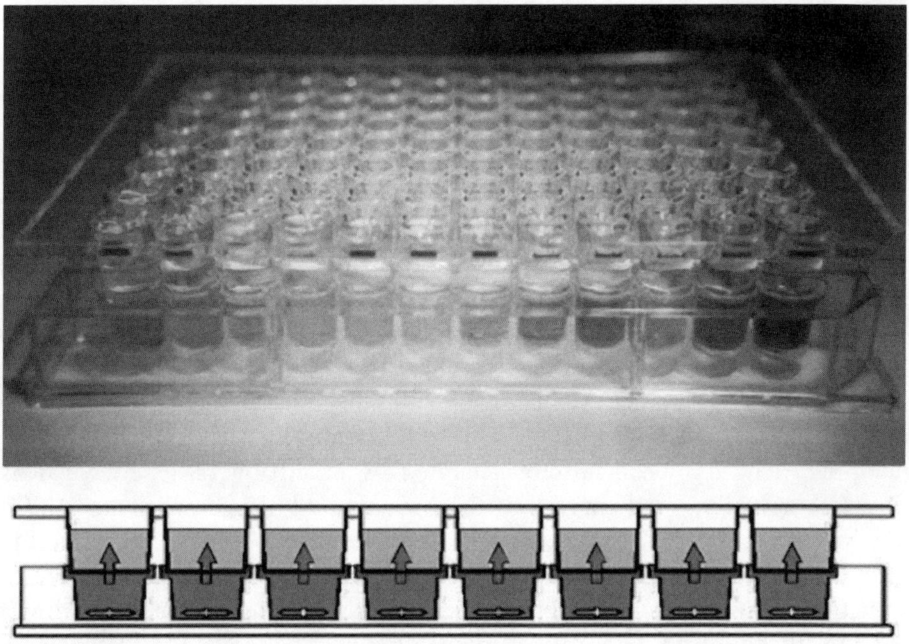

Fig. 2. PAMPA sandwich: perspective view and cross-sectional view. Individual-well stirrers (lower view) are optional.

3. Assay Variables

PAMPA experiments are performed in a "sandwich-like" apparatus similar to that used in cell-based assays such as Caco-2 and MDCK (**Fig. 2**). When two microplates are joined to form a sandwich, one is referred to as the "donor" plate and the other as the "acceptor" plate. Permeability is determined by observing the disappearance of compound from the donor and the appearance in the acceptor. The distinction of donor and acceptor is not decided by plate placement because permeability can be measured equally well with the donor compartment on the top or bottom of the sandwich. The compartment that contains drug at the start of the experiment is referred to as the donor.

3.1. Plate and Filter Properties

The precise fit between the two sandwich plates (**Fig. 2**) enables the compound to transfer between compartments, passing through the filter barrier only. The choice of filter material can have a profound affect on the experimental conditions and results. The original Kansy PAMPA method uses a hydrophobic filter with a small pore size of 0.45 μm, a thickness of 125 μm, and a nominal porosity of 0.7. These filters may require incubation times of several hours before measurable amounts of compound appear in the acceptor compartment.

3.2. Equations for Calculation of Effective Permeability

Wohnsland and Faller *(22,24)* and Sugano et al. *(25–28)* defined effective permeability equations used in PAMPA, assuming zero loss of test compound to the lipid phase and to the plastic surfaces of the wells (mass balance assumed to be confined to the aqueous phase). The equations presented by Avdeef (*36,38*; **Subheading 14.**) directly incorporate the additional effects of (a) membrane retention (complete mass balance) and (b) pH gradients.

3.3. Apparent and Nominal Filter Porosity

Faller's group was the first to factor filter porosity into their permeability equation by multiplying the filter area by the nominal porosity of 0.2. This made their permeability scale five times greater than that of others who neglect the porosity correction when using filters of the same porosity (in effect, assuming porosity to be unit value). Bermejo et al. *(39)*, Nielsen and Avdeef *(40)*, and Ruell et al. *(41)* incorporated filter porosity in the effective permeability equation but in a way different from that of Faller. All other PAMPA practitioners have assumed unit porosity. Nielsen and Avdeef *(40)* introduced the concept of apparent filter porosity: if more lipid is deposited on the filter than can be accommodated by the volume of the pores (**Fig. 3**), the *apparent* porosity, ε_a, is different from the *nominal* porosity, ε. For example, Faller's group *(20,22)* deposited 0.75 μL of hexadecane on top of 10-μm thick polycarbonate filters (**Fig. 1A**), which had the nominal porosity $\varepsilon = 0.2$. The lipid volume substantially exceeded the pore volume. The resulting thickness of the excess lipid layer is 29 μm, giving a total apparent membrane thickness of 39 μm. The excess lipid significantly alters the contribution of the pores to the overall resistance in the membrane barrier. Analysis of the geometry suggests that instead of using the nominal porosity, $\varepsilon = 0.2$, it would have been appropriate to apply the apparent porosity, $\varepsilon_a = 0.50$, a 150% increase over the nominal value. In such cases, the apparent porosity is calculated from the following equation *(40)*:

$$\varepsilon_a = [V/A + h\,(1 - \varepsilon)]/[V/A + h\,(1/\varepsilon - \varepsilon)], \qquad (1)$$

where V (cm^3) is volume of lipid deposited, A (cm^2) is the filter area, h (cm) is the filter thickness, and ε is the nominal filter porosity. Most PAMPA practitioners use the metrics and the IPVH filter suggested by Kansy: $V = 4$ μL, $A = 0.3$ cm^2, $h = 125$ μm. The nominal filter porosity of Millipore's IPVH filters (**Fig. 1B**) is $\varepsilon = 0.7$. The resulting thickness of the excess lipid layer is 46 μm,

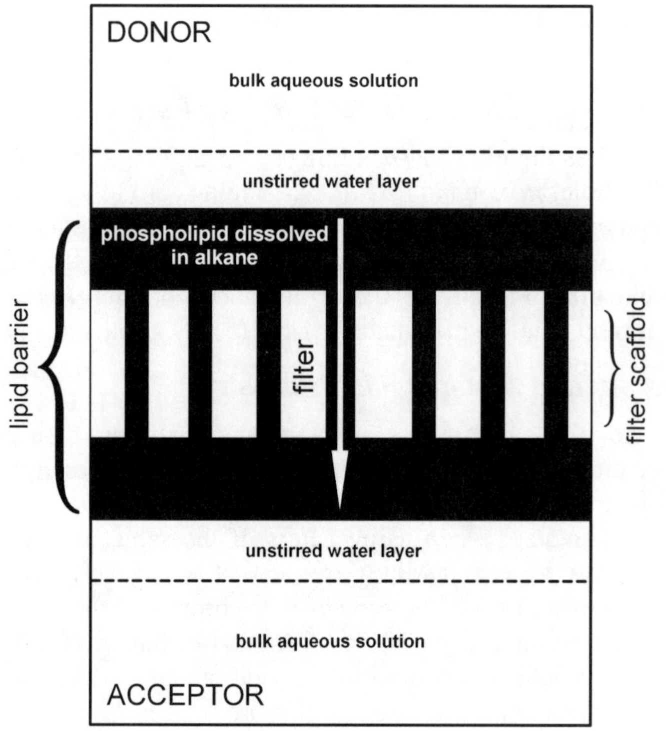

Fig. 3. PAMPA lamella schematic. The region shaded in black denotes the lipid solution, which is added in excess of the volume needed to fill all the pores of the filter scaffold, denoted in white within the black-shaded composite lipid barrier. The water adjacent to each side of the lipid barrier is the unstirred water layer (*see* text).

giving a total apparent membrane thickness of 171 μm. Applying these metrics to **Eq. 1** yields $\varepsilon_a = 0.76$, a 9% increase from the nominal value.

3.4. Lipid Composition

In PAMPA experiments, test compounds need to transfer by passive diffusion through the membrane environment created on the filter plate. Because pure phospholipids are solids that will not disperse into filters, a nonpolar solvent is normally used to dissolve the phospholipid prior to filter coating. This allows experimenters flexibility in the choice of lipid, provided the lipid can be dissolved in an inert solvent. The use of alcohols or water-soluble polar solvents is not recommended as these can leach out of the filter during the assay along with the phospholipids. Most researchers focus on hydrocarbon solvents such as *n*-dodecane. Pure hydrocarbons can dissolve only small amounts of lipid (<10% wt/v). Some investigators have chosen simple lipid systems such as phosphatidylcholine dissolved in dodecane as the model membrane barrier. This choice is inspired by the prevalence of phosphatidylcholine in mammalian membranes. In fact, the first lipid substance tested successfully was a very simple commercial egg lecithin formulation, which was shown to provide results as good as the more expensive synthetic lipids. The egg lecithin was doped with cholesterol to mimic the high presence of this compound in mammalian membranes. Other trends have developed since then. For example, Faller's group *(22,24)* has demonstrated that some solvents alone (e.g., hexadecane) can provide adequate results for simple permeability testing. In searching for the ideal PAMPA model to predict human jejunal permeability, Avdeef *(38)* reported the evaluation of about 50 different lipid compositions. Further attempts to replicate in vivo conditions using highly biomimetic lipid compositions have also been made. Sugano and coworkers *(25–28)* demonstrated the use of complex lipid combinations similar to those found in vivo (**Subheading 8.**). The high cost of these lipids may prohibit their widespread adoption, but the Sugano lipid formulation demonstrates the open-system nature of PAMPA. Finally, a new lecithin-based lipid combination, referred to as the gastrointestinal tract (GIT) lipid formulation (Double-Sink), has been described by Avdeef and coworkers (*36,38–41* and **Subheading 9.**). Excellent correlations between PAMPA permeability based on this membrane and several absorption parameters have been demonstrated. Furthermore, this new lipid is very cost-effective. The structure of the lipid phase in PAMPA membranes is not known. Normal bilayers, inverted hexagonal phases, cubic phases, water trapped in oil, and mixtures of these classic types of structures may actually be present.

3.5. Composition of Donor and Acceptor Well Solutions

The properties of buffer solutions used in the donor wells are very important to the experiment. A key problem found when implementing PAMPA is the low solubility of many research compounds, with some soluble only in the low micromolar range. This fact is often not fully appreciated by experimenters because PAMPA papers tend to emphasize results based on catalog drug compounds with good aqueous solubility. These drugs can be assayed at concentrations up to 500 μM *(25–28)* without difficulty, but when low-solubility compounds are encountered, the analytics may become problematic. Two approaches have been suggested to overcome this problem: the use of excipients and cosolvents. Kansy et al., who used solutions of glycocholic acid in pH 6.5 buffer to solubilize compounds, first described the use of excipients in PAMPA experiments *(20)*. Other solubilizing agents have been tested (**Subheading 12.**), including cosolvents (**Subheading 11.**), to overcome the problems of low sample solubility. The composition of the acceptor well solution plays an equally important role in the outcome of permeability experiments. In many reported cases, donor and acceptor solutions are of the same composition. This is contrary to the in vivo GIT conditions in which compounds, after passing through the cells of the intestinal wall, are immediately removed from the receiver site by blood flow assisted by their binding to serum proteins. This sink state maintains the largest possible concentration gradient across the membrane and thus hastens the transfer across the intestinal barrier. In PAMPA experiments, adding carrier proteins and other agents that bind compounds in aqueous solution can be used (**Subheading 9.**). The detection method most often applied in PAMPA is direct UV spectroscopy so proteins and other agents having swamping UV absorbance need to be avoided. Avdeef *(36,38)* recently described a nonselective binding agent added to the acceptor well buffer to create a sink condition simulating the presence of serum proteins and blood flow. Acceptor solution agents that strongly bind the test compounds can greatly reduce the time needed for permeability experiments.

3.6. Buffer pH and Permeability-pH Profiles

Another variable often changed in PAMPA experiments is the buffer pH. Avdeef *(21,32)*, Faller and Wohnsland *(22,24)*, and Sugano et al. *(25–28,42)* discussed in detail the pH dependence in PAMPA measurements. The idea behind this is the widely accepted pH partition hypothesis, which predicts that pH conditions favoring a neutral compound distribution will result in higher permeability than conditions favoring charged species. Because test compounds are often ionizable (acid, bases, or ampholytes), the hypothesis becomes significant in designing suitable permeability experiments. With knowledge of a compound's ionization constant(s), the buffer pH favoring neutral species may easily be predicted based on simple equilibrium theory *(41)*. To overcome this difficulty and get the highest permeability that may be reached in the GIT, Faller and Wohnsland *(22,24)* described a unified approach to working with different types of compounds, ionizable or not. The approach is to measure permeability at two or more widely separated but GIT-relevant pH levels and then use the highest permeability measured to characterize the compound. Zhu et al. *(29)* also applied this technique.

4. Unstirred Water Layers Affect the Measured Permeability

Transport across an artificial membrane barrier is a combination of diffusion through the membrane and diffusion through the unstirred water layers (UWL) at the two sides of the membrane (**Fig. 3**). Convective forces (e.g., from stirring) and diffusion quickly translocate solute molecules in the bulk aqueous phase. However, their transport through the UWL is governed solely by diffusion, which can be very time-consuming if the UWL is very thick or if

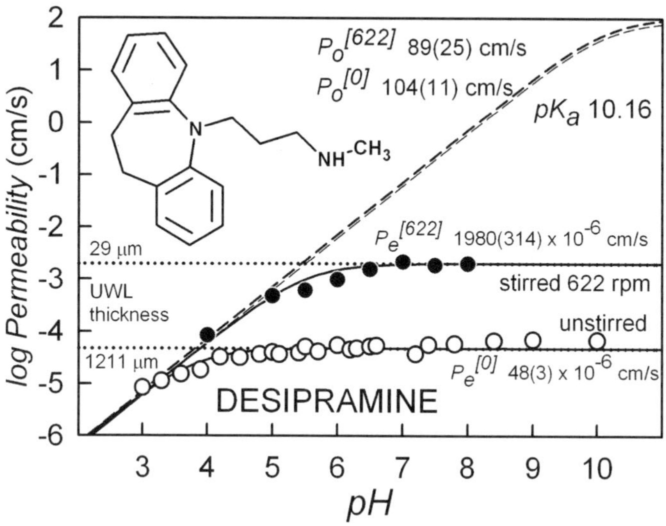

Fig. 4. The log permeability vs pH plots of desipramine. The open circles denote data collected under unstirred DS-PAMPA conditions, and the filled circles refer to data collected while each donor well was stirred at 622 rpm. The two dashed curves are the calculated membrane permeability, based on stirred and unstirred data. The maximum level in the dashed curves reveals the intrinsic permeability value, 89–104 cm/s.

the solute molecules are very large. If the thickness of the UWL is much greater than the thickness of the phospholipid membrane barrier, the water layer becomes the rate-limiting component in the transport of *lipophilic* molecules. It is important, when modeling in vivo transport of compounds, to match the dimensions of the UWL in the in vitro and in vivo assays. Because of the efficient mixing near the surface of the GIT, the in vivo UWL is estimated to be 30 to 100 µm thick ***(43)***. The UWL in the blood-brain barrier (BBB) is <1 µm, given that the diameter of the capillaries is about 6 µm and the tight fit of the distorted circulating erythrocytes gives efficient mixing ***(44)***. However, in unstirred in vitro permeation cells, the UWL can be 1500 to 4000 µm thick, depending on permeation cell geometry and dimensions ***(24,38,40,41)***. If the assays ignore the UWL effect with lipophilic test compounds, the resulting permeability values will not correctly indicate the in vivo conditions of permeability and will merely reveal properties of water rather than membrane permeation. For example, desipramine, with a pK_a 10.16, should be nearly a million times more permeable at pH 11.0 than at pH 5.0 as a result of the higher concentration of neutral species present in solution at the higher pH. As seen from **Fig. 4** (DS-PAMPA model, **Subheading 9.**), this does not appear to be the case. The average effective permeability, P_e, is *constant* in that pH interval at $(48 \pm 3) \times 10^{-5}$ cm/s (open circles, **Fig. 4**). The dashed curves represent the expected membrane permeability-pH profile in the absence of the unstirred water layer contribution. At high pH, the membrane curve levels off at 104 ± 11 cm/s, about two million times greater than what was measured directly. The *effective* (measured) permeability reaches its maximum value at about pH 5, and there is no increase when pH is raised further regardless of the increased concentration of the neutral species. Above pH 5.0, the observed transport is limited by the diffusion layer, and the effective permeability is that of the unstirred water layer, not the membrane. The thickness of the unstirred water layer in the unstirred PAMPA example is 1211 μm (**Fig. 4**).

5. Stirring Reveals More of the Membrane Permeability and Shortens Assay Time

When the solution in a permeation cell is stirred, the thickness of the unstirred water layer decreases ***(23,24,38,39,45,46)***, and the UWL plays a lesser role in the overall in vitro transport process. The layer can be made thinner with more vigorous stirring, but it cannot be made to vanish. To mimic the in vivo UWL, stirring must reduce the nascent thickness from 1500 to 4000 μm to less than 100 μm. The hydrodynamic equation ***(45)*** relating thickness of the UWL to the stirring speed is

$$h = (D_{aq}/K)\, \upsilon^{-\alpha}, \tag{2}$$

where D_{aq} is the aqueous diffusivity of the test compound, υ is the stirring speed (rpm), and K and α are empirical hydrodynamic constants. Adson et al. ***(45)*** reported values of $K = 4.1 \times 10^{-6}$ cm/s and $\alpha = 0.8$ based on data for testosterone in a stirred Caco-2 assay. Avdeef et al. ***(46)*** reported the values $K = 23.1 \times 10^{-6}$ cm/s and $\alpha = 0.709$ for PAMPA, based on the average behavior of 13 different lipophilic molecules, stirred from 49 to 622 rpm. For desipramine (D_{aq} 5.9×10^{-6} cm^2/s), according to the latter parameters and **Eq. 2**, to obtain a UWL of 30 μm, one would have to stir at 528 rpm. This is experimentally achievable in PAMPA. However, to achieve <1 μm UWL thickness (expected at the BBB), one would have to stir at >103,000 rpm!

Figure 4 shows the effective permeability-pH profile of desipramine in an assay in which each well is stirred at 622 rpm ***(46)***. The stirring raised the effective permeability at high pH from the unstirred value of $(48 \pm 3) \times 10^{-6}$ cm/s (open circles) to $(1980 \pm 314) \times 10^{-6}$ cm/s (filled circles). As dramatic as that increase is, the effective permeability at pH 11 is still UWL limited. The true membrane value of (89 ± 25) cm/s (top of the dashed curve) is about 50,000 times greater. The UWL was reduced from 1211 μm to 29 μm as a result of the stirring. A most welcome aspect of stirring solutions in PAMPA is that lipophilic molecules can be characterized with 15-min permeation assay times, a notable decrease from the 15 h originally used by Kansy et al. *(4)*.

6. Determining Intrinsic Permeability: Logarithmic Scale vs Direct Scale

In the above desipramine examples, we referred to intrinsic permeability, P_o, values of 104 ± 11 cm/s determined from unstirred assays and 89 ± 25 cm/s from assays stirred at 622 rpm. These two values are essentially the same, given the variance in their measurement. Such high values cannot be directly measured because speed over 100,000 rpm is not experimentally practical. These enormous values were calculated by the pK_a^{flux} method *(32,36,38,41)*, an extension of the approach first described by Gutknecht's group *(7–9)*. The method is based on using the observed shift in the apparent pK_a from its true value (pH at the bend in the dashed curve, **Fig. 4**) to its "flux" value (pH at the bend in the solid curves). This method can be applied to stirred or unstirred solutions and, within experimental error limits, yields the same intrinsic permeability, regardless of the stirring speed used. This is the expected permeability of the uncharged molecule if all contributions from the UWL were removed. The intrinsic permeability values that can be determined in PAMPA span nearly 10 orders of magnitude *(32,38,46)*. It is useful to consider the logarithmic scale when evaluating such large ranges of a property. It is interesting to note that the difference between 104 and 89 in the above examples is only 0.07 log units. It is estimated that the uncertainty in the universal pH buffers prepared by robotic control is not better than about ±0.1 *(38)*.

7. PAMPA Models for the Blood–Brain Barrier (BBB)

Di et al. *(31)* used 2% wt/vol porcine brain tissue extract dissolved in dodecane as their model lipid to successfully differentiate CNS+ from CNS– compounds. Given that the thickness of the UWL is <1 μm, it would be interesting to extend the method of Di and coworkers to apply intrinsic permeability constants, obtained from stirred PAMPA assays. The *p*ION group is currently developing its own BBB model, in which measured membrane permeability coefficients at pH 7.4, corrected for the UWL effect, are coupled with *in silico* predicted P-gp substrate specificity coefficients, using the Algorithm Builder software from Pharma Algorithms *(47)*. Predicting BBB is considerably more challenging than predicting intestinal absorption.

8. BM-PAMPA

The very productive and inventive group of Sugano and coworkers *(25–28,42)* explored a biomimetic lipid model (BM-PAMPA) containing several different phospholipids, closely resembling the mixture found in reconstituted brush border lipids *(48)*, and demonstrated dramatically improved intestinal absorption property predictions. The best-performing composition consisted of a lipid mixture of 0.8% wt/vol phosphatidylcholine, 0.8% phosphatidylethanolamine, 0.2% phosphatidylserine, 0.2% phosphatidylinositol, and 1.0% cholesterol dissolved in 1,7-octadiene. Various other diene solvents were explored, but the octadiene performed best *(26)*. (The researchers noted that the use of 1,7-octadiene in the assay requires safety precautions.) A similar exploration of solvents was made by Anderson's group *(11–15)* in searching for the characteristic barrier domain in purified egg lecithin bilayer lipid membranes; 1,9-decadiene was identified to precisely mimic the barrier selectivity *(14)*. The importance of the effect of pH on the observed permeability was recognized early *(25)* and was explored in depth *(42)*. The permeability characteristics of weak bases timolol and propranolol were studied in the pH interval of 3 to 10 *(42)*. The BM-PAMPA results suggested that the positively charged forms of the two bases were permeable at low pH, apparently in violation of the pH partition hypothesis. Similar low-pH anomalies were reported for the weak base quinine by Avdeef *(38)*. These very interesting observations deserve further study. Sugano et al. *(25)* also studied the effect of dimethylsulfoxide (DMSO), PEG400, and ethanol, up to 30%, in their PAMPA assays. In their regular assays, 5% vol/vol DMSO was present in both donor and acceptor wells. In general, water-miscible cosolvents are expected to decrease the membrane-water partition coefficients. In addition, the decreased dielectric constants of the cosolvent-water solutions should give rise to a higher proportion of the ionizable molecule in the uncharged state. These two effects oppose each other. Mostly, increasing levels of cosolvents were observed to lead to decreasing permeability. However, ethanol made the weak acid ketoprofen (pK_a of 4.12) more permeable with increasing cosolvent levels, an effect consistent with the increasing pK_a with the decreasing dielectric constant of the cosolvent mixtures, which leads to a higher proportion of uncharged species at a given pH. However, the same reasoning cannot be used to explain why the weak base propranolol (pK_a of 9.53) decreased in permeability with increasing amounts of ethanol. This may be because of the increased solubility of propranolol in water with the added ethanol in relation to the solubility in the membrane phase. The result is a lowered membrane/mixed-solvent partition coefficient lowering the flux as a result of the diminished sample concentration gradient in the membrane. It is generally appreciated that PAMPA only predicts passive permeability. However, in vivo transport of small molecules can also involve the paracellular route *(45)*. Molecules with molecular weights <250 Da can sieve through the aqueous pores in the tight junctions connecting the epithelial cells of the intestine. The direction taken by Sugano's group *(27,28)* involved combining measured BM-PAMPA permeability with *in silico* calculated paracellular permeability, using the Renkin function and electrostatics analysis. They used an empirical fitting approach, similar to that described by Adson's group ***(45)*** in their study of Caco-2 paracellular permeability. The pore size and electrical potential lining the tight junctions, which best correlated Sugano's BM-PAMPA data with in vivo absorption data, were about 5.61 Å and 75 mV, respectively ***(28)***. Adson's group found 12 Å and 17.7 mV, based on the cellular model. Our group is applying this "half-measured/half-calculated" approach to predict transport properties of the BBB, as described in the preceding section.

9. DS-PAMPA

DS-PAMPA is one of the newest PAMPA variants described in the literature ***(38–40,46,49)*** and has gained considerable attention in the industry. In this experiment, the traditional conditions developed by Kansy and Faller have been replaced by two gradient systems (Double-Sink). For example, traditional PAMPA experiments maintain the same buffer pH in the donor and acceptor wells (iso-pH conditions). However, in DS-PAMPA, pH gradients between the donor and acceptor compartments are introduced. The rationale for this procedure is the underlying physiology of the absorption process in the human body. After a compound is ingested, it travels through the stomach and the intestines to be absorbed. The human body exposes the drug to different pH conditions throughout the GIT, and the blood, the first target of the compounds for systemic delivery, is maintained at pH 7.4. To mimic this environment in vitro, DS-PAMPA uses a pH gradient between the aqueous compartments. The donor compartment pH can be set from 3 to 10 (but commonly from 5.0 to 7.4), depending on the compound, and the acceptor compartment is maintained at pH 7.4. This difference can drive transport for weak acid compounds by enabling those with low pK_a (e.g., naproxen, at 4.32) to enter the membrane at low pH in the donor well and then become trapped in the acceptor well in their charged form, creating a virtual sink condition. This gradient-pH state is the first sink condition. The second sink condition takes advantage of chemical scavengers in the acceptor well to make transport of lipophilic compounds across the membrane unidirectional ***(38)***. In iso-pH experiments without scavengers, equilibrium will be established between the two compartments, and a test compound will eventually divide into equal amounts in both compartments, minus what is retained by the membrane to complete mass balance. However, in vivo static equilibrium is not maintained as both blood flow and serum proteins constantly shift the equilibrium to favor permeation (in the absence of efflux transporter effects). Scavengers in the acceptor well simulate this in vitro. Lipophilic scavengers ***(38)*** serve to increase the volume of distribution of the acceptor compartment. They can bind compounds similar to the way proteins do. In theory, they can shift the equilibrium so much that the entire amount of test compound is eventually moved to the acceptor compartment. They also drastically reduce the permeation time of the experiment, apart from the effect of stirring mentioned above. They do so by desorbing compound from the membrane into solution. The lipophilic scavengers are superior to proteins and other chaperone molecules because they (1) are chemically very stable; (2) are relatively nonspecific in what they bind; (3) do not promote bacterial growth in buffers, which facilitates preparation and storage; and (4) absorb minimally in the 230- to 500-nm region of the UV spectrum. The use of unstirred DS-PAMPA has reduced assay time. Typical assays need not be run longer than 4 h for most compounds. A dramatic additional decrease in assay time can be achieved with stirring (*see* **Subheading 5.**). A further benefit of the Double-Sink method is that membrane retention of compounds is greatly reduced ***(38)***. This finding is not trivial because research compounds tend to be highly lipophilic (octanol-water log $P > 4$). This lipophilicity makes most compounds accumulate in the membrane instead of transporting into the acceptor compartment. Studies performed by Avdeef's group ***(38)*** suggest that membrane loading of drugs must reach a critical level before compound can be seen in the acceptor well. In some cases, this critical level requires almost all the compound available!

10. Correlations of PAMPA with Caco-2 and Rat *In Situ* Perfusion Assays

Bermejo et al. ***(39)*** described remarkable correlations between DS-PAMPA and rat *in situ* perfusion and Caco-2 permeability data based on 17 fluoroquinolones, including three congeneric series with a systematically varied alkyl chain length at the 4'*N* position of the piperazine residue. **Figure 5** shows the correlation between the rat data and PAMPA. The permeability values span more than three orders of magnitude. The intrinsic permeability, P_o, was determined from the pH dependence of the effective permeability (pK_a^{flux} method). The DS-PAMPA method employed stirring, adjusted such that the UWL thickness matched the 30-µm value estimated to be in the human small intestine. Increasing the alkyl chain length in the congener series resulted in increased PAMPA permeability, about 0.36 log units per methylene group, except that of the first (H-to-Me), which was about 1.2 log units. The *in situ* closed-loop technique used for obtaining permeability values in rat showed a UWL thickness of about 103 µm. The rat-PAMPA correlation ($r^2 = 0.87$) was better than that of rat-Caco-2 ($r^2 = 0.63$), whereas the Caco-2-PAMPA correlation indicated that $r^2 = 0.66$. Caco-2 correlations can be improved if the data are first corrected for the UWL effect.

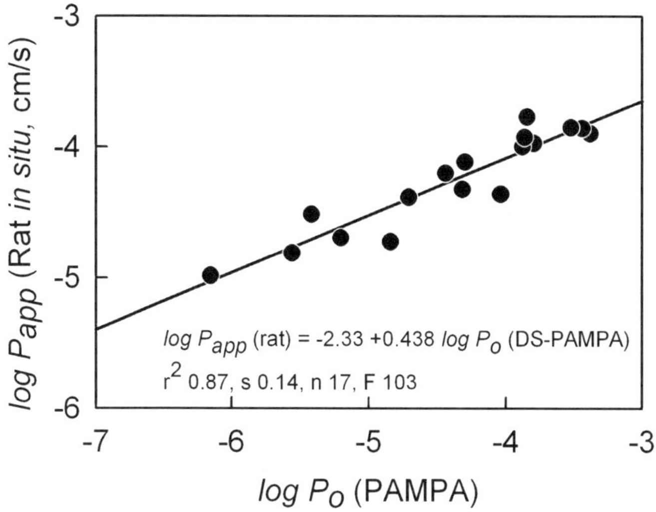

Fig. 5. Rat *in situ* perfusion permeability compared to DS-PAMPA intrinsic permeability for 17 substituted fluoroquinolones, adapted from the work of Bermejo et al. ***(39)***.

11. Cosolvent Use Overcomes the Problems of Studying Very Sparingly Soluble Molecules

Ruell et al. ***(49)*** described a cosolvent procedure, based on the use of 20% v/v acetonitrile in a universal pH buffer. For the first time, it was possible to measure the permeability of molecules such as amiodarone, which has an intrinsic aqueous solubility of about 6 ng/mL. Its measured intrinsic permeability was determined as 1.32 cm/s, which is close to the DS-PAMPA values determined for propranolol and verapamil. A procedure was devised in which values determined in 20% acetonitrile are extrapolated to cosolvent-free conditions ***(49)***.

12. Use of PAMPA in Formulation Research

PAMPA has shown unexpected versatility. For example, it has been used to determine partition coefficients in alkane-water ***(22,24)*** and octanol-water ***(37)*** mixtures. Liu et al. ***(50)*** designed a PAMPA screening method for solubilizers, such as Brij® 35, Cremophor EL, ethanol, and Tween-80, used in conjunction with compounds of low aqueous solubility. Because many solubilizers were found to interfere with UV detection, the liquid chromatography/mass spectrometry (LC/MS) approach was used, rather then the usual direct UV spectroscopy. The effect of the solubilizers on the observed permeability was characterized in a search for effective excipients in preformulation applications.

13. Outlook

The PAMPA method has demonstrated its versatility in many instances since 1998. It is a remarkable "open-system" approach, in which practitioners may formulate their own lipid barriers for any number of different applications, not all focused on permeability screening. The method can be a low-cost, very fast, and particularly helpful add-on to cellular permeability assays, such as Caco-2. It readily provides information about passive-transport permeability, not complicated by other mechanisms, such as active transport and metabolism. Its continuing development in BBB permeation applications is expected to produce further exciting progress. Low solubility of test compounds is not an obstacle to permeability measurement, as has been demonstrated with the cosolvent method. Continuing improvements in PAMPA will make it the method of choice for primary screening of permeability, as suggested by Lipinski *(1)*. These are still the early days of PAMPA, which in some ways resemble those of high-performance liquid chromatography (HPLC) in the 1980s. As suggested by Faller's work *(24,37)* and the rising interest in preformulation applications, PAMPA may one day even displace the use of octanol-water partition coefficients in pharmaceutical and agrochemical research and become the new surrogate for lipophilicity with broad-based biological applications.

14. PAMPA: Experimental Methods and Technical Notes

Described below is the general experimental method that single-pH experiments use in manual mode. It can also be used with single pH and cosolvent because the cosolvent may simply be added to the buffer.

14.1. Summary of Operations

Stock plate with test compounds is prepared. Universal buffer solution (System Solution) is prepared. Universal buffer is added to the deep-well plates. Samples from stock plate are diluted and mixed in the deep-well plate. Diluted sample mixtures are added to the donor plate (bottom). Acceptor/filter plate (top) is painted with lipid. Painted acceptor/filter plate is placed on top of the donor plate. Acceptor plate (top) is filled with universal buffer solution. Concentration of the diluted sample mixtures is measured. The sandwich incubates.

14.2. Materials

The following required materials may be obtained from *p*ION INC (Woburn, MA) in a kit called PAMPA BUNDLE PACKAGE. (The part numbers refer to those of *p*ION.)

PAMPA Sandwich (PN 110163). 96-Well deep-well plate (PN 110023). 96-well UV plate (PN 110024). Bottle of universal buffer solution concentrate (*p*ION System Solution, PN 110151). Phosphatidylcholine, 2% wt/vol in dodecane, packed under nitrogen in a flame-sealed glass ampoule (BLM-0 lipid, PN 110615). Ampoule breaker (PN 110617).

Also needed are the following: A handheld disposable-tip pipettor, preferably one that has an eight-tip head, suitable for use with the microplate; and a sealed container with wet sponge or, alternatively, the Gut Box™ Environmental Chamber containing a built-in stirrer, oxygen and carbon dioxide scrubbers, and humidity control (PN 110205).

14.3. Apparatus Needed

Recommended: SPECTRAmax 190 (or SPECTRAmax Plus) microplate-scanning UV spectrophotometer from Molecular Devices (Sunnyvale, CA). *Alternatives:* HPLC/UV, LC/MS, or other apparatus for concentration measurement.

14.4. Assay Protocol

The following general protocol is used to measure PAMPA effective permeability, P_e, of a set of test molecules, using the BLM model lipid ***(23,41)***. It assumes that 32 compounds are measured in triplicate, filling the entire 96-well microplate. This number may vary depending on the blank method used with the detection system. The values needed (for the equation below) from the measurement of $C_D(0)$ and $C_A(t)$ are concentration-proportional numbers, not necessarily absolute concentration values. It is further assumed that the System Solution (universal pH buffer) is prepared according to the instructions in Subheading 14.12. and is placed in a trough to be picked up by an eight-tip pipettor, and BLM lipid from one vial has been placed in a V-shaped trough for pickup by an eight-tip pipettor.

If a UV spectrophotometer is used for quantitation, sample concentration of 10 to 500 μ*M* should be used (typical value is 50 μ*M*). In choosing the concentration, the strength of the UV chromophore and the solubility of the compound should be considered.

1. Prepare 3 × 32 drug solutions of a 10- to 500-μM concentration using the System Solution (universal buffer), and place 400 to 500 μL mixed solution in each well of the deep-well plate.
2. Transfer 150 μL of drug solution from each well of the deep-well plate to the corresponding wells of a clean UV plate. Measure $C_D(0)$ as the blank corrected area under the curve or absorbance at a suitable wavelength in the range 250 to 500 nm.

3. Dismantle the empty PAMPA sandwich, carefully keeping the filter plate (acceptor) covered with the lid until use.
4. Transfer 200 µL of drug solution from each well of the deep-well plate to the corresponding bottom (donor) plate well.
5. Dispense 5 µL of BLM lipid solution onto each filter of the acceptor (top) plate of the PAMPA sandwich.
6. Carefully place the acceptor plate on top of the donor plate and ensure that no air bubbles are trapped under the membrane.
7. Add 200 µL of System Solution (universal buffer) to each of the acceptor (top) plates of the PAMPA sandwich.
8. Cover the sandwich with the plate lid and incubate in a humidity chamber for 16 h (less time is required if the sandwich is stirred using the Gut-Box™ or if very lipophilic samples are tested).
9. When the UV reading is complete, wash and dry the UV plate or use a new clean one for the next measurement.
10. After the incubation period, carefully transfer 150 µL of solution from the acceptor (top) plate of the sandwich to the clean UV plate. Measure $C_A(t)$ as in **step 2**.
11. Discard the sandwich.
12. To calculate the effective permeability, insert in the formula below the actual incubation time *t*, in hours, $C_A(t)$ as any concentration-proportional number and $C_D(0)$ as a corresponding concentration-proportional number. The ratio $C_A(t)/C_D(0)$ should not exceed 0.495.

$$P_e = -\frac{218.3}{t}\log_{10}\left[1 - 2\frac{C_A(t)}{C_D(0)}\right]10^{-6}\ \text{cm / s.}$$

14.5. The General Equation for Iso-pH PAMPA

Avdeef *(32,36,38)* derived the general single-pH permeability equation, which also takes membrane retention factor, *R*, into account:

$$P_e = -\frac{2.303}{A(t-\tau_{ss})}\left(\frac{V_A V_D}{V_A + V_D}\right)\log_{10}\left[1 - \left(\frac{V_A + V_D}{V_D(1-R)}\right)\frac{C_A(t)}{C_D(0)}\right],$$

where A = area of filter (cm^2); t = time (here in seconds, not hours); τ_{ss} = steady-state time (s); V_A and V_D are the acceptor and donor volumes (cm^3), respectively; and $C_A(t)$ and $C_D(0)$ are the measured acceptor and donor sample concentrations (mol/cm^3) at time t and time 0, respectively. The membrane retention factor, *R*, is defined as $1 - [C_D(t) + C_A(t)\,V_A/V_D]/C_D(0)$. To take advantage of this equation, $C_D(t)$ needs to be measured as well. This can best be done by inserting the necessary steps in the above assay protocol after **step 10**.

14.6. General Experimental Method for Gradient-pH Experiments

In the gradient-pH method, the acceptor solution is maintained at pH 7.4, and the donor pH is varied from pH 3.0 to 10.0. The typical range used is 5.0 to 7.4, which corresponds to the pH of the upper intestinal tract. The benefits of an assay designed under gradient-pH conditions are (1) less retention, R, and thus more sensitivity; (2) shorter permeation times and thus higher throughput possible; and (3) more realistic modeling of the in vivo pH gradients found in the small intestinal tract and thus better predictions of oral absorption. Gradient-pH methods and calculations of permeability have been described in detail by Avdeef ***(36,38)***.

14.7. Dealing With Compounds With Low Aqueous Solubility

Many compounds barely have the aqueous solubility needed to measure permeability. In such experiments, at least 10-μ*M* concentrations are needed. Because particles in solution scatter light, it is important to make certain that compounds are completely dissolved in the assay medium. Either filtering or adding cosolvents to samples can meet this need (**Subheading 11.**).

14.8. Filtering Samples

Filtering samples is a tedious process but is often necessary. The choices are limited to either using 96-well filter plates or individual-well filtration methods. In either case, the deep-well plate should be carefully examined for particles in wells. When in doubt, filter the sample. A possible alternative would be to centrifuge the sample (2000*g* for 15 min) and work only with the supernatant.

14.9. Cosolvents

Cosolvents may be used. Be aware that cosolvents will affect the membrane-buffer partition coefficients. They may also change the pH of the buffer used, affecting the ionization of the compounds. Care should also be used when choosing cosolvent because some may dissolve the filters or plastic plates. When using a cosolvent, proceed as described in the general method, except the cosolvent should be added directly to the buffer. The System Solution (universal buffer) from *p*ION (PN 110151) normally works well with up to 10% cosolvent. After that, too much buffering capacity is generally lost, and the buffer capacity is less linear with the volume of NaOH added to adjust pH (*see* **Subheading 14.12.**).

14.10. Liquid Chromatography/Mass Spectrometry

Sometimes compounds have very low UV absorbance at the typical concentrations used. In such cases, concentration of acceptor and donor wells may be measured using LC/MS and used in the permeability equation. The disadvantages of LC/MS vs UV detection is the time and work involved for the user. UV data collection and processing is much faster.

14.11. Impure Compounds

A small amount of impurity may be tolerated (<10%). If not, an appropriate use of HPLC/UV or LC/MS detection systems for the concentration measurement is a possibility. The PAMPA BUNDLE is equally well suited for all detection systems, especially because phosphate is avoided in the universal buffer.

14.12. pION System Solution (Universal pH Buffer)

The PAMPA BUNDLE uses a unique aqueous universal buffer called the *p*ION System Solution, especially designed for permeability and solubility measurement and other applications in which concentration measurements using spectrophotometric methods (such as UV/vis, HPLC/UV) are needed at a specific pH. The phosphate-free universal buffer has been used in LC/MS-based assays as well ***(23,50)***. A buffer is needed that is based on components that will not interact with the molecules being studied. For that reason, phosphate is not used because of its strong tendency to cause precipitation of salts of positively charged drug substances ***(51)***. Also, boric acid is avoided because it is known to interact with glycosides. Making the UV detection system produce the highest possible sample signal and the smallest possible signal from the background buffers, the UV absorption of the buffer components had to be kept low. Citric acid and several other common buffers should not be used because of their appreciable UV absorption. The pH vs the volume of alkaline titrant relationship must be as linear as possible, to allow easy adjustment of the pH to any needed value in the range 3.0 to 10.0. None of the commonly known universal buffers ***(52,53)*** fits the desired profile. The System Solution has been designed with five different ionization groups, evenly spaced in pK_a values, to produce a very constant buffer capacity in the interval of pH 3.0 to 10.0. The ionic strength of the System Solution is about 10 m*M*. No NaCl or KCl has been added to boost the ionic strength to higher values. The System Solution is normally shipped as a concentrate in 50-mL plastic bottles. The concentrate contains a small amount of bacteriostatic preservative to prevent growth during storage. Still, the concentrate should be kept refrigerated but not frozen. To prepare the System Solution at its minimum pH (~2.8), you will need the following: 2-L volumetric flask or 2-L graduated cylinder; System Solution concentrate bottle (50 mL); and 2-L storage bottle for the prepared System Solution. Pour the entire 50 mL of concentrate into an empty and clean 2-L volumetric flask or 2-L graduated cylinder. Note the lot number of the concentrate. Add distilled or deionized water to a total volume of 2 L and shake the capped flask/cylinder well to mix the solution. Add the solution to the 2-L storage bottle, cap, and label the bottle with date, lot number, and pH ~2.8. Once diluted, the buffer is stable for up to a week (sometimes much longer, depending on laboratory conditions) in the refrigerator. Bacterial growth may be experienced and would be indicated by a higher baseline in a blank UV spectrum. It is recommended that the buffer be filtered through a 0.2-µm filter to remove the growth. If in doubt about the purity of the buffer, simply filter it or discard it and make up a fresh solution. When using just one pH value for all the PAMPA wells, the System Solution is set for that pH value as described below. To set the pH of the System Solution to pH_{TARGET}, you will need the following: calibrated pH meter, magnetic stirrer, large stir bar, stir bar retriever, up to 120 mL of 0.5 *M* carbonate-free NaOH (do not use NaOH pellets to prepare the solution—purchase a ready-made standardized solution from a reliable source), 100-mL graduated cylinder, and 1-mL disposable-tip pipettor.

To make up 2 L of System Solution, proceed as follows:

1. Place the 2-L storage bottle containing the System Solution on top of the magnetic stirrer. Place a sufficiently large, clean magnetic stir bar in the 2-L bottle and turn on the stirrer.
2. Using distilled or deionized water, rinse the calibrated pH electrode and place it in the System Solution bottle. Secure it with a clamp or carefully hold by hand.
3. Read the pH. This value is referred to as pH_{START}.
4. Choose the pH for the assay to be run, and use Table 1 to find the approximate volume of 0.5 *M* NaOH needed to bring 2 L of System Solution from pH_{START} to pH_{TARGET}.

   Example: If the wanted pH is 7.4 and pH_{START} was measured at 2.8, look up in the pH_{START} = 2.8 column of **Table 1** the needed volume of 0.5 *M* NaOH. You will see that it would take about 63 mL of 0.5 *M* NaOH to take the solution from pH 2.8 to pH 7.4.
5. Using the graduated cylinder, measure out about 60 mL of 0.5 *M* NaOH (about 5% less than indicated in Table 1, so as not to overshoot the target), and add the NaOH to the System Solution.
6. Take a new pH reading using the pH meter. Fine-tune the pH value using the 1-mL disposable-tip pipettor until the desired pH_{TARGET} of 7.4 has been reached. Allow at least 2 min for the final pH reading to stabilize. For future use, note on the 2-L bottle label the actual total volume of NaOH that was added to 2000 mL for this lot number to reach pH_{TARGET}.

Table 1
Approximate Volumes of 0.5 *M* NaOH To Be Added to 2000 mL System Solution to Reach a Certain pH

pH_{START} = 2.6		pH_{START} = 2.8		pH_{START} = 3.0	
pH_{TARGET}	Vol (mL)	pH_{TARGET}	Vol (mL)	pH_{TARGET}	Vol (mL)
2.8	2				
3.0	5	3.0	2		
3.2	8	3.2	5	3.2	2
3.4	11	3.4	8	3.4	5
3.6	13	3.6	11	3.6	8
3.8	16	3.8	13	3.8	11
4.0	19	4.0	16	4.0	13
4.2	22	4.2	19	4.2	16
4.4	25	4.4	22	4.4	19
4.6	27	4.6	25	4.6	22
4.8	30	4.8	27	4.8	25
5.0	*33*	*5.0*	*30*	*5.0*	*27*
5.2	36	5.2	33	5.2	30
5.4	38	5.4	36	5.4	33
5.6	41	5.6	38	5.6	36
5.8	44	5.8	41	5.8	38
6.0	47	6.0	44	6.0	41
6.2	*50*	*6.2*	*47*	*6.2*	*44*
6.4	52	6.4	50	6.4	47
6.6	55	6.6	52	6.6	50
6.8	58	6.8	55	6.8	52
7.0	61	7.0	58	7.0	55
7.2	63	7.2	61	7.2	58
7.4	*66*	*7.4*	*63*	*7.4*	*61*
7.6	69	7.6	66	7.6	63
7.8	72	7.8	69	7.8	66
8.0	75	8.0	72	8.0	69
8.2	77	8.2	75	8.2	72
8.4	80	8.4	77	8.4	75
8.6	83	8.6	80	8.6	77
8.8	86	8.8	83	8.8	80
9.0	88	9.0	86	9.0	83
9.2	91	9.2	88	9.2	86
9.4	94	9.4	91	9.4	88
9.6	97	9.6	94	9.6	91
9.8	100	9.8	97	9.8	94
10.0	102	10.0	100	10.0	97

Acknowledgments

We thank Drs. Manfred Kansy, Holger Fischer, Bernard Faller, Kiyohiko Sugano, Ed Kerns, Li Di, Jeanne Phillips, and Profs. Bradley Anderson and Marival Bermejo for sharing with us some of their latest research of relevance to PAMPA. Dr. Christian Schobert has guided us in areas relevant to agrochemical research. Prof. Norman Ho has been very helpful in discussions related to the biophysics of membrane transport. Thanks also are extended to colleagues at *p*ION (especially Per Nielsen and Cynthia Berger) and Sirius Analytical Instruments (especially John Comer and Karl Box) for many helpful discussions.

References

1. Lipinski, C. A. (2002) Observation on current ADMET technology: no uniformity exists. Paper presented at the annual meeting of the Society of Biomolecular Screening, 24 September, The Hauge, The Netherlands.
2. Di, L. and Kerns, E. H. (2003) Profiling drug-like properties in discovery research. *Curr. Opin. Chem. Biol.* **7,** 402–408.
3. Kerns, E. H. and Di, L. (2003) Pharmaceutical profiling in drug discovery. *Drug Disc. Today* **8,** 316–323.
4. Kansy, M., Senner, F., and Gubernator, K. (1998) Physicochemical high throughput screening: parallel artificial membrane permeability assay in the description of passive absorption processes. *J. Med. Chem.* **41,** 1007–1010.
5. Mueller, P., Rudin, D. O., Tien, H. T., and Westcott, W. C. (1962) Reconstitution of cell membrane structure in vitro and its transformation into an excitable system. *Nature* **194,** 979–980.
6. Tien, T. H. and Ottova, A. L. (2001) The lipid bilayer concept and its experimental realization: from soap bubbles, kitchen sink, to bilayer lipid membranes. *J. Mem. Sci.* **189,** 83–117.
7. Gutknecht, J. and Tosteson, D. C. (1973) Diffusion of weak acids across lipid membranes: effects of chemical reactions in the unstirred layers. *Science* **182,** 1258–1261.
8. Gutknecht, J., Bisson, M. A., and Tosteson, F. C. (1977) Diffusion of carbon dioxide through lipid bilayer membranes. Effects of carbonic anhydrase, bicarbonate, and unstirred layers. *J. Gen. Physiol.* **69,** 779–794.
9. Walter, A. and Gutknecht, J. (1984) Monocarboxylic acid permeation through lipid bilayer membranes. *J. Mem. Biol.* **77,** 255–264.
10. Antonenko, Y. N., Denisov, G. A., and Pohl, P. (1993) Weak acid transport across bilayer lipid membrane in the presence of buffers. *Biophys. J.* **64,** 1701–1710.
11. Xiang, T.-X. and Anderson, B. D. (1993) Diffusion of ionizable solutes across planar lipid bilayer membranes: boundary-layer pH gradients and the effect of buffers. *Pharm. Res.* **10,** 1654–1661.
12. Xiang, T.-X. and Anderson, B. D. (1994) Substituent contributions to the transport of substituted p-toluic acids across lipid bilayer membranes. *J. Pharm. Sci.* **83,** 1511–1518.

13. Mayer, P. T., Xiang, T.-X., and Anderson, B. D. (2000) Independence of substituent contributions to the transport of small-molecule permeants in lipid bilayers. *AAPS PharmSci.* **2,** 1–13.
14. Mayer, P. T. and Anderson, B. D. (2002) Transport across 1,9-decadiene precisely mimics the chemical selectivity of the barrier domain in egg lecithin bilayers. *J. Pharm. Sci.* **91,** 640–646.
15. Mayer, P. T., Xiang, T.-X., Niemi, R., and Anderson, B. D. (2003) A hydrophobicity scale for the lipid bilayer barrier domain from peptide permeabilities: nonadditivities in residue contributions. *Biochemistry* **42,** 1624–1636.
16. Mountz, J. M. and Tien, H. T. (1978) Photoeffects of pigmented lipid membranes in a micropourous filter. *Photochem. Photobiol.* **28,** 395–400.
17. Thompson, M., Lennox, R. B., and McClelland, R. A. (1982) Structure and electrochemical properties of microfiltration filter-lipid membrane systems. *Anal. Chem.* **54,** 76–81.
18. Cools, A. A. and Janssen, L. H. M. (1983) Influence of sodium ion-pair formation on transport kinetics of warfarin through octanol-impregnated membranes. *J. Pharm. Pharmacol.* **35,** 689–691.
19. Camenisch, G., Folkers, G., and van de Waterbeemd, H. (1997) Comparison of passive drug transport through Caco-2 cells and artificial membranes. *Int. J. Pharm.* **147,** 61–70.
20. Kansy, M., Fischer, H., Kratzat, K., Senner, F., Wagner, B., and Parrilla, I. (2001) High-throughput artificial membrane permeability studies in early lead discovery and development, in *Pharmacokinetic Optimization in Drug Research*, (Testa, B., van de Waterbeemd, H., Folkers, G., and Guy, R., eds.), Verlag Helvetica Chimica Acta, Zürich/Wiley–VCH, Weinheim, pp. 447–464.
21. Avdeef, A. (2001) High-throughput measurements of solubility profiles, in in *Pharmacokinetic Optimization in Drug Research*, (Testa, B., van de Waterbeemd, H., Folkers, G., and Guy, R., eds.), Verlag Helvetica Chimica Acta, Zürich/Wiley–VCH, Weinheim, pp. 305–326.
22. Faller, B. and Wohnsland, F. (2001) Physicochemical parameters as tools in drug discovery and lead optimization, in in *Pharmacokinetic Optimization in Drug Research*, (Testa, B., van de Waterbeemd, H., Folkers, G., and Guy, R., eds.), Verlag Helvetica Chimica Acta, Zürich/Wiley–VCH, Weinheim, pp. 257–274.
23. Avdeef, A., Strafford, M., Block, E., Balogh, M. P., Chambliss, W., and Khan, I. (2001) Drug absorption in vitro model: filter-immobilized artificial membranes. 2. Studies of the permeability properties of lactones in *piper methysticum forst. Eur. J. Pharm. Sci.* **14,** 271–280.
24. Wohnsland, F. and Faller, B. (2001) High-throughput permeability pH profile and high-throughput alkane/water log P with artificial membranes. *J. Med. Chem.* **44,** 923–930.
25. Sugano, K., Hamada, H., Machida, M., Ushio, H., Saitoh, K., and Terada, K. (2001) Optimized conditions of bio-mimetic artificial membrane permeability assay. *Int. J. Pharm.* **228,** 181–188.

26. Sugano, K., Hamada, H., Machida, M., and Ushio, H. (2001) High throughput prediction of oral absorption: improvement of the composition of the lipid solution used in parallel artificial membrane permeability assay. *J. Biomol. Screen.* **6,** 189–196.
27. Sugano, K., Takata, N., Machida, M., Saitoh, K., and Terada, K. (2002) Prediction of passive intestinal absorption using bio-mimetic artificial membrane permeation assay and the paracellular pathway model. *Int. J. Pharm.* **241,** 241–251.
28. Sugano, K., Nabuchi, Y., Machida, M., and Aso, Y. (2003) Prediction of human intestinal permeability using artificial membrane permeability. *Int. J. Pharm.* **257,** 245–251.
29. Zhu, C., Jiang, L., Chen, T.-M., and Hwang, K.-K. (2002) A comparative study of artificial membrane permeability assay for high-throughput profiling of drug absorption potential. *Eur. J. Med. Chem.* **37,** 399–407.
30. Veber, D. F., Johnson, S. R., Cheng, H.-Y., Smith, B. R., Ward, K. W., and Kopple, K. D. (2002) Molecular properties that influence the oral bioavailability of drug candidates. *J. Med. Chem.* **45,** 2615–2623.
31. Di, L., Kerns, E. H., Fan, K., McConnell, O. J., and Carter, G. T. (2003) High throughput artificial membrane permeability assay for blood-brain barrier. *Eur. J. Med. Chem.* **38,** 223–232.
32. Avdeef, A. (2001) Physicochemical profiling (solubility, permeability, and charge state). *Curr. Top. Med. Chem.* **1,** 277–351.
33. Kerns, E. H. (2001) High throughput physicochemical profiling for drug discovery. *J. Pharm. Sci.* **90,** 1838–1858.
34. Kerns, E. H. and Di, L. (2002) Multivariate pharmaceutical profiling for drug discovery. *Curr. Top. Med. Chem.* **2,** 87–98.
35. Ruell, J. (2003) Membrane-based drug assays. *Mod. Drug Disc.* Jan., 28–30.
36. Avdeef, A. (2003) High-throughput measurements of permeability profiles, in *Drug Bioavailability: Estimation of Solubility, Permeability, Absorption and Bioavailability*, (van de Waterbeemd, H., Lennernäs, H., and Artursson, P., eds.), Wiley–VCH, Weinheim, pp. 46–70.
37. Faller, B. (2003) High-throughput physiochemical profiling : potential and limitations, in *Analysis and Purification Methods in Combinatorial Chemistry*. Wiley & Sons, New York, in press.
38. Avdeef, A. (2003) *Absorption and Drug Development*. Wiley-Interscience, New York.
39. Avdeef, A., Ruiz, A., Nalda, R., Ruell, J. A., Tsinman, O., Gonzalez, I., et al. (2004) PAMPA—a drug absorption in vitro model: 7. Comparing rat *in situ*, Caco-2, and PAMPA permeability of fluoroquinolones. *Eur. J. Pharm. Sci.*, **21,** 429–441.
40. Nielsen, P. E. and Avdeef, A. (2004) PAMPA—a drug absorption in vitro model: 8. Apparent filter porosity and the unstirred water layer. *Eur. J. Pharm. Sci.* **21,** in press.
41. Ruell, J. A., Tsinman, K. L., and Avdeef, A. (2004) PAMPA—a drug absorption in vitro model: 5. Unstirred water layer in Iso-pH mapping assays and pK_a^{flux}-optimized design (pOD-PAMPA). *Eur. J. Pharm. Sci.* **20,** 393–402.

42. Sugano, K., Nabuchi, Y., and Aso, Y. (2003) Transport mechanism of basic compounds through bio-mimetic artificial membrane. Poster presented at the Acad. Pharma. Sci. Technol. (APSTJ) Meeting, April, Kyoto, Japan.
43. Lennernäs, H. (1998) Human intestinal permeability. *J. Pharm. Sci.* **87,** 403–410.
44. Partridge, W. M. (1991) *Peptide Drug Delivery to the Brain.* Raven Press, New York.
45. Adson, A., Burton, P. S., Raub, T. J., Barsuhn, C. L., Audus, K. L., and Ho, N. F. H. (1995) Passive diffusion of weak organic electrolytes across Caco-2 cell monolayers: uncoupling the contributions of hydrodynamic, transcellular, and paracellular barriers. *J. Pharm. Sci.* **84,** 1197–1204.
46. Avdeef, A., Nielsen, P., and Tsinman, O. (2004) PAMPA—a drug absorption in vitro model: 11. Matching the in vivo unstirred water layer thickness by individual-well stirring in microtitre plates. *Eur. J. Pharm. Sci.* **21,** in press.
47. Pharma Algorithms, Toronto, Canada: www.ap-algorithms.com.
48. Proulx, P. (1991) Structure-function relationships in intestinal brush border membranes. *Biochim. Biophys. Acta* **1071,** 255–271.
49. Ruell, J. A., Tsinman, O., and Avdeef, A. (2004) Acid-base cosolvent method for determining aqueous permeability of amiodarone, itra conazole, tamoxifen, ter fenadine and other very insoluble molecules. *Chem. Pharm. Bull.* **52,** in press.
50. Liu, H., Sabus, C., Carter, G. T., Avdeef, A., and Tischler, M. (2003) Solubilizer selection in the parallel artificial membrane permeability assay (PAMPA) for *in vitro* permeability measurement of low solubility compounds. *Pharm. Res.* **20,** 1820–1826.
51. Streng, W. H., Hsi, S. K., Helms, P. E., and Tan, H. G. H. (1984) General treatment of pH-solubility profiles of weak acids and bases and the effect of different acids on the solubility of a weak base. *J. Pharm. Sci.* **73,** 1679–1684.
52. Perrin, D. D. and Dempsey, B. (1974) *Buffers for pH and Metal Ion Control.* Chapman & Hall, London.
53. Avdeef, A. and Bucher, J. J. (1978) Accurate measurements of the concentration of hydrogen ions with a glass electrode: calibrations using the Prideaux and other universal buffer solutions and a computer-controlled automatic titrator. *Anal. Chem.* **50,** 2137–2142.

4

In Situ Single-Pass Perfused Rat Intestinal Model for Absorption and Metabolism

Eun Ju Jeong, Yan Liu, Huimin Lin, and Ming Hu

Summary

The single-pass perfused rat intestinal model is an *in situ* perfusion method that can be used to determine regional disposition of drugs. It is useful for selecting a development candidate from a series of active compounds and for studying mechanisms of absorption and excretion. It is also useful for determining if a compound may be appropriate for a sustained-release control formulation. The Food and Drug Administration (FDA) recognized the model system as a useful model to classify a compound's absorption characteristics in the Biopharmaceutics Classification System. This model may be modified to determine the contribution of intestine versus liver in the disposition of a specific compound, both of which may be useful to determine the enteric and enterohepatic recycling of drugs.

Key Words: Perfusion; *in situ*; intestine; rat; regional absorption; regional metabolism; Biopharmaceutics Classification System.

1. Introduction

The perfused rat intestinal model is an *in situ* single-pass intestinal perfusion model widely used for studying absorption of drugs and, more recently, natural occurring chemicals such as flavonoids. It is one of the two models recognized by the FDA to perform absorption studies so that we can characterize a drug or drug candidate according to the Biopharmaceutics Classification System. The special feature of this model is that the blood supply to the perfused segment of intestine is maintained throughout the experimental period, which could last for more than 8 h, although a typical study lasts 2 to 3 h.

From: *Methods in Pharmacology and Toxicology*
Optimization in Drug Discovery: In Vitro Methods
Edited by: Z. Yan and G. W. Caldwell © Humana Press Inc., Totowa, NJ

Because of this special feature, the model is especially suited for the study of active transport and intestinal metabolism.

The model was originally developed in mid-1980s at Dr. Gordon L. Amidon's laboratory at the Department of Pharmaceutical Sciences, College of Pharmacy, University of Michigan (Ann Arbor, MI) ***(1,2)***. This model differs from the more classic "through-and-through" perfusion method of Doluisio et al. ***(3)***. Originally, the model used one segment of the intestine per experiment and perfused a compound with or without an inhibitor at a particular pH to determine the absorption characteristics of a compound ***(1,2)***. Initially, emphasis was on the achievement and maintenance of a laminar flow condition, which is important to determine the true "membrane permeability or intestinal wall permeability (or P_w)" of a compound. The determination of P_w is important when it is necessary to estimate K_m values of a carrier-mediated transport process or to compare the true membrane permeabilities of a series of related compounds ***(1,2)***. It was later shown that there is a correlation between jejunal P_w and percent absorption in humans ***(4)***.

Another use of the perfused rat intestinal model was to determine absorption of drugs in different regions of the intestine ***(5,6)***. Regional perfusion studies are important to determine the absorption mechanism because the carrier responsible for the transport of a drug often has different levels of expression at different segments of the intestine. For example, the peptide carrier responsible for the absorption of many oral antibiotics and angiotensin-converting enzyme inhibitors is expressed at the highest level in the jejunum and at the lowest level in the colon. Regional perfusion studies are also important for determining if a drug candidate could be used in sustained-release formulations that are expected to release its content in regions where absorption is slow or nonexistent.

Recently, we have started to modify this model via several different ways. The first is to perform simultaneous perfusion of all four segments of the intestine that includes the duodenum, jejunum, ileum, and colon ***(7)***. This modification significantly reduced the number of animals necessary for obtaining similar results using single-segment perfusion. The second is to measure segment-dependent production of metabolites, which is particularly useful for determining the excretion of metabolites in different regions of the intestine. It was determined that the intestinal excretion of phase II metabolites of flavones and isoflavones is dependent on both the enzyme activities and capability of the efflux transporters ***(8)***. The third is to determine the contribution of the intestine vs the liver in the excretion of phase II metabolites by adding cannulation of the bile duct in addition to intestinal perfusion ***(8)***. The last is to determine the extent of intestinal metabolism by measuring the portal vein concentration of the parent compound and its conjugates. Compared with other available absorption models that are currently used in pharmaceutical companies, the perfused rat intestinal model is a good transition model between an in vitro model such as the Caco-2 model, intestinal strips, and in vivo pharmacokinetic models.

Compared with previously mentioned in vitro models, the perfused rat intestinal model is less adapted at determining the transport mechanism of drugs, especially the basolateral efflux. However, the perfused rat intestinal model maintains the blood supply to the perfused segment, which allows us to study absorption, metabolism, or both, even when a compound is slowly absorbed or metabolized, which cannot be achieved using intestinal strips with a viability of 30 to 90 min. The perfused rat intestinal model is expected to have correct expression levels of various nutrient transporters and enzymes, which are normally underexpressed in the Caco-2 model. Another use of the perfused rat intestinal model is that it can be used to determine regional absorption, metabolism, or both. Regional absorption and metabolism is useful information for designing sustained-release dosage forms. Lack of absorption from a particular segment of the intestines or extensive first-pass metabolism at another segment of the intestine may be used to determine if it is worthwhile to design a sustained-release dosage form. It may also be used to design dosage forms that are intended to escape gut first-pass metabolism. In summary, the perfused rat intestinal model and its variants could be used to determine the absorption mechanisms of a drug or drug candidate, absorption and metabolism in different regions of the intestine, and contribution of intestinal metabolism to the overall metabolism of a particular compound.

2. Materials

2.1. Chmicals

1. Hank's balanced salt solution (modified) (HBSS) (Sigma).
2. D-Glucose (JRH Bioscience).
3. HEPES (JRH Bioscience).
4. Sodium bicarbonate ($NaHCO_3$; Sigma).
5. Sodium chloride (NaCl) (J. T. Baker).
6. Polyethylene glycol (PEG) 4000 (Union Carbide).
7. [^{14}C]-PEG4000 (store at –20°C) (PerkinElmer Life Sciences).

2.2. Reagents

1. Anesthetizing agent mix (hereafter called drug mix): 100 mg/mL ketamine HCl injection (Fort Dodge Animal Health); 20 mg/mL xylazine (Bayer); and 100 mg/mL acepromazine maleate (store at 4°C) (Butler). Prepare a mixture of all three agents

according to the following formula: 7.5 mL ketamine, 0.75 mL acepromazine, and 1.9 mL xylazine.
2. Saline (0.9% NaCl) (autoclaved or USP grade).
3. HBSS buffer (pH 6.5 or 7.4): 9.801 g/L HBSS powders, 0.372 g/L $NaHCO_3$, 3.502 g/L glucose, 5.963 g/L HEPES, 1.164 g/L NaCl.

Preparation note: Dissolve all powders in 1 L previously autoclaved double-distilled water, stir, and adjust the pH to 6.5 or 7.4 using the NaOH solution. Store at 4°C in an autoclaved water after filtration through a 0.22-μm filter (Millipore). An *unopened* bottle will last 6 mo. 2-(*N*-morpholino) ethane-sulfonic acid (MES) at same molar concentration should be used for buffers of pH 6.0 or less.

2.3. Equipment

1. PHD 2000 Infuse/Withdraw Pump (Harvard Apparatus).
2. Water bath with cooling capability: refrigerated water bath.
3. Heating lamp (purchased from a hardware store).
4. Electric heating blanket (purchased from a pharmacy).
5. Scissors (one coarse for cutting skin and muscle and one fine to cut the intestine). Do not use the fine scissors to cut skin or muscle.
6. Flat head and pointed (not too sharp) twisters (stainless steel).
7. Liquid scintillation counter.

2.4. Other Materials

1. Tubing (Teflon or other tubing may be used to further decrease adsorption.)
   Silicon tubing, OD 0.5 in., thickness 1/16 in. (VWR)
   Silicon tubing, OD 1/4 in., thickness 1/16 in. (VWR)
   PE350 tubing, OD 0.157 in., ID 0.125 in. (Becton Dickinson)
2. Syringe: Plastic, glass, and stainless steel are available for different compounds. We recommend plastic syringes because they are disposable and inexpensive. However, some chemicals may stick to plastic (*see* **Note 1**).

2.5. Animals

Male Sprague-Dawley rats, 300–375 g, 70–90 d old (*see* **Note 2**). Female Sprague-Dawley rats, 230–280 g, 80–90 d old (*see* **Note 3**).

3. Methods

3.1. Intestinal Perfusion Steps and Comments

Intestinal perfusion is a rather complex procedure, which is described below and demonstrated using **Scheme 1** and **Fig. 1**.

The following are detailed steps for the perfusion procedure:

1. Starve rats on or before 5 PM (but no more than 16 h) on the preceding day. Leave fresh water for rats overnight (*see* **Note 4**).

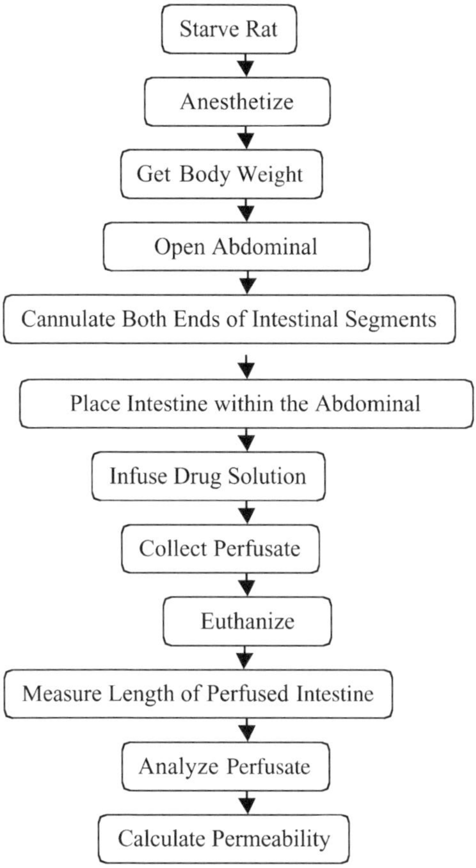

Scheme 1. Flowchart of intestinal perfusion steps.

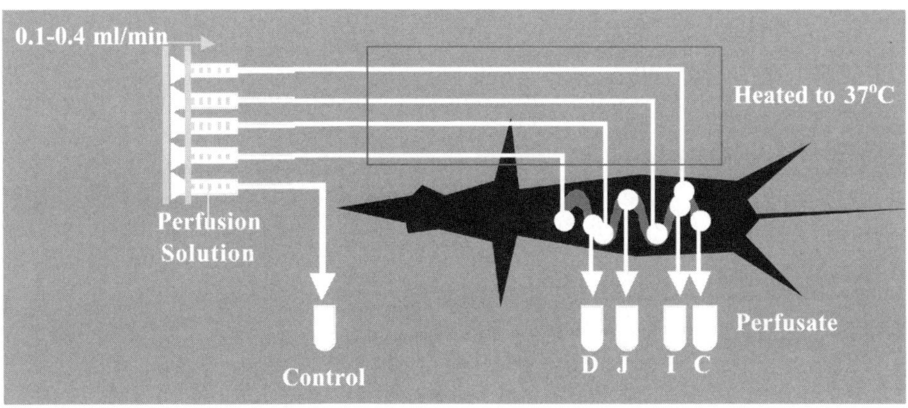

Fig. 1. Schematic of four-site simultaneous *in situ* perfusion model of rat intestine.

2. Anesthetize rats with ip or im (leg quarter muscles) injection of drug mix at about 0.25 mL per 300 g of rat (*see* **Note 5**).
3. Weigh rats and record total body weight. Rats should not react to tail pinch before cutting into the abdominal cavity to ensure compliance with the Institutional Animal Care and Use Committee (IACUC) protocol (*see* **Note 6**).
4. First cut into the skin and then open the abdominal cavity by a middle incision of 3–4 cm and locate the jejunum (other possible sites of perfusion include the duodenum, ileum, and colon) (*see* **Note 7**).
5. Cannulate a segment of the jejunum (about 10–15 cm) using PE350 tubing (precut to length). The cannulae are secured with a surgical silk suture (*see* **Note 8**).
6. Place a portion of the intestine within the abdominal cavity after the cannulation. Lay the rest of the intestinal segment flat on the abdominal surface of the rats. The whole area is then covered by a paper towel wetted with normal saline. A piece of plastic wrap is put on the towel to keep the intestinal segments moist (*see* **Note 9**).
7. Keep the circulating water bath at 37°C to maintain the temperature of the perfusate constant (*see* **Note 10**).
8. Set the infuse pump to a desired flow rate. Clear the intestine for about 30 min by using the perfusate containing the compound of interest and the nonabsorbable water flux marker (commonly, [^{14}C]-PEG-4000 and 0.1 m*M* cold PEG4000 are used) in a desired buffer (e.g., HBSS) (*see* **Note 11**).
9. Collect the perfusate at 30-min intervals afterward until all four samples are collected (*see* **Note 12**).
10. Euthanize the rats using an overdose of phenobarbital (10 mg/mL) after perfusion (*see* **Note 13**).
11. Measure the length of perfused intestine by wetting them with normal saline (4°C) and carefully laying them flat without stretching (*see* **Note 14**).
12. Prepare the collected perfusate for further measurements. We commonly centrifuge the samples at 16,000*g* for 30 min at room temperature to pellet any proteins, cells, or cellular debris before samples are injected into high-performance liquid chromatography (HPLC). Normally, no additional cleanup procedure is required (*see* **Note 15**).
13. In addition to perfusate samples, one could cannulate the bile, jugular vein, and portal vein and harvest the organs of tested animals at the end of each experiment if so desired (*see* Chen et al. *[8]*). The bile was also collected from the cannulae of the bile duct (PE10 tubing) from time zero to the end of the studies. After rats are euthanized, organs are harvested at the end of the each study. Weights of heart, lung, liver, spleen, kidney, intestine, colon, and cecum are measured, and the amount of the test compound in each organ is determined by an appropriate method.

3.2. Sample Analysis

After adding 5 mL of scintillation cocktail to a portion (usually 0.5–1 mL) of perfusate, mix them thoroughly and measure the radioactivity of the perfusate using the liquid scintillation counter. Determine the concentration of the drug and its metabolites using an appropriate method such as HPLC.

3.3. Calculation of Permeability

This method measures the steady-state uptake of a compound from the perfusate by determining the rate of disappearance from the perfusate and uses the rate of disappearance to calculate an unbiased intestinal wall permeability (P_w). At steady state, the P_w of a compound is calculated using the following equations:

$$P_w^* = \frac{P_{eff}^*}{1 - P_{eff}^* / P_{aq}^*} \tag{1}$$

where

$$P_{eff}^* = \frac{1 - C_m / C_o}{4G_z} \tag{2}$$

$$P_{aq}^* = \left(A \ (GZ)^{1/3}\right)^{-1} \tag{3}$$

$$\begin{aligned} A &= 10.0\ G_z + 1.01 \qquad && 0.004 \le G_z \le 0.01 \\ A &= 4.5\ G_z + 1.065 \qquad && 0.01 \le G_z \le 0.03 \\ A &= 2.5\ G_z + 1.125 \qquad && 0.03 \le G_z \end{aligned} \tag{4}$$

In **Eqs. 2–4**, C_o and C_m are inlet and outlet concentrations, respectively; G_z, or the Graetz number $\left(G_z = \frac{\pi DL}{2Q}\right)$, is a scaling factor that incorporates flow rate (Q), intestinal length (L), and diffusion coefficients (D) to make the permeability dimensionless; and A is a correction factor for the aqueous resistance of the intestine. C_m was adjusted for water flux, as indicated by the concentration of [^{14}C]-PEG4000, a nonabsorbable marker compound. For experiments performed in the small intestine, the data points are discarded if the water flux exceeds 0.55%/cm of intestine. For experiments in the colon, this limit may be relaxed to 1.5%/cm because of the slow flow rate (sometimes necessary as a result of slower absorption) and rapid water absorption. For calculating the permeability parameters, we usually use the Microsoft Excel program. **Figure 2** presents a typical sheet for calculating permeability for one rat.

Experiment date:
Sample analyzed date:
Site of perfusion: **Duo, Jej, Ile, Col**
Birthday of the Rats:
Sex: female

Inhibitor (no)
Concentration:
Drug Name:

Rat characteristics

Rat#1	W(gm)	L(cm)	Q(ml/min)	Gz	A	Pa*
Duo	225	10	0.382	0.0288	1.1946	2.7311
Jej	225	10	0.382	0.0288	1.1946	2.7311
Ileu	225	8	0.382	0.0230	1.1687	3.0072
Colon	225	12	0.382	0.0346	1.2114	2.5344

Check volume change with 14C-PEG 3350

	CPMA						%H_2O change			
T(min)	Duo	Jej	Ileu	Colon	Original	BLK	Duo	Jej	Ileu	Colon
30-60	2615	2505	2456	2443	2525	28	3.46	-0.83	-2.88	-3.41
60-90	2531	2494	2511	2424	2525	28	0.23	-1.29	-0.56	-4.24
90-120	2578	2566	2499	2353	2525	28	2.05	1.61	-1.06	-7.41
120-150	2516	2465	2525	2438	2525	28	-0.37	-2.46	-0.03	-3.62
Avg.	2560	2508	2498	2414	2525	28	1.34	-0.74	-1.13	-4.67

Sample's peak area ratio from HPLC(T=13.1)

	Peak area					corrected peak height			
T(min)	Duo	Jej	Ileu	Colon	Original	Duo	Jej	Ileu	Colon
30-60	499	510	431	130	645	482	514	443	135
60-90	502	539	461	121	645	501	546	464	126
90-120	588	544	469	138	645	576	536	474	149
120-150	602	521	506	99	645	605	534	507	103
Avg.	548	529	467	122	645	541	533	472	128
					%ABS	16	17	27	80

Calculate permeability

	Peff*=(1-Cm/C0)/4Gz				Pw*=Peff*/(1-Peff*/Pa*)			
T(min)	Duo	Jej	Ileu	Colon	Duo	Jej	Ileu	Colon
30-60	2.19	1.75	2.71	6.87	10.93	4.89	27.50	-4.02*
60-90	1.94	1.32	2.43	6.98	6.65	2.56	12.68	-3.98*
90-120	0.92	1.47	2.30	6.67	1.39	3.17	9.73	-4.09*
120-150	0.54	1.49	1.86	7.30	0.67	3.26	4.86	-3.88*
Avg.	1.39	1.51	2.32	6.96	4.91	3.47	13.69	-3.99
S.D.	0.79	0.18	0.36	0.26	4.82	1.00	9.76	0.08

* See Note 4.2.13

Fig. 2. Worksheet of sample perfusion in the intestine.

3.4. Interpretation of Permeability Data

The P_w values are a much better representation of the intestinal membrane permeability than P_{eff} because the permeability contribution of the unstirred water layer (P_{aq}) is factored out. It was indicated by previous publications ***(4)*** that compounds with a P_w larger than 1 are generally well absorbed (>75%). However, P_w^* could approach infinity as P_{aq}^* dominates the P_{eff}^* when the drug permeates rapidly. Under such circumstances, a change in P_w^* does not significantly affect the overall permeation, whereas a change in P_{aq}^* does.

4. Notes

1. It is prudent to measure drug concentration in the perfusate before it is loaded into the syringe, as well as after it has flowed out of the cannulation tubing, to check for binding to the various perfusion apparatuses.
2. The smallest rats we have used are about 200 g. Generally, rats around 300 g are the best as to survival, volume of blood samples available, and reasonable price. Occasionally, our suppliers have run out rats in this range when we tried to order. Therefore, it may be necessary to reserve the rats. Rats from 300–325 g could be used as the ideal weight to set up the validation. The oldest rats we used were around 450 g and probably 120–150 d old.
3. Female rats are smaller than male rats of the same age.
4. We recommend at least 16 to 18 h of starving. Make sure that the rats are kept in a suspending cage because they will eat their own feces.
5. The dose may be divided if rats are unusually sensitive. Additional drug mix at 0.02 to 0.05 mL per injection may be given after 15 min and during the perfusion experiments. Drug mix should not be used for more than 8 wk. Occasionally, rats may become sensitive to drugs that have been stored for a long time, perhaps as a result of the formation of the degradation product. The use of needles that are much bigger than 25 gage may cause unnecessary stress to the rats and bleeding.
6. We also found that rats tend to die prematurely if they are in too much stress (e.g., excessive bleeding during surgery and experiment).
7. The midline is a visible white line on the rat abdominal muscle. After the segment of interest is located, the rest of the intestine should be put back into the abdominal cavity.
8. This procedure makes the assumption that two adjacent sites are used. It is possible to perfuse all four regions of the intestine simultaneously, but colon perfusion tends to be more difficult because of the need to rid off the feces. A standard 24-h or 48-h fasting will not clean the colon of its feces, although a 48-h fasting is better than a 24-h fasting. A longer fasting may produce rats that are weaker (more likely to die during surgery) or excitable. Cannulation is the most difficult part of the surgery for beginners. The best thing to do is to ensure that the intestinal segment is not overhandled. Do not use sharp objects to grab the intestine because intestine bruises extremely easily. Use your hand to gently handle the intestine and insert the cannulae, after an opening equivalent to one-third to one-half of the intestinal radius is cut using fine scissors. Do not use big or dull scissors.
9. The goal here is to keep the bleeding to a minimum, to have an obstruction-free perfusate flow, and to keep the intestine warm and moist. The use of 37°C normal saline to wet the towels is recommended before putting towels on the intestine.
10. The water bath should be turned on first thing in the morning, as with the heating blanket.

11. This step serves to clean the intestine and lets the absorption proceed to a steady state. If there is an insufficient amount of drug, one can use buffer to wash out the foodstuff and then start with a perfusion of the compound (empty the intestine first with an air push). The second method will take more time and is definitely more time-consuming. If the flow rate is less than 0.1 mL/min, the wash perfusion time may have to be longer (e.g., 45 min).
12. We normally collect four samples and calculate the permeability individually. We typically want at least 1 mL of perfusate. Therefore, a longer sampling time may be necessary if the perfusion rate is less than 0.1 mL/min.
13. This euthanasia protocol is recommended by the IACUC.
14. In this step, an operator's error may be significant. It is necessary to develop a standard way of measuring the length. Consistency is more important than absolute accuracy here because everything cancels out at the end. Be consistent and document exactly how the intestinal segment is measured to avoid a large difference between operators. Weighing the intestine after the experiment is more tedious and no more accurate because it is difficult to remove the fluid inside and fat outside. Finally, half of the intestinal segment (by weight) may be homogenized and/or solubilized to determine the amount bound to the enterocytes. The other half may be fixed using a histological procedure to observe any damage to the mucus.
15. It is often necessary to prepare the samples against chemical and microbiological instability. These samples have bacteria that can consume your chemical at room temperature (most autosamplers) in less than a day. We commonly acidify the samples to pH 2.0 or less. Sometimes, antioxidants are added too.

5. Practice and Familiarization

This is not a particularly difficult method but will need practice to get consistent results. For the surgery to work well, one probably need three to six tries of three to four rats each trial using standard compounds such as propranolol, phenylalanine, and testosterone. Make sure the water flux is monitored during each trial run. You will find that the water flux improves and the amount of blood in the samples decreases as you get better at handling the intestine. Water flux needs to be controlled carefully because some investigators have shown that it affects absorption. Excessive water flux is often a sign of toxicity of a compound in the perfusate when the operator has become familiarized with the technique.

6. Preliminary Studies

Preliminary studies must be first conducted to determine the chemical stability of the test compound in buffers of various pHs. The best buffer is the one that has been passed through a segment of the intestine. Stability of the test compounds may be enhanced through the use of a stabilizing agent (e.g., acidification of the samples). Stability studies should also be performed using freshly prepared intestinal homogenate (concentration of protein 10 mg/mL). One can study the stability at different pH or at pH 7.4. Spiking concentrated solution into the homogenate is acceptable for the starting solution. One should harvest the enterocytes if possible.

7. Preparation To Be Done the Day Before or Earlier

Check the water bath, the tubings connecting the water bath and the inlet tubing (this apparatus is used to keep the perfusate warm), the electric heating blanket, and the heating lamp. Set up and clean up the perfusion pump, and make sure it functions properly. Make sure HBSS buffer, saline, and the precipitation solution are enough for next day's experiments. There is not sufficient time to do both on the same day without compromising the quality and efficiency. Assemble needed materials and supplies: tubings for collecting the perfusate (prelabel all tubes); scissors, forceps, and suture (precut to length); disposable gloves; and preparation of tables for surgery. At or before 4 PM, place rats in suspension cages for fasting, and do not forget to get plastic bags and tags to hold animal carcasses.

8. Special Cleanup Procedures

All perfusion tubing should be washed with 70% ethanol the day of the experiment and air-dried to prevent growth of microbials in the perfusate tubing. All surgical equipment must be washed so that bloodstains are removed. The equipment may be air-dried or immersed in 75% ethanol. The second method is not recommended if equipment is not used again within 1 wk.

References

1. Sinko, P. J. and Amidon, G. L. (1988) Characterization of the oral absorption of beta-lactam antibiotics: I. Cephalosporins: determination of intrinsic membrane absorption parameters in the rat intestine *in situ*. *Pharm. Res.* **5,** 645–650.
2. Hu, M., Sinko, P. J., DeMeere, A. L. J., Johnson, D. A., and Amidon, G. L. (1988) Membrane permeability parameters for some amino acids and β-lactam antibiotics: application of the boundary layer approach. *J. Theor. Biol.* **131,** 107–114.
3. Doluisio, J. T., Billups, N. F., Dittert, L. W., Sugita, E. T., and Swintosky, J. V. (1969) Drug absorption: I. An *"in situ"* rat gut technique yielding realistic absorption rates. *J. Pharm. Sci.* **58,** 1196–1200.
4. Amidon, G. L., Sinko, P. J., and Fleisher, D. (1988) Estimating human oral fraction dose absorbed: a correlation using rat intestinal membrane permeability for passive and carrier-mediated compounds. *Pharm. Res.* **5,** 651–654.
5. Hu, M. and Amidon, G. L. (1988) Passive and carrier-mediated intestinal absorption components of captopril. *J. Pharm. Sci.* **77,** 1007–1011.

6. Hu, M., Roland, K., Ge, L., Chen, J., Li, Y., Tyle, P., and Roy, S. (1998) Determination of absorption characteristics of AG337, a novel thymidylate synthase inhibitor, using a perfused rat intestinal model. *J. Pharm. Sci.* **87,** 886–890.
7. Liu, Y. and Hu, M. (2002) Absorption and metabolism of flavonoids in the caco-2 cell culture model and a perused rat intestinal model. *Drug Metab. Dispos.* **30,** 370–377.
8. Chen, J., Lin, H., and Hu, M. (2003) Metabolism of flavonoids via enteric recycling: role of intestinal disposition. *J. Pharmacol. Exp. Ther.* **304,** 1228–1235.

5

In Vitro Permeation Study With Bovine Brain Microvessel Endothelial Cells

Seong-Hee Park, Sung-Hack Lee, Yaming Su, and Patrick J. Sinko

Summary

Drug permeability through cell monolayer is known to correlate well with *in situ* intestinal permeability and/or oral bioavailability. Several mammalian cell lines such as Caco-2, MDCK, MDCKII, and LLC-PK have been used to predict in vivo intestinal absorption of drugs. However, there are no well-characterized cell lines available representing the blood–brain barrier. In this chapter, the authors describe the primary culture of bovine brain microvessel endothelial cells (BMECs) lining the interface between the blood and the brain as the model for screening central nervous system (CNS) drug candidates. The culture procedures and measurement of permeability in BMEC can be applied to other model cell lines such as Caco-2, MDCK, and MDCKII cells.

Key Words: Permeability; bovine brain microvessel endothelial cells (BMECs).

1. Introduction

The brain microvessel endothelial cell (BMEC) model is widely used in the screening of central nervous system (CNS) drug candidates to determine permeability to the blood–brain barrier (BBB). In addition, BBB penetration can be a great merit in the drug discovery process of chemotherapeutic agents to cure brain tumors or anti-AIDS drugs to kill the human immunodeficiency virus (HIV) virus residing in brain. BMEC is also used as an in vitro model to elucidate the mechanism of drug transport across the BBB. BMEC is one of the first in vitro methods that uses endothelial cells lining the interface between the blood and the brain. BMEC forms confluent monolayers, and these monolayers exhibit many of the characteristics of BBB, which means that this endot-

From: *Methods in Pharmacology and Toxicology*
Optimization in Drug Discovery: In Vitro Methods
Edited by: Z. Yan and G. W. Caldwell © Humana Press Inc., Totowa, NJ

helial cell line can be cultured to maintain physiological characteristics such as few pinocytic vesicles and tight intercellular junctions. Expression of alkaline phosphatase, γ-glutamyl transpeptidase, angiotensin-converting enzyme, and drug transporters such as P-glycoprotein (P-gp) and multidrug resistance-associated proteins (MRPs) play an important role in making the BMEC model used to study BBB transport and investigate the correlation between BMEC permeability and central nervous system (CNS) uptake. Utilization of BMEC in uptake, permeability, and metabolism experiments is reported, but we will not cover the metabolism study in this chapter. Uptake study is not described here because the uptake study is very similar to the transport study, except for using a normal well instead of a transwell. This protocol describes the process of the isolation and culture of BMECs, as well as its application to permeability assays.

2. Materials

1. Phosphate-buffered saline (PBS) (0.01 *M*). Dissolve the following components together, adjust pH to 7.4, and sterile filter it when needed.

Component	Molecular weight	1 L (g)	Concentration (m*M*)
NaCl	58.44	7.54	129
KCl	74.56	0.186	2.5
Na_2HPO_4	141.96	1.05	7.4
KH_2PO_4	136.09	0.177	1.3

2. Amphotericin B (ampho B). Add 10 mL of sterilized deionized water to a sterilized vial containing 100 mg of amphotericin B. This is a 10-mg/mL solution of ampho B, which must be stored in the refrigerator. Dilute this with culture medium to make a 2.5-μg/mL solution (i.e., put 0.25 mL ampho B into 1 L of Eagle's minimum essential medium (MEM) or 0.125 mL into 500 mL of MEM).
3. Polymixin B (poly B). To get a 20-mg/mL solution of poly B, dissolve 400 mg of polymixin B with PBS into a total volume of 20 mL. Sterile-filter this, put it into a sterilized vial, and store it in the refrigerator. Dilute this 1:400 with culture medium to get a final concentration of 50 μg/mL (i.e., 1.25 mL per 500 mL of MEM).
4. Penicillin-G (pen) and streptomycin (strep). To get 50-mg/mL solutions, dissolve 1.25 g of penicillin G and streptomycin with PBS into a total volume of 25 mL. Sterile filter these solutions and put them into sterilized vials. Dilute these 1:500 with solutions needed to get a final concentration of 100 μg/mL (i.e., 1 mL of each solution per 500 mL of dextran).
5. Pen/strep. We generally get a combination of these already mixed and lyophilized in a buffer that only needs to be reconstituted in sterilized water. Provided the vial reads 10,000 U/mL penicillin and 10,000 μg/mL streptomycin, just add

20 mL of sterilized water into the vial. This will give you a solution containing 10,000 μg/mL of each. When using this solution, you must dilute it 1:100 into whatever solution you are making to get a final concentration of 100 μg/mL; that is, it takes 5 mL of this added to 500 mL of medium, which is quite a lot (and expensive), so if you plan to use pen/strep for medium, add it in the powder form when initially making it up.

6. Gentamycin. To get a 50-mg/mL solution, dissolve 1.25 g of gentamycin into a total volume of 25 mL with PBS. Sterile-filter this, put it into a sterilized vial, and store it in the refrigerator. Use this solution for making up the isolation solutions by diluting 1:1000 into solutions to get a final concentration of 50 μg/mL (i.e., 0.5 mL of this solution into 500 mL of dextran).
7. MEM, pH 7.4.

Component	Amount	Final concentration	Source
MEM	1-L package	1X	Gibco®, 61100-061
HEPES	11.29 g	50 m*M*	Sigma®, H-9136
Ampho B	0.25 mL	2.5 μg/mL	Sigma®, A-9528
Poly B	2.5 mL	50 μg/mL	Sigma®, P-1004
Pen/strep (or gentamycin)	10 mL	100 U (or μg)/mL	Sigma®, P-4333

Directions: Mix all components but ampho B in 900 mL of deionized water and adjust pH to 7.2. Stir this for a while, and then bring it up to a final volume of 1 L. Sterile filter this solution, put it into a 1-L sterilized bottle, and add ampho B. Store it in the refrigerator.

8. 12.5% Dispase (protease): Sigma®, P-3417. Mix 2.5 g of dispase (Boehringer-Mannheim®, 165 859 Dispase II from *Bacillus polymyxa*, grade II) with 20 mL of MEM, pH 7.4 in a 50-mL centrifuge tube (the vials of dispase from Sigma® have 5 g in them, so it is easier to just use the entire vial and dissolve it into 40 mL of MEM [pH 7.4] and then split it in half later). Dissolve the dispase by placing the tube in the shaker bath at 37°C for 30 min. Remove the vial and centrifuge it for 30 min in the tabletop centrifuge at maximum speed. Sterile filter the supernatant into a new sterilized centrifuge tube (aliquot it into 20-mL portions if you made extra), and store it in the freezer. When you use this, you will empty the entire contents into a 500-mL container with brain suspension, yielding a final concentration of 0.5% (w/v).
9. MEM, pH 9.0~10.0. Make this exactly the same way, but adjust pH to around 9.5 (this takes longer to sterile filter). Store it in the refrigerator (*see* **Note 1**).
10. 10X MEM: Gibco®, BRL 11700-010. Dissolve one package of 10X MEM into a total volume of 500 mL of deionized water. Put this into a 500-mL bottle. Autoclave this solution for 20 min on the slow or liquid cycle and then store it in the refrigerator.
11. HEPES, pH 7.6: Sigma®, H-9136. If the formula weight of HEPES is 238.3, then

dissolve 119.15 g of HEPES into a total volume of 500 mL of deionized water to make a 1.0-*M* solution of HEPES. Adjust pH to 7.6, sterile-filter it, and put it in the refrigerator. HEPES comes in several different salts or in free base, so check the formula weight to make sure that you are making it up correctly.

12. 13% Dextran.

Component	Amount
Deionized water	422 mL
Dextran: Sigma®, D-3759	65 g
10X MEM	50 mL
1 *M* HEPES, pH 7.6	25 mL
Ampho B	0.125 mL
Poly B	1.25 mL
Pen/strep (or gentamycin)	5 mL (0.5 mL)

Directions: Dissolve dextran in deionized water and autoclave this solution. When cool, add the other components (sterile) and store this in the refrigerator. You will know if the other components are added by the color. If it is only the dextran and water, it will be slightly yellow. If the other components are added, then it will be red. Do not add only some of the other components without explicitly writing that on the label.

13. Collagenase/dispase (coll/disp): Sigma®, C-3180. To make up 5 mL of a stock solution of coll/disp (Boehringer-Mannheim®, 269 638 from *Vibrio alginolyticus/ B. polymyxa*) that is 4 mg/mL in MEM, pH 7.4, either dissolve 20 mg of coll/disp into 5 mL MEM, pH 7.4, or weigh out 100 mg of coll/disp and dissolve it in 25 mL of MEM, pH 7.4. To dissolve it, place this mixture into the shaker bath at 37°C for 30 min. Sterile-filter this solution into a sterile centrifuge tube (aliquot it into 5-mL portions if you made extra), and store this in the freezer. When ready to use, thaw this quickly and dilute the 5-mL portion up to 20 mL with MEM, pH 7.4, to get a final concentration of 1 mg/mL.
14. 50% Percoll.

Amount	Component
75 mL	Percoll (well mixed): Sigma®, P-4937/1644
52 mL	Sterilized water
15 mL	10X MEM
7.5 mL	HEPES, pH 7.6
0.4 mL	Poly B
0.1 mL	Ampho B
1.5 mL (0.15 mL)	Pen/strep (or gentamycin)

Directions: Mix all of these sterile components, and mix them well (if the percoll is not mixed well prior to adding, the percoll could settle toward the bottom, and the density gradient will be messed up). Put 35 mL of the mixture into a 40-mL centrifuge tube (will fill 4), and spin these for 1 h at 39,200*g*, which corresponds to 18,250 rpm in a SS34 rotor. Following centrifugation, be very careful with the gradients so that they do not get messed up before use.

15. Rat tail collagen: Collaborative Research®, 40236.
16. Fibronectin. We want a 50-µg/mL working solution of fibronectin, but this is rather hard to weigh out (only 1 mg/20 mL PBS), so instead we make 5X concentrated stock solutions that is 250 µg/mL. Sterile filter this solution and put into a sterilized vial. Dilute 1:5 when the working solution is needed (i.e., mix 5 mL stock fibronectin and 20 mL sterile PBS). After using the first-hand fibronectin, place it into another vial. When this vial becomes sufficiently full, sterile-filter this and use it. After using this refiltered second-hand fibronectin, discard the solution (*see* **Note 2**).
17. Heparin. Heparin should be made up as a 50-mg/mL solution. Dissolve 2.5 g of heparin in 50 mL of PBS. It is not very soluble, so you will have to stir it for a while. Sterile filter this solution into two 25-mL sterilized vials (*see* **Note 3**).
18. Complete culture medium (2 L).

Component	Amount	Final concentration	Source
MEM	1-L package	50%	Gibco®, 61100-061
Ham's F12	1-L package	50%	Gibco®, 21700-075
HEPES	4.76 g	10 m*M*	Sigma®, H-9136
Sodium bicarbonate	2.18 g	13 m*M*	Sigma®, S-5761
Pen/strep (or gentamycin)	20 mL	100 U (or µg)/mL	Sigma®, P-4333

Directions: Mix all components in 1800 mL of deionized water. Stir this solution for a while to dissolve. Adjust pH to be approx 7.3 (later sterile-filtering will change the pH to 7.4). Add deionized water to a final volume of 2 L. Sterile-filter this solution and transfer it into sterilized bottles.

19. Plating medium. To 450 mL of complete culture medium, add the following: 50 mL of horse serum (platelet poor), 1.25 mL of poly B, 0.125 mL of ampho B, and 2.5 mL of endothelial cell growth factor (ECGF) (optional).
    Use this to wash the cells prior to plating. When ready to resuspend to plate, add 0.03 mL heparin of 50 mg/mL for every 10 mL of plating medium (*see* **Note 4**).
20. Changing medium. To 450 mL of complete culture medium, add the following: 50 mL of horse serum, .25 mL of heparin (final concentration: 125 µg/mL), 0.125 mL of ampho B (optional), and 2.5 mL of ECGF (optional). Whenever you need this media, add 0.03 mL heparin for each 10 mL of changing medium (*see* **Note 4**).

21. Assay media 1 (1% bovine serum albumin [BSA]).

Component	Final concentration
NaCl	150 m*M*
KCl	4 m*M*
$CaCl_2$	3.2 m*M*
$MgCl_2$	1.2 m*M*
HEPES	15 m*M*
Glucose	5 m*M*
BSA	1%

Directions: Mix all components in 0.9 L of deionized water. Adjust pH to 7.4 and fill it up to 1.0 L.

22. Transendothelial assay buffer (assay media 2)

Component	Final concentration
NaCl	122 m*M*
$NaHCO_3$	25 m*M*
D-Glucose	10 m*M*
KCl	3 m*M*
$MgSO_4$	1.2 m*M*
K_2HPO_4	0.4 m*M*
$CaCl_2$	1.4 m*M*
HEPES	10 m*M*

Directions: Add ingredients to 0.9 L of deionized water with mixing. Adjust pH of this solution with sodium hydroxide to 7.4, and fill it up to 1.0 L. Store in the refrigerator when not in use ***(1)***.

3. Methods

This section will be divided into two parts: (1) isolation of brain microvessels and (2) seeding cells onto transwells and the transport study. The method described here for BMEC is essentially based on the procedures developed by Bowman et al. ***(2)*** and, subsequently, Audus and Borchardt ***(3,4)***, with minor modifications. The key modifications from the original Bowman method include changing the times of incubation for cells with enzymes and quantitatively defining the amount of the enzyme (collagenase/dispase) required for enzymatic digestion of microvessels to help ensure the successful and consistent isolation of a pure population of healthy BMECs.

3.1. Isolation of Brain Microvessels

1. Obtain two or three fresh bovine brains from a local slaughterhouse, place them in 300 mL of ice-cold MEM, pH 7.4, immediately, and transport to the laboratory on ice. Do not use any brains that are bruised. Ideally, the tissue should be soft and have a pink hue. All the subsequent procedures for collecting brain gray matter are then performed preferably on ice in a laminar flow hood and under aseptic conditions.
2. Remove the brain stems and the cerebellums and separate the hemispheres. Transfer the hemispheres to a large plate. Remove brain surface vessels and the outer membrane (meninges) with hands or a pair of forceps. Start to peel from the anterior median edge (where the two lobes meet) over to the lateral edge. Transfer the cleaned brains to another beaker containing cold MEM, pH 7.4.
3. Scrape the cortical brain gray matter from the brain using a sterile surgical blade or a sterile razor blade. Collect the gray matter in a sterile beaker containing approx 50 mL of ice-cold MEM, pH 7.4. (After 250 mL of gray matter has been collected, discard the remainder of the brain material.)
4. Mince the gray matter into 1- to 2-mm cubes with a sterile multirazor blade (five razor blades glued together). Collect the minced gray matter into a 500-mL preweighed sterile Nalgene® bottle and weigh the gray matter. (Drain off the excess MEM, pH 7.4, before mincing) (*see* **Note 5**).
5. Add 12.5% dispase to the minced gray matter at a ratio of 4 mL of dispase per 50 g of gray matter, and incubate for 30 min in a 37°C shaker water bath at about 100 oscillations/min. The enzyme treatment results in a dispersal of the tissue releasing low pH cell materials and reducing the pH of the incubation medium with the first 30 min. After 30 min, remove the bottle from the water bath, and add to it a volume of MEM, pH 9.4, equal to the weight of the gray matter, to give final dispase concentration of 0.5%. This restores the pH of the medium to the neutral range where dispase is active and cell damage in the presence of prolonged low pH conditions will be minimized. Incubate in the 37°C water bath for an additional 2 h with shaking.
6. Remove the bottle from the water bath after no more than a 2.5-h dispase digestion, distribute the content equally into two preweighed 250-mL sterile centrifuge bottles, and centrifuge the suspension in the JA-14 rotor for 10 min at 3700 rpm (2000*g*) at room temperature. At the end of centrifugation, there are three distinct layers formed in the bottles: a red pellet and a large pink-colored semisolid layer—both of which contain microvessels—and a brown-colored liquid supernatant containing enzyme solution. *Remove and discard only the liquid supernatant, being careful not to disturb the soft pellet.*
7. Resuspend the red pellet in the thick pinkish mush. Split the contents of each of these suspensions into two 250-mL centrifuge tubes. Divide the 12.5% dextran equally among the four 250-mL centrifuge tubes and balance the tubes to within

2 g. Centrifuge the suspension in the JA-14 rotor for 10 min at 7730 rpm (9000*g*) at room temperature. After centrifugation, there is a large red pellet containing microvessels and erythrocytes, a clear supernatant, and a semisolid brown-colored layer on the top of the supernatant and on the side of the bottle. Pour off all of the liquid supernatant and semisolid layer, and wipe out the remaining supernatant and semisolid material on the side of the bottles with sterile cotton swabs. The step isolates a crude population of microvessels that are further purified in the remaining steps.

8. The purpose of this step is to enzymatically remove the basement membrane, pericytes, and any remaining adherent cell types from microvessels using a collagenase/dispase preparation. The ratio of collagenase/dispase to microvessels is 2.5 mg collagenase/dispase per gram of microvessels, and a final collagenase/dispase concentration at 0.5 mg/mL was found to be the optimal condition. Dilute the 5 mL of 4 mg/mL collagenase/dispase up to 20 mL in MEM, pH 7.4, to get a final concentration of 1 mg/mL. Use this to resuspend the four red pellets (use 2 mL each for resuspending and 3 mL to rinse each tube) (*see* **Note 6**).
9. Percoll gradient preparation. Add 35 mL of well-mixed 50% percoll solution to each of four 40-mL centrifuge tubes, and centrifuge them for 1 h at 18,000*g* at 4°C in a J-20 rotor. At the end of the spin, remove the tubes containing percoll gradients very carefully and store at 4°C so that they do not get messed up before use.
10. After collagenase/dispase incubation, dilute the microvessel suspension with MEM, pH 7.4, to 50 mL and centrifuge for 10 min at 2000 rpm at room temperature on the tabletop centrifuge to terminate enzymatic digestion and sediment the microvessels.
11. Remove and discard the supernatant from the tube. Resuspend the microvessel pellet in 10 mL of MEM, pH 7.4. Some of the microvessel pellets may not be resuspendable because of the formation of large fibrous aggregates. Therefore, to release the microvessels trapped in the aggregates, transfer the large fibrous aggregates to another tube, and wash them in 30 mL of MEM, pH 7.4. Remove and discard the washed fibrous aggregates. Combine the 30-mL microvessel resuspension with the 10-mL original microvessel resuspension in one 50-mL centrifuge tube. Centrifuge for 10 min at 2000 rpm at room temperature on the table-top centrifuge.
12. Resuspend the microvessel pellet in 8 mL of MEM, pH 7.4. This microvessel resuspension contains microvessels, endothelial cells, and other components, including red blood cells, a small amount of other cell types (including pericytes), and cell debris. To separate the microvessels and endothelial cells from those components, apply 2 mL of the suspension onto the top of each of the four preformed percoll gradients (*see* **step 9**), and spin for 10 min at 3500*g* in the JA-20 rotor. At the end of the centrifugation, there are three layers of bands formed: band 1, the top white layer containing cell debris and contaminating cell types; band 2, which is under band 1 and is a diffuse layer with red clumps containing

microvessel fragments and some endothelial cells; and band 3, a red band near the bottom containing red blood cells.

13. Collect band 2 from the four percoll gradients into four 50-mL centrifuge tubes using a 5-mL syringe with an 18-gage needle attached. Dilute the cell suspension in each tube with MEM-F12 to 50 mL, and centrifuge for 10 min on the tabletop centrifuge at a setting of 2000 rpm at room temperature to remove percoll (*see* **Note 7**).
14. Pour off the supernatant and resuspend the pellets in a culture medium supplemented to 20% horse serum and 10% dimethylsulfoxide (DMSO). (Usually, you just need to combine 30 mL of culture medium with 4 mL of horse serum and 4 mL of DMSO because the plating medium already contains 10% serum. Resuspend the pellets in this and then dilute with the culture medium up to 40 mL.) Aliquot 1.5 mL into each cryovial and store at –80°C. These cells may be stored for longer periods of time under liquid nitrogen.
15. Count the cells after being frozen so the cells that ruptured upon freezing will not be counted. Thaw a vial of cells, rinse them three times with plating medium, and resuspend them in 1.5 mL of plating medium. After incubation with trypan blue, count the cells in a hemacytometer.

The cells isolated by this procedure are generally 85% to 90% viable by trypan blue exclusion. The yield of microvessel endothelial cells for the gray matter of about two bovine brains is variably 30 to 200 million cells, depending on the efficiency of the isolation procedure and, more often, the age and condition of the starting tissues (*see* **Note 8**). Isolates of single cells have very poor plating efficiency and generally will not proliferate to form confluent monolayers *(1)*.

3.2. Seeding Cells Onto Transwells and the Transport Study

1. Seed at 6.6×10^4 cells/cm^2 onto 24-mm diameter transwell filter inserts coated with collagen and fibronectin, with a filter pore size of 0.4 μm. The plating media are not changed for the first 3 d, and the media are changed every other day with the changing media. It takes usually 14 d for BMEC to be confluent.
2. Discard the remaining media, rinse the transwells with PBS three times, and fill the inserts and wells with transendothelial assay buffer.
3. Measure TEER using Endohm-snap (World Precision Instruments). Resistances of blank filters were subtracted from those of filters with cells before final TEER values were calculated. Radiolabeled [^{14}C]-mannitol standards can also be used to verify monolayer integrity.
4. After a 30-min equilibration period, the experiment is initiated by changing the existing media of the donor side with a dosing solution dissolved in the assay buffer. Place the assay plate in an incubator maintaining 37°C.
5. At defined time periods, samples of each side (10% of the each side volume) are

removed from the receptor side initially devoid of test compound (e.g., basolateral side for apical to basolateral flux studies). An equal volume of assay buffer is added to replace the volume lost. Samples are also removed from the donor compartment at the beginning and end of the sampling period without replacement to ensure that the donor concentration does not change by more than 10%.

6. At the end of the experiment, the cells on the membrane can be scraped for measuring the accumulation inside the cells after washing three times with ice-cold buffer.
7. The apparent permeability coefficient (P_{app}) expressed in cm/s is determined as follows:

$$P_{app} = \frac{dC}{dt} \times \frac{V}{A \times C_o}$$

where dC/dt is the change in concentration on the receiving side over time (µ*M*/s), V is the volume of the solution in the receiving compartment (cm^3), A is the surface area of the membrane (1 cm^2), and C_o is the initial concentration in the donor chamber (µ*M*).

4. Notes

1. Use HEPES sodium salt (MW 250 Sigma®, H-0763) instead of HEPES (MW 238 Sigma®, H-9136). When you sterile filter it, be patient. If you try to increase the speed of the peristaltic pump too much, you will only create an unwanted messy situation.
2. There is a liquid form of fibronectin (human or bovine) available from Sigma® that is much easier to deal with than the lyophilized fibronectin, which is very difficult to dissolve in PBS. Try using the liquid form first (final concentration: 0.04 mg/mL in MEM-F12).
3. This is notorious for becoming contaminated, so check it out each time you use it (look at it under the light and make sure you do not see anything floating in it).
4. If you include the serum, ampho B, poly B, and heparin all in one bottle, you will get a precipitate. Therefore, you will see a precipitate on your plates during the first 3 d in incubation.
5. We usually can get approx 250 to 300 g of wet gray matter from two brains. The procedure was optimized for 250 g wet tissue.
6. Do not throw out any pellets at this stage! Combine all of the resuspended pellet solution in one sterile 50-mL centrifuge tube. Place this in the shaker bath at 37°C and 100 oscillations/min for approx 2 to 2.5 h.
7. Not a complete medium containing horse serum. Serum contains platelets, which cause microvessels to stick together.
8. It has been the purpose of this procedure to isolate microvessel fragments.

References

1. Cardelli-Cangiano, P., Cangiano, C., James, J. H., Jeppsson, B., Brenner, W., and Fischer, J. E. (1981) Uptake of amino acids by brain microvessels isolated from rats after portal canal anastomosis *J. Neurochem.* **36,** 627–632.
2. Bowman, P. D., Ennis, S. R., Rarey, K. E., Betz, A. L., and Goldstein, G. W. (1983) Brain microvessel endothelial cells in tissue culture: a model for study of blood-brain barrier permeability. *Ann. Neurol.* **14,** 396–402.
3. Audus, K. L. and Borchardt, R. T. (1986) Characteristics of the large neutral amino acid transport system of bovine brain microvessel endothelial cell monolayers. *J. Neurochem.* **47,** 484–488.
4. Audus, K. L. and Borchardt, R. T. (1987) Bovine brain microvessel endothelial cell monolayers as a model system for the blood-brain barrier. *Ann. NY Acad. Sci.* **507,** 9–18.

6

An Enzymatic Microplate Assay for Testing P-Glycoprotein Substrates and Inhibitors

S. Orlowski, J. Nugier, and Eric Ezan

Summary

P-Glycoprotein (P-gp) is a multidrug transporter responsible for resistance to anticancer chemotherapy and physiologically involved in absorption, distribution, and excretion of a large number of hydrophobic xenobiotics. P-gp exhibits both an adenosine triphosphatase (ATPase) activity correlated with its drug transport function and a basal ATPase activity in the absence of any drug. The authors have developed an enzymatic test based on modulation of these ATPase activities, which makes it possible to detect specific interactions between drugs and P-gp. They took into account the existence of multiple binding sites on P-gp to finalize an optimized strategy that involves the assay of the P-gp ATPase stimulated by three reference substrates (verapamil, vinblastine, and progesterone) in addition to its basal ATPase activity. This assay uses a coupled enzyme system with spectrophotometric detection for measurement on P-gp-containing native membrane vesicles. This assay may be performed on 96- or 384-well microplates and is therefore suitable for high-throughput screenings.

Key Words: Absorption; distribution; elimination; multidrug resistance; detoxification; high-throughput screening; P-glycoprotein; ATPase; active transport.

1. Introduction

P-Glycoprotein (P-gp) is an active plasma membrane transporter involved in cellular detoxification and drug pharmacokinetics (i.e., absorption, distribution, metabolism, and excretion [ADME] processes) of numerous amphiphilic and hydrophobic compounds *(1)*. Therefore, it is clearly desirable to determine, rather early in the course of its industrial development, whether a newly

From: *Methods in Pharmacology and Toxicology*
Optimization in Drug Discovery: In Vitro Methods
Edited by: Z. Yan and G. W. Caldwell © Humana Press Inc., Totowa, NJ

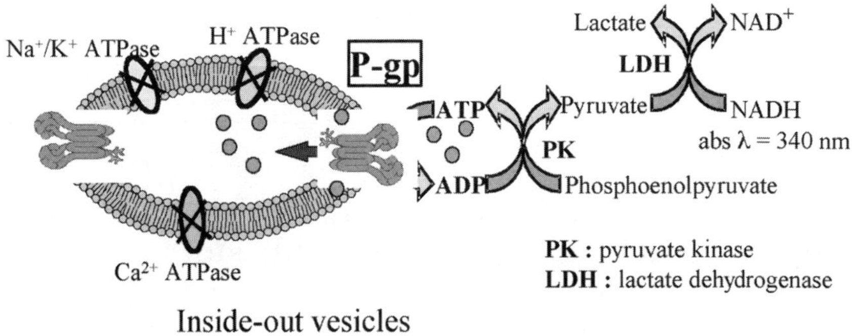

Fig. 1. Functional scheme of the coupled enzyme assay of ATPase activity. The enzymatic cascade consists of an ATP-regenerating system using pyruvate kinase (0.1 mg/mL) and phosphoenolpyruvate (initially at 1 m*M*) and a coupled system for spectrophotometric detection using lactate dehydrogenase (0.1 mg/mL) and NADH (initially at 0.5 m*M*). MgATPase activities of the membrane vesicle suspensions are measured at 37°C by continuous monitoring of NADH absorbency at 340 nm. NADH consumption corresponds stoichiometrically to ADP production by the ATPases to be measured, provided that PK and LDH are not limiting for the whole enzymatic reaction. The ATPases are born by inside-out native membrane vesicles, and the ATP hydrolyzing sites therefore face the reaction medium. The main ionic pumps present in these membranes are inhibited by the simultaneous presence of azide, ouabain, and EGTA.

synthesized molecule interacts with P-gp to be eventually handled for a transmembrane active flux across a biological barrier. P-gp exhibits high drug-dependent adenosine triphosphate (ATP) hydrolysis activity that is a reflection of its drug transport ability *(2)*. As a consequence, the test of stimulation or inhibition of P-gp ATPase activity by a drug can be used to probe the potential interaction of this drug with P-gp *(3,4)*.

The assay described in this chapter allows in vitro screening for testing drug interactions with P-gp, based on the study of ATPase activity modulations measured on native membrane vesicles containing high amounts of P-gp ***(5–7)*** (*see* **Note 1**). P-gp ATPase activity is measured by a spectrophotometric method monitoring adenosine 5'-diphosphate (ADP) formation in the vesicle suspension medium through the indirect measurement of stoichiometric beta-nicotinamide adenine dinucleotide reduced (NADH) consumption by the decrease of its absorption at 340 nm ***(6,8)***. The scheme of the coupled enzyme assay is presented in **Fig. 1** (*see* **Note 2**).

The basal ATPase activity of P-gp is defined as its MgATP hydrolysis activity determined in the absence of any added drug. Modulation of basal ATPase activity can be induced by adding various compounds at different concentrations ***(9,10)***. The compounds tested can also modulate the ATPase activity of P-gp first stimulated by other drugs ***(11,12)***. This assay combines the determination of the modulations of P-gp basal activity and P-gp activity stimulated by three compounds (verapamil, progesterone, and vinblastine) known to be P-gp substrates to improve the reliability of the interaction test ***(13)*** (*see* **Note 3**). Data are analyzed by comparing the variations of the basal and stimulated activities induced by a tested compound to the corresponding activities determined in the absence of this compound. Such a convenient experimental setup with a rather simple data treatment makes this test well suitable for high-throughput screening (HTS) use.

2. Materials

1. P-gp-containing membrane vesicles (SPI-Bio, Massy, France) (*see* **Note 4**).
2. Verapamil, progesterone, and vinblastine (Sigma, St. Louis, MO).
3. Pyruvate kinase and lactate dehydrogenase (Boehringer Mannheim, Darmstadt, Germany).
4. Phosphoenolpyruvate, NADH, and Na_2ATP (vanadium-free) (Sigma, St. Louis, MO).
5. Ion pump ATPase activity inhibitors: ouabain, sodium azide, and EGTA (Sigma, St. Louis, MO).
6. 96-Well plate (Nunc Maxisorb, Denmark).

In addition to standard laboratory equipment, the following material is required:

Precision micropipets (20, 200, and 1000 mL) with corresponding tips.
Multipipettor with 0.5- and 1.0-mL combitips.
Multichannel pipettors 5 to 50 mL and 50 to 300 mL.
Spectrophotometer plate reader (340-nm filter).
Microplate incubator at 37°C, with gentle stirring.
Microplate shaker.
Distilled or deionized water.
Polypropylene tubes.

3. Methods

3.1. Preparation of Reagents

The quantities prepared are available for testing 10 compounds at four concentrations in duplicates, for one out of the four ATPase activities assayed, in one 96-well microplate (*see* **Note 5**). A complete test comprising the assay of both the basal and the three stimulated activities needs four times more reagents (*see* **Note 6**).

1. The enzymatic buffer, 30 mM Tris-HCl, pH 7.8, at 20°C, 100 mM NaCl, 10 mM KCl, 2 mM $MgCl_2$, and 1 m*M* dithiothreitol (DTT). Store at 4°C for no more than 1 mo.

2. The ion pump inhibitors, called "nonspecific ATPase inhibitors," which are mixed at the following concentrations in a volume of 3 to 4 mL of enzymatic buffer: ouabain at 3.33 m*M*, sodium azide at 66.7 m*M*, and EGTA at 6.67 m*M*. These reagents may be prepared from solutions at 1 mg/mL and may be stored at –20°C once prepared. They will be diluted 6.67-fold in the final assay (final concentration 0.5 m*M*, 10 m*M*, and 1 m*M*, respectively).
3. The reference compounds (separately, 2 mL per compound) at 600 µ*M* for verapamil (in 2% v/v dimethylsulfoxide [DMSO]), 1200 µ*M* for progesterone (in 20% v/v EtOH), and 100 µ*M* for vinblastine (in 1% v/v DMSO). These reagents may be prepared from solutions at 1 mg/mL in ethanol and stored at –20°C in aliquots once prepared. They will be diluted 20-fold in the final assay (final concentration 30 µ*M*, 60 µ*M*, and 5 µ*M*, respectively).
4. The coupled enzymes (PK/LDH solution): pyruvate kinase (PK) at 1 mg/mL and lactate dehydrogenase (LDL) at 1 mg/mL, which can be mixed in a volume of 1 to 1.5 mL of enzymatic buffer. These reagents may be stored at –20°C in aliquots once prepared. They will be diluted 10-fold in the final assay (final concentration 0.1 mg/mL).
5. Phosphoenolpyruvate (PEP) and NADH, each at 10 m*M* (1–1.5 mL of enzymatic buffer), separately. These reagents may be stored at –20°C in aliquots once prepared. They will be diluted 20-fold in the final assay (final concentration 0.5 m*M*).
6. MgATP at 20 mM, prepared from Na_2ATP and $MgCl_2$ by equimolar mixing. This reagent may be stored at –20°C in aliquots once prepared. It will be diluted 20-fold in the final assay (final concentration 1 m*M*).
7. Compounds to be tested, which should be diluted at the desired concentrations in the enzymatic buffer. Recommended final concentrations are 50, 5, 0.5, and 0.05 µ*M*. Because the compounds will be diluted 10-fold in the final assay, the initial concentrations will be 500, 50, 5, and 0.5 µ*M*. The final solvent concentrations (ethanol or DMSO) should be less than 0.5% v/v for DMSO and less than 5% v/v for EtOH.
8. P-gp-containing membrane vesicle suspension at 0.1 mg/mL (final concentration 5 µg/mL).

3.2. Reagent Distribution and ATPase Activity Measurement

3.2.1. Typical Plate Setting

To avoid any degradation, all samples and reagents should be maintained at 4°C (ice bath) during their distribution.

1. Identify in a plate setting the following wells (it is recommended to perform the assays in duplicate to increase assay precision):

   Blank: used for the spectrophotometer reference (contains only the enzymatic buffer).

   Nonspecific absorption decrease or "nonspecific activity": apparent activity in the absence of membranes.

	1	2	3	4	5	6	7	8	9	10	11	12
A	Blank	Vinblastine	Drug 2	Drug 6	Drug 10	Drug 14	Drug 18	Drug 22	Drug 26	Drug 30	Drug 34	Drug 38
B	Blank	Vinblastine	Drug 2	Drug 6	Drug 10	Drug 14	Drug 18	Drug 22	Drug 26	Drug 30	Drug 34	Drug 38
C	Non Specific Activity	Verapamil	Drug 3	Drug 7	Drug 11	Drug 15	Drug 19	Drug 23	Drug 27	Drug 31	Drug 35	Drug 39
D	Non Specific Activity	Verapamil	Drug 3	Drug 7	Drug 11	Drug 15	Drug 19	Drug 23	Drug 27	Drug 31	Drug 35	Drug 39
E	Total Activity	Progesterone	Drug 4	Drug 8	Drug 12	Drug 16	Drug 20	Drug 24	Drug 28	Drug 32	Drug 36	Drug 40
F	Total Activity	Progesterone	Drug 4	Drug 8	Drug 12	Drug 16	Drug 20	Drug 24	Drug 28	Drug 32	Drug 36	Drug 40
G	Basal Activity	Drug 1	Drug 5	Drug 9	Drug 13	Drug 17	Drug 21	Drug 25	Drug 29	Drug 33	Drug 37	Drug 41
H	Basal Activity	Drug 1	Drug 5	Drug 9	Drug 13	Drug 17	Drug 21	Drug 25	Drug 29	Drug 33	Drug 37	Drug 41

Fig. 2. Typical plate setup. Drugs 1 to 41 indicate the wells corresponding to the tested drug at various concentrations in the absence or presence of the three reference compounds (verapamil, progesterone, or vinblastine).

Total activity: ATPase activity in the absence of nonspecific inhibitors.

Basal activity: residual activity in the presence of nonspecific inhibitors, mainly due to P-gp.

Activity stimulated by the reference compounds: P-gp activity in the presence of verapamil, progesterone, or vinblastine, the three reference P-gp substrates.

Activity in the presence of the tested compounds, called *samples*: P-gp activity induced by the tested compounds, in the presence of verapamil, progesterone, or vinblastine or none of these three reference compounds.

A typical plate setup is presented in **Fig. 2**. It is recommended to perform the basal activity wells in four replicates, using the two wells "Drug 1" for this purpose, because this activity will be used as a reference.

2. Switch on the spectrophotometer and the incubator at 37°C (*see* **Note 7**).
3. Distribute the reagents according to the following sequence (and use different tips to pipet the various reagents to avoid possible cross-contamination) (*see* **Fig. 3**): 200 µL of enzymatic buffer in blank wells.

   In each other well and using a multipipettor distributor, dispense the following: 80 µL of enzymatic buffer + 20 µL of PK/LDH solution + 10 µL of PEP solution + 10 µL of NADH solution.

   Dispense in nonspecific activity wells the following: 30 µL of nonspecific ATPase inhibitor solution + 30 µL of enzymatic buffer.

Assay protocol - one concentration						
Steps	Blank	Non Specific Activity	Total Activity	Basal Activity	Refence compound	Samples
Step 1: distribute,						
Enzymatic buffer	200 µl	80 µl	80 µl	80 µl	80 µl	80 µl
PK/LDH solution		20 µl	20 µl	20 µl	20 µl	20 µl
PEP solution		10 µl	10 µl	10 µl	10 µl	10 µl
NADH solution		10 µl	10 µl	10 µl	10 µl	10 µl
Enzymatic buffer*		30 µl	60 µl	30 µl	20 µl	10 µl*
Non-specific ATPase inhibitor solution		30 µl		30 µl	30 µl	30 µl
Reference compound*					10 µl	10 µl*
Step 2:	Shake the plate 10 seconds & read the plate at 340 nm.					
Step 3:	Incubate the 96-well plate for 30 minutes at 37°C.					
Step 4: add,						
Enzymatic buffer		10 µl				
Membrane vesicles			10 µl	10 µl	10 µl	10 µl
Step 5:	Incubate the 96-well plate for 5 minutes at 37°C.					
Step 6: dispense,						
tested compound						20 µl
Step 7:	Incubate the 96-well plate for 5 minutes at 37°C.					
Step 8: dispense,						
MgATP		10 µl	10 µl	10 µl	10 µl	10 µl
Step 9:	Incubate the 96-well plate for 20 minutes at 37°C.					
Step 10:	Shake the plate 10 seconds & read the plate at 340 nm. Keep on incubating the plate					
Final volume	200 µl	200 µl	200 µl	200 µl	200 µl	200 µl

*: you may either test your compound *versus* the basal activity. If so, add 10 µl of enzymatic buffer. If you wish to test your compound with a reference compound add 10 µl of this reference.

Fig. 3. Protocol of reagent distribution.

Dispense in total activity wells the following: 60 µL of enzymatic buffer.
Dispense in basal activity wells the following: 30 µL of nonspecific ATPase inhibitor solution + 30 µL of enzymatic buffer.
Dispense in reference compound wells the following: 30 µL of nonspecific ATPase inhibitor solution + 10 µL of reference compound (verapamil, progesterone, or vinblastine) + 20 µL of enzymatic buffer.
Dispense in all the other wells, the "samples," the following:
30 µL nonspecific ATPase inhibitor solution + 10 µL of either enzymatic buffer (for testing compounds on basal activity) or reference compound (for testing compounds on stimulated activity).

4. Shake the plate 10 s and read the plate at 340 nm to verify NADH absorbance in each well. The absorbance should be around 1.9 U.
5. To homogenize the plate temperature, incubate the 96-well plate for 30 min at 37°C under gentle stirring.
6. Add 10 µL of enzymatic buffer in nonspecific activity wells and 10 µL membrane vesicles in all the other wells except the blank wells. Just before distribution, vortex suspension to homogenize membrane vesicles and eliminate aggregates.
7. Incubate the 96-well plate for 5 min at 37°C.
8. Dispense in the sample wells 20 µL of tested compound at each concentration, and incubate for 5 min at 37°C (*see* **Note 8**).
9. Dispense 10 µL of MgATP in every well except the blank wells, and incubate the plate for 20 min at 37°C.
10. Shake the plate 10 s and read the plate at 340 nm. Then keep on incubating the plate at 37°C and read 20 min later.

3.2.2. Alternative Plate Setting for "Cumulative Measurements"

To spare the reagents or increase the number of the assays in one microplate, it is possible to test the different concentrations of a considered compound in the same well. To do so, after **step 7**, the following should be done:

1. Add 5 µL of the drug at the lowest concentration (e.g., 0.05 µ*M*, final concentration) and incubate for 5 min at 37°C. Then, dispense 10 µL of MgATP in every well except the blank wells, and incubate the plate for 10 min at 37°C. Shake the plate 10 s and read the plate at 340 nm. Then, keep on incubating the plate at 37°C and read 20 min later.
2. Add 5 µL of the drug at a second concentration (e.g., 0.5 µ*M*, final concentration), incubate the plate 5 min at 37°C, shake the plate, and read the plate immediately and 20 min later.
3. Add 5 µL of the drug at a third concentration (e.g., 5 µ*M*, final concentration), incubate the plate 5 min at 37°C, shake the plate, and read the plate immediately and 20 min later.

4. Add 5 μL of the drug at a fourth concentration (e.g., 50 μ*M*, final concentration), incubate the plate 5 min at 37°C, shake the plate, and read the plate immediately and 20 min later.

Make sure to take into account the final volume (and the previous concentration tested) to determine the final concentration of the compound. For example:

Add 5 μL of a compound at 1.85 μ*M* for a 0.05-μ*M* final concentration (final volume 185 μL).
Add 5 μL of a compound at 17.2 μ*M* for a 0.5-μ*M* final concentration (final volume 190 μL).
Add 5 μL of a compound at 176 μ*M* for a 5-μ*M* final concentration (final volume 195 μL).
Add 5 μL of a compound at 1.79 μ*M* for a 50-μ*M* final concentration (final volume 200 μL).

3.3. Data Analysis and Interpretation

3.3.1. Calculations

1. Make sure that your plate reader has subtracted the absorbance readings of the blank wells from the absorbance readings of the rest of the plate.
2. Calculate the average absorbance, the standard deviation, and the coefficient of variation for each duplicate (normal range: 0.1%–1.5%).
3. On the mean value, determine the absorption decrease rate ΔmAU/min between 0 and 20 min for each drug concentration. Calculate the corresponding activity (nmol/mg/min): (ΔmAU/min $\times$ 26 10^{-2})/protein concentration. This figure comes from the Beer-Lambert law ($A = \varepsilon \times L \times C$), which is precisely the following:

Activity(nmol/mg/min) = Abs(mAU/min) $\times$ 1000/[6230 (NADH extinction coefficient in $mol^{-1} \cdot l \cdot cm^{-1}$) $\times$ 0.62 (optical pathway in cm)]/protein concentration (mg/mL).

$$\text{Activity(nmol/mg/min)} = \text{Abs(mAU/min)} \times 26\ 10^{-2} \times \text{protein concentration}^{-1}.$$

4. Subtract the nonspecific activity of wells without the vesicle from each other well.
5. Calculate relative activity induced by each compound concentration compared to the reference activity (basal or stimulated activity). *Example:*
   Basal activity: 160 nmol/mg/min.
   Verapamil-stimulated activity: 400 nmol/mg/min.
   Drug X at 5 μM in the absence of verapamil: 180 nmol/mg/min.
   Thus, drug X at 5 μM relative to the basal activity: 1.1.
   Drug X at 5 μM in the presence of verapamil: 288 nmol/mg/min.
   Thus, drug X at 5 μM relative to verapamil: 0.6.

3.3.2. Quality Criteria of the Assay

The nonspecific activity should be under 1.5 mAU/min. The ratio between total and basal activity should be higher than 2. The basal activity should be in the range of 150 to 250 nmol/mg/min. The typical level of basal ATPase activity is somehow dependent on the batch of membranes used. The stimulated activities induced by vinblastine, progesterone, and verapamil, relative to the basal activity, should be in the range of 1.2 to 1.7, 1.5 to 2.5, and 2.2 to 3.2, respectively.

3.3.3. Test Conclusions

A tested molecule is concluded to interact specifically with P-gp if it significantly (>30%) modulates either one of the four ATPase activities assayed (i.e., basal or stimulated by verapamil, progesterone, or vinblastine) ***(13)***. In the latter example, although the drug tested does not change the basal activity (less than 30%), it modulates significantly the activity stimulated by verapamil and can thus be considered as interacting with P-gp (*see* **Note 9**).

Conversely, a tested molecule that has no effect on any of the four ATPase activities assayed can be considered as not interacting with P-gp. Actually, this case represents the opportunity for a compound to escape from the digestive absorption barrier and biliary/renal active excretion. The ATPase-based test is thus of value for screening molecules in the aim to evidence those that can bypass P-gp handling.

From a more general practical view, the ATPase-based test can be used to address different questions of interest for the pharmaceutical industry. For example, this test is well suited for conveniently evaluating in vitro the possibility of whether newly developed (or already known medicines) molecules will suffer from ADME processes that can limit their bioavailability after administration in vivo. Actually, in the case of evidencing an interaction of the tested molecule with P-gp, it can be expected that this molecule will be subjected to a P-gp-mediated transmembrane flux across biological barriers (a molecule that is called a "substrate") and will present a risk for being responsible for drug interactions with other medicines mediated by P-gp (a molecule that is called an "inhibitor"). These are two connected properties of molecules transported by P-gp but sometimes are distinct because they depend respectively on the passive transmembrane diffusion rate and on mutual relationships between the two drugs of interest when they bind on the transport sites of P-gp (*see* **Note 10**). Although it could be interesting to recognize these two functional properties, it should be pointed out that the ATPase-based assay is not used to distinguish a molecule tested to be a substrate or an inhibitor; instead, it probes a specific interaction of this molecule with P-gp. Anyway, a molecule interacting with P-gp is highly likely to be considered as a substrate, an inhibitor, or even often both (*see* **Note 11**), and this appears to be of importance for the industrial development of this compound with respect to ADME processes (crossing of the intestine absorption barrier or the blood–brain barrier) as well as drug interactions ***(13)***.

The ATPase-based test can also be used to discover molecules aimed at specifically modulating the P-gp function according to typical properties. A first step is to search for molecules characterized by a very high affinity for interacting with P-gp, which is obviously a criterion for a fair specificity against P-gp (with few side effects, from the perspective of a clinical administration). This can be obtained by testing molecules at very low concentrations, even lower than in the test in its typical form as presented previously, within a range such as 1 nM to 1 μ*M*, for example. Also, it could be of interest to search for molecules capable of inhibiting P-gp transport of virtually all its substrates, that is, to find a broad-spectrum inhibitor for P-gp. According to the energetic coupling between drug-stimulated ATPase and drug transport presented by P-gp, such an inhibitor will inhibit all the stimulated ATPase activities assayed, and this can be detected by the simultaneous inhibition of the three P-gp ATPase activities stimulated by the reference substrates of the ATPase test (no matter what the effect is on the basal activity).

3.4. Assay Troubleshooting

No activity: no vesicle or no MgATP in well, or P-gp degradation.
All activities are low: verify that incubator temperature is at 37°C.
Control values for vinblastine, progesterone, and verapamil out of the typical range: check their concentrations.
Nonspecific activity value too high: presence of an NADH oxidant substance.
High dispersion of duplicates: poor pipetting technique or low vortex of membrane vesicle suspensions.

4. Notes

1. The advantage of the ATPase-based test is to provide information about specific interaction (binding) between P-gp and tested molecules in a simpler manner than using transport tests performed on living cells (Caco-2, MDCK, and so on). As a matter of fact, this assay avoids using any radiolabeled compounds or specific techniques such as high-performance liquid chromatography–mass spectrometry (HPLC-MS) to measure each drug in different compartments. Obviously, this assay should be considered as a first screening step performed on a number of candidate molecules. The precise characterization of some selected molecules of interest should be completed by a direct transport assay.
2. Measurement of ATPase activity using the coupled enzyme technique presents some advantages: real-time recording, a reaction that does not need to be stopped,

no radioactivity used, stationary ATP concentration in the reaction medium, and a rather low protein requirement.

3. It should be pointed out that if the ATPase test is performed only by assaying the drug effect on the basal activity, false-negative results may be encountered, which could be why a rather bad correlation exists between ATPase and transport measurements ***(14,15)***. Indeed, among the number of compounds interacting with P-gp, it has been demonstrated that some of them do not change the basal ATPase activity level. However, these compounds do alter the ATPase activity stimulated by known P-gp substrates, such as verapamil, progesterone, and vinblastine, revealing their interaction with P-gp.
4. These P-gp-containing membranes are prepared from highly resistant MDR cells, the DC-3F/ADX line, which are Chinese hamster lung fibroblasts that have been spontaneously transformed and selected from the parent-sensitive cell line DC-3F by stepwise selection against increasing concentrations of actinomycin D ***(6)***. Membranes are kept for several months frozen at –80°C in aliquots to prevent freeze-thaw cycles. P-gp is highly overexpressed in the DC-3F/ADX cells, where it represents about 15% of the total membrane proteins, compared to the parent DC-3F cells, where it cannot be detected by the C219 or C494 antibodies specific to P-gp. In addition, P-gp is the only membrane protein that is so overexpressed, as evidenced by sodium dodecyl sulfate–polyacrylamide gel electrophoresis (SDS-PAGE), which shows only one major band at 150 to 160 kDa, and as shown by a densitometric analysis of the electrophoresis gel. Thus, it cannot be excluded that other ABC proteins, as well as other membrane ATPases, are present in the vesicles, but their amount should be limited to low expression levels, as found in the parent DC-3F cells (in particular, we checked by immunodetection the absence of MRP1, unpublished data). Control experiments using membrane vesicles prepared from the DC-3F cells can be performed to ensure the role of P-gp in the ATPase signal observed on the vesicles from DC-3F/ADX cells. The mainly inside-out orientation of these vesicles allows the P-gp ATPase sites on the cytoplasmic face of the plasma membrane to be exposed to the external medium. In these membranes, there is no need to substract the vanadate-resistant ATPase activity because its low level is negligible compared to the basal activity of P-gp ***(6)***.
5. The same test can be performed on 386 wells, allowing one to reach an HTS format. Simply adapt the procedure described to the final volume of the reaction medium, which is 0.1 mL in this case.
6. It is possible to completely test five compounds (at four concentrations) in one plate by omiting duplicates and distributing the reference P-gp substrates in the adequate wells.
7. Temperature regulation displayed by spectrophotometers are often unefficient for setting a homogeneous temperature in all the wells. A remote thermoregulated incubator is preferred because enzyme activities are highly dependent on the reaction medium temperature.
8. A possible absorption at 340 nm of the compound tested is of no matter because activity measurement is based on the absorption decrease rate.

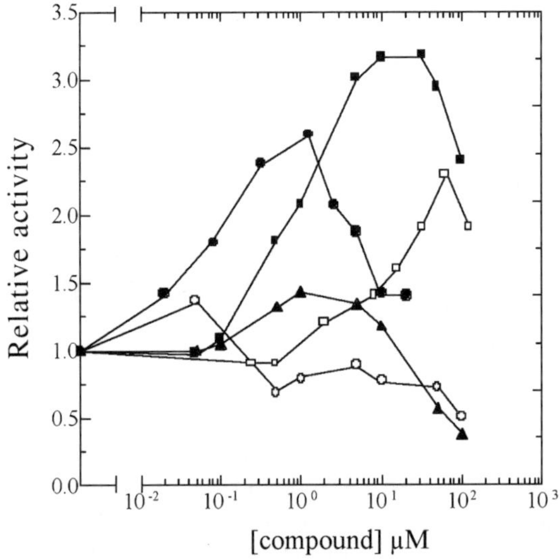

Fig. 4. ATPase activities of P-gp-containing membrane vesicles from DC-3F/ADX cells in the presence of different compounds interacting with P-gp. The ATPase assay medium (at 37°C) contained 10 m*M* sodium azide, 0.5 m*M* ouabain, 1 m*M* EGTA, and 5 μg/mL P-gp-containing membrane vesicle suspensions in 96-well microplates in the presence of increasing concentrations of verapamil (filled squares), nicardipine (filled circles), vinblastine (filled triangles), progesterone (hollow squares), or cyclosporin A (hollow circles). The relative ATPase activity is normalized with respect to the basal activity.

9. As a matter of fact, P-gp is described as having different binding sites for the various drugs it recognizes ***(16)***. We have chosen verapamil, progesterone, and vinblastine as reference-stimulating substrates because these drugs bind to distinct sites on P-gp and, because they are complementary, can thus "probe" with a high probability the interaction of a number of other ligands on P-gp. The typical action of these three compounds on the P-gp basal activity is shown in **Fig. 4**. The two other classic P-gp substrates, nicardipine and cyclosporin A, also presented in this figure, have been shown to be redundant with the three references we have chosen for probing the multiple binding sites on P-gp ***(13)***.
10. Semantics about "substrate" and "inhibitor" must be clarified here. A true, enzymatic P-gp substrate is a molecule that can bind to and be translocated by P-gp; this molecule is referred to be a substrate for P-gp-mediated cellular transport if P-gp is able to create a detectable concentration gradient across the cell membrane for this molecule, owing to its slow enough transmembrane passive diffusion rate ***(17)***. This property is tested by assaying the flux of this molecule on cultured cells. A true, enzymatic P-gp inhibitor is a molecule that can decrease the catalytic turnover rate of P-gp; at the cellular level, an inhibitor of P-gp-

mediated transport of drug X is a molecule that can decrease the measured flux of this given drug X across the cell membrane. In that case, and as a consequence of the characteristic multispecific recognition property presented by P-gp, the considered molecule can or cannot be transported itself, and if it is, it can or cannot compete with drug X. This property is determined by the molecular properties for the binding of the two molecules on P-gp, according to their mutual exclusivity or nonexclusivity for being translocated by P-gp, as well as the resulting turnover rate of this translocation (and this depends on the nature of X) ***(16)***. It thus appears that at the cellular level—the only one relevant for a pharmaceutical approach—the properties "substrate" and "inhibitor" refer to distinct aspects of the P-gp function, which are independent and nonexclusive ***(14,15)***.

11. The comparison of data obtained from cell systems and membrane fractions has been recently reported to check the correlation between ATPase assays and transport measurements evidencing either P-gp substrates or inhibitors ***(13,15,18)***. The key point of these studies (performed on 12, 41, and 66 compounds tested, respectively) is that it appears that all the compounds that scored as positive in the ATPase test are never false positive regarding the cell transport measurements. Thus, this suggests that all compounds positive for the ATPase assay are substrates or inhibitors. Conversely, in the last study, it appears that 67% of the compounds positive for cell transport measurements are scored positive for the ATPase test (considering only the basal activity). In our hands, this fraction represents 78% when only considering modulations of the basal ATPase activity but is 95% when including modulations of the activities stimulated by the reference P-gp substrates ***(13)***.

References

1. Schinkel, A. H. (1997) The physiological function of drug-transporting P-glycoproteins. *Semin. Cancer Biol.* **8,** 161–170.
2. Sauna, Z. E., Smith, M. M., Müller, M., Kerr, K. M., and Ambudkar, S. V. (2001) The mechanism of action of multidrug-resistance-linked P-glycoprotein. *J. Bioenerg. Biomembrane* **33,** 481–491.
3. Orlowski, S., Valente, D., Garrigos, M., and Ezan, E. (1998) Bromocriptine modulates P-glycoprotein function. *Biochem. Biophys. Res. Commun.* **244,** 481–488.
4. Schmid, D., Ecker, G., Kopp, S., Hitzler, M., and Chiba, P. (1999) Structure-activity relationship studies of propafenone analogs based on P-glycoprotein ATPase activity measurements. *Biochem. Pharmacol.* **58,** 1447–1456.
5. Sarkadi, B., Price, E. M., Boucher, R. C., Germann, U. A., and Scarborough, G. A. (1992) Expression of the human multidrug resistance cDNA in insect cells generates a high activity drug-stimulated membrane ATPase. *J. Biol. Chem.* **267,** 4854–4858.
6. Garrigos, M., Belehradek, J., Jr., Mir, L. M., and Orlowski, S. (1993) Absence of cooperativity for MgATP and verapamil effects on the ATPase activity of P-glycoprotein containing membrane vesicles. *Biochem. Biophys. Res. Commun.* **196,** 1034–1041.

7. Al-Shawi, M. K. and Senior, A. E. (1993) Characterization of the adenosine triphosphatase activity of Chinese hamster P-glycoprotein. *J. Biol. Chem.* **268,** 4197–4206.
8. Scharschmitd, B. F., Keeffe, E. B., Blankenship, N. M., and Ockner, R. K. (1979) Validation of a recording method for measurement of membrane-associated Mg- and NaK-ATPase activity. *J. Lab. Clin. Med.* **93,** 790–799.
9. Garrigos, M., Mir, L. M., and Orlowski, S. (1997) Competitive and non-competitive inhibition of the multidrug-resistance-associated P-glycoprotein ATPase: further experimental evidence for a multisite model. *Eur. J. Biochem.* **244,** 664–673.
10. Litman, T., Zeuthen, T., Skovsgaard, T., and Stein, W. D. (1997) Structure-activity relationships of P-glycoprotein interacting drugs: kinetic characterization of their effects on ATPase activity. *Biochim. Biophys. Acta* **1361,** 159–168.
11. Orlowski, S., Mir, L. M., Belehradek, J., Jr., and Garrigos, M. (1996) Effects of steroids and verapamil on P-glycoprotein ATPase activity: progesterone, desoxycorticosterone, corticosterone and verapamil are mutually non-exclusive modulators. *Biochem. J.* **317,** 515–522.
12. Borgnia, M. J., Eytan, G. D., and Assaraf, Y. G. (1996) Competition of hydrophobic peptides, cytotoxic drugs, and chemosensitizers on a common P-glycoprotein pharmacophore as revealed by its ATPase activity. *J. Biol. Chem.* **271,** 3163–3171.
13. Garrigues, A., Nugier, J., Orlowski, S., and Ezan, E. (2002) A high-throughput screening microplate test for the interaction of drugs with P-glycoprotein. *Anal. Biochem.* **305,** 106–114.
14. Scala, S., Akhmed, N., Rao, U. S., Paull, K., Lan, L.-B., Dickstein, B., et al. (1997) P-glycoprotein substrates and antagonists cluster into two distinct groups. *Mol. Pharmacol.* **51,** 1024–1033.
15. Polli, J. W., Wring, S. A., Humphreys, J. E., Huang, L., Morgan, J. B., Webster, L. O., et al. (2001) Rational use of in vitro P-glycoprotein assays in drug discovery. *J. Pharmacol. Exp. Ther.* **299,** 620–628.
16. Orlowski, S. and Garrigos, M. (1999) Multiple recognition of various amphiphilic molecules by the multidrug resistance P-glycoprotein: molecular mechanisms and pharmacological consequences coming from functional interaction between various drugs. *Anticancer Res.* **19,** 3109–3124.
17. Ferté, J. (2000) Analysis of the tangled relationships between P-glycoprotein-mediated multidrug resistance and the lipid phase of the cell membrane. *Eur. J. Biochem.* **267,** 277–294.
18. Adachi, Y., Suzuki, H., and Sugiyama, Y. (2001) Comparative studies on in vitro methods for evaluating in vivo function of MDR1 P-glycoprotein. *Pharm. Res.* **18,** 1660–1668.

7

Evaluation of Drug–Transporter Interactions Using In Vitro Cell Models

Yaming Su and Patrick J. Sinko

Summary

Drug transporters have been isolated from many tissues, including the intestines, liver, kidney, blood–brain barrier, and placenta, in animals and humans. There is increasing evidence that they play a very important role in drug absorption and disposition. By gaining a better understanding of the characteristics of drug transporters, drugs and prodrugs can be designed with improved bioavailability by targeting delivery to low-affinity, high-capacity absorptive transporters (e.g., hPept1) while avoiding secretory efflux transporters (e.g., P-glycoprotein [P-gp]). Delineation of drug-transporter interactions is also helpful for predicting in vivo pharmacokinetics and transporter-mediated drug-drug interactions. The identification of membrane transporters that influence the absorption, disposition, and safety of drugs is very important in drug discovery and development. In this chapter, protocols are summarized for some widely used cell models for characterizing the drug-transporter interactions.

Key Words: Transporter; P-gp; PepT1; CHO cells; *Xenopus laevis* oocytes.

1. Introduction

The oocyte from the South African clawed frog *Xenopus laevis* has been widely used as an expression system for functional studies of membrane proteins. In this system, in vitro transcribed poly(A)-cRNA (complementary ribonucleic acid) is microinjected into the cytoplasm of the oocyte and, on the next day, the function of the encoded protein can be measured. The advantages of transporter cRNA-injected oocytes (transportocytes) as an overexpression system are that the expression of endogenous transporters (e.g., P-gp) is very low and the posttranslational modification of the protein is similar to mammalian cells.

From: *Methods in Pharmacology and Toxicology*
Optimization in Drug Discovery: In Vitro Methods
Edited by: Z. Yan and G. W. Caldwell © Humana Press Inc., Totowa, NJ

Mammalian cell lines transiently or stably transfected with membrane transporter complementary deoxyribonucleic acid (cDNA) are also widely used to investigate interactions between drugs and transporters, including determination of the affinity, capacity, and other transport parameters. The typical cell lines used to overexpress transporter proteins are Madin-Darby canine kidney (MDCK), Hela, HEK293, and Chinese hamster ovary (CHO) cells ***(1)***. Compared to cRNA-injected *X. laevis* oocytes, this cellular model is easier to construct, and the results are relatively more consistent. If the transfected cDNA is for a cell uptake transporter (e.g., OATPs, PepT1), the transfected cells can be used directly for uptake studies. However, if an efflux transporter (e.g., MRP2, P-gp) is transfected into the cells, the direction of the transporter will prevent cell uptake studies from being performed. Therefore, three options exist. First, inside-out cell membrane vesicles can be prepared and drug uptake can then be measured directly. Although membrane vesicle techniques do not require unusual or highly specialized equipment, the technique is considered to be an "art," and considerable practice is required to prepare consistent batches. A second option is to preload the cells, usually in suspension, with drug and then monitor drug efflux into the surrounding medium. There are limitations to this technique, with the most significant being the sensitivity of the bioanalytical assay because small amounts of drug are effluxed from the cells into a relatively large volume of suspension solution. The third alternative is to use cells seeded on supports and grown as a monolayer. This popular method can be used to study the bidirectional transport of drugs.

This protocol describes the use of the peptide transporter (PepT1) in the uptake of a nonpeptide prodrug, valacyclovir (vacv), by using PepT1 cRNA injected oocytes ***(1)*** and PepT1 cDNA transiently transfected CHO cells ***(2)***. The construction of the transporter plasmid, the in vitro transcription to cRNA, and the microinjection of cRNA into oocytes are not included in this protocol.

2. Materials

2.1. Materials Needed for the Uptake Experiment Using Transportocytes

1. Valacyclovir (Glaxo Wellcome, Inc., Research Triangle Park, NC).
2. [^{3}H] Valacyclovir was custom prepared by Moraveck Biochemicals (Brea, CA).
3. Modified bath's solution: 88 m*M* NaCl, 1 m*M* KCl, 2.4 m*M* $NaHCO_3$, 0.82 m*M* $MgSO_4$, 0.33 m*M* $Ca(NO_3)_2$, 0.41 m*M* $CaCl_2$, and 10 m*M* HEPES adjusted to pH 7.4 using 5 *N* NaOH.
4. Medium A: 100 m*M* NaCl, 2 m*M* KCl, 1 m*M* $CaCl_2$, 1 m*M* $MgCl_2$, and 10 m*M* 2-[*N*-morpholino]ethanesulfonic acid (MES) adjusted to pH 5.5 using 5 *N* NaOH.
5. 10% Sodium dodecyl sulfate (SDS).
6. ScintiVerse® scintillation fluid (Fisher, Fairlawn, NJ).
7. 24-Well cell culture plate (BD, Franklin Lakes, NJ).

8. Transfer pipet.
9. Scintillation counter.

2.2. Materials Needed for the Uptake Experiment Using PepT1 Transiently Transfected CHO Cells

1. Cell culture medium: Dulbecco's modified Eagle's medium (DMEM) containing 90% DMEM, 10% fetal bovine serum (FBS), 1% nonessential amino acids, 100 U/mL penicillin, and 100 μg/mL streptomycin (Invitrogen, Carlsbad, CA).
2. 0.05% Trypsin (Invitrogen, Carlsbad, CA).
3. Lipofectamine reagent (Invitrogen, Carlsbad, CA).
4. 1X Phosphate-buffered saline (PBS): 3 mM Na_2HPO_4, 1 mM KH_2PO_4, 155 mM NaCl.
5. Opti-MEM I reduced serum medium (Invitrogen, Carlsbad, CA).
6. Hank's balanced salt solution (Invitrogen, Carlsbad, CA).
7. Bicinchoninic acid (BCA) protein assay reagent (Pierce, Rockford, IL).
8. CHO cells (ATCC, Rockville, MD).
9. 24-Well cell culture plate (BD, Franklin Lakes, NJ).

3. Methods

3.1. Methods for Uptake Experiment Using Transportocytes

The methods described below outline methods to study (1) the time-course of drug uptake, (2) the concentration dependency of drug uptake in PepT1 cRNA-injected oocytes, and (3) the inhibition of uptake of glycylsarcosine by vacv. Although these three elements are the most common study protocols, numerous other protocols can be employed to ascertain critical information about drug-transporter interactions.

3.1.1. Time Course of vacv Uptake

The objective of time-course experiments is to determine the minimum time required to get reliable drug uptake.

1. Prepare the test compound. vacv was diluted in medium A as a concentration of 0.2 mM spiked with [^{3}H]vacv. If the stock compound is diluted in dimethylsulfoxide (DMSO), methanol, or acetonitril, the final concentration of those solvents should be 1% to 2% or less (*see* **Note 1**).
2. Using the transfer pipet, place 8–12 oocytes into 1 well of a 24-well cell culture plate, with approx 500 μL of Barth's media (*see* **Note 2**).
3. Using a vacuum pump fitted with a pipet tip, remove the Barth's media as much as possible; be careful not to disrupt the oocytes.
4. Immediately add approx 500 μL of room temperature medium A by using the transfer pipet.
5. Repeat the previous step twice to wash the oocytes. If Na^+ dependency is under investigation, medium A should be replaced by Na^+ free medium as the uptake medium and used to wash the oocytes.
6. After washing three times with medium A, add 500 μL of 0.2 mM vacv.

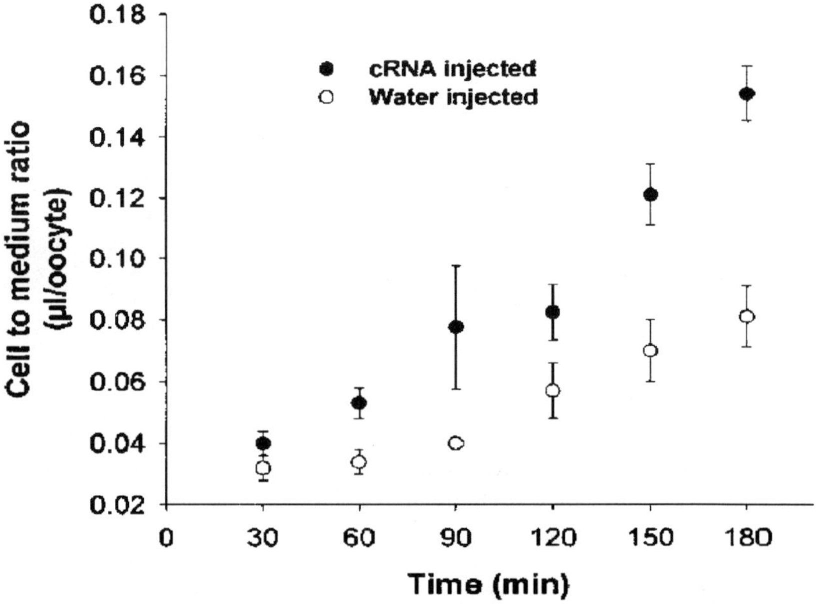

Fig. 1. Time-course of uptake of vacv by PepT1 cRNA-injected oocytes. Uptake of vacv was measured after the indicated time period. The cell-to-medium ratio, which was obtained by dividing the uptake amount by the concentration in the medium, in cRNA- or water-injected oocytes is shown. Each point represents the mean (±) SEM of 6–10 oocytes.

7. The PepT1 cRNA or water-injected oocytes were incubated with 0.2 m*M* vacv for 30, 60, 90, 120, 150, and 180 min at room temperature.
8. At the end of indicated incubation time, use a vacuum pump to remove the test compound (*see* **Note 3**).
9. Wash the oocytes three times by adding approx 1 mL of ice-cold medium A.
10. Using a vacuum pump fitted with a pipet tip, remove all of the solution.
11. Immediately after washing, take the oocytes one at a time using a transfer pipet and place them in separate scintillation vials (*see* **Note 4**).
12. To lyse the oocytes, add 150 µL of 10% SDS buffer to each scintillation vial.
13. Incubate the scintillation vials on a rocker for 30 min at room temperature (*see* **Note 5**).
14. Add 4 mL of scintillation fluid to each vial. Cap each vial and mix.
15. Assay using the scintillation counter. A typical time course of uptake of vacv by PepT1 cRNA-injected oocytes is shown in **Fig. 1**.

Several experimental parameters, such as the number of washes, will require pilot studies to determine the optimal parameter value (in this case, the optimal number of washes). Washing too many times could lead to the leaching of drug from the oocyte, resulting in an underestimate of drug uptake, whereas too little washing would result in a higher amount of drug associated with the oocyte as a result of binding, leading to an overestimate of drug uptake.

3.1.2. Concentration Dependence of vacv Uptake

1. Prepare vacv solutions with various concentrations from 0.1 to 2.5 m*M*. If the apparent K_m of transport can be estimated, then an equal number of concentrations above and below the K_m should be studied. Failure to do this may result in the inability to estimate V_{max} and K_m in a reliable manner.
2. Follow the procedure used in **Subheading 3.1.1.** Perform the uptake study at 60 min by using different concentrations of vacv.
3. The saturable uptake of vacv is analyzed using the following equation when the interactions of the drug with the transporter are competitive in nature:

$$V = \frac{V_{max}\,[S]}{K_m + [S]}$$

where *V* and *S* are the uptake rate and vacv concentration, respectively. V_{max} and K_m represent the maximum uptake rate and Michaelis constant, respectively. The kinetic parameters can be estimated by using a weighted nonlinear least squares analysis program, (in this case Scientist, Micromath Scientific Software). The weighting scheme used in the analysis was 1/SEM. Although many investigators use linearization techniques such as Lineweaver-Burk or Eadie-Hofstee analysis to analyze nonlinear data, the resulting kinetic parameters are biased and unreliable. Therefore, special weighting schemes must be employed if a linearization technique is used to numerically analyze the data. A typical concentration dependence plot of vacv uptake is shown in **Fig. 2**.

3.1.3. Inhibition of the Uptake of Glycylsarcosine (a Typical PepT1 Substrate)

In the following procedure, the inhibitory activity of vacv on PepT1 was investigated.

1. Prepare 0.02 m*M* of glycylsarcosine solutions spiked with [^{3}H]glycylsarcosine and aliquot them.
2. Add different amounts of vacv to each aliquot of the glycylsarcosine solution to make vacv concentrations at 0, 0.05, 1, 10, and 25 m*M*. Once again, the concept of selecting concentrations to span the K_m and *Ki* of the substrate and inhibitor should be used. A common approach is to hold either the inhibitor or substrate concentrations constant and vary the other one. This simplifies the data analysis.
3. Follow the procedure used in **Subheading 3.1.1.**, and perform the uptake study at 60 min.
4. The saturable inhibition of the uptake of glycylsarcosine by various concentrations of vacv was analyzed using the following equation:

$$V = \frac{V_{max} * S}{K_m\,(1 + ([I]\,/\,Ki))\,S}$$

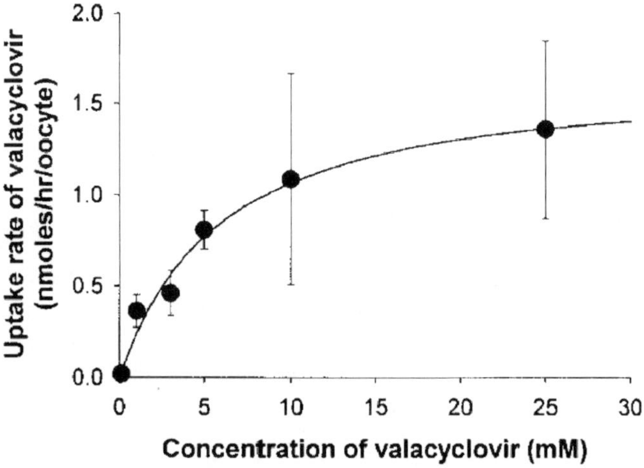

Fig. 2. Concentration dependence of vacv uptake. Uptake of vacv was measured at various concentrations (0.1, 1, 3, 5, 10, and 25 m*M*) at room temperature for 60 min. The reported uptake rate was calculated by subtracting the uptake rate in water-injected oocytes from PepT1-injected oocytes. Each point represents the mean ± SEM of 6–10 oocytes. The fitted line represents the carrier-mediated uptake estimated from the kinetic parameters as explained in the text.

where V, V_{max}, S, and K_m are the uptake rate, maximum uptake, concentration, and Michaelis constant for glycylsarcosine, respectively. $[I]$ and Ki represent the concentration of vacv and the inhibition constant of vacv, respectively. The kinetic parameters were estimated using nonlinear least squares analysis, as described previously. A typical inhibition curve is shown in **Fig. 3**.

3.2. Uptake Experiments Using PepT1 Transiently Transfected CHO Cells

The methods described below outline (1) transfection of CHO cells with PepT1 cDNA and (2) vacv uptake studies using transfected CHO cells.

3.2.1. Transfection of CHO Cells

1. Prepare the pcDNA3 vector using PepT1 cDNAs.
2. One day before transfection, trypsinize and count the cells, plating them in 24-well plates at 1×10^5 cells per well. Cells are seeded in 0.5 mL of DMEM medium containing 10% FBS (*see* **Note 6**).
3. For each well of cells to be transfected, dilute 0.8 µg of PepT1 cDNA into 50 µL of Opti-MEM I medium. Dilute 1.5 µL of lipofectamine reagent into 50 µL of Opti-MEM I medium and incubate for 5 min. The diluted lipofectamine reagent

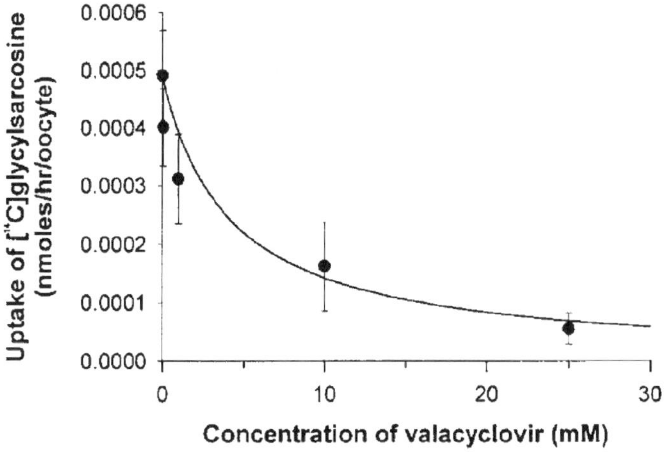

Fig. 3. Inhibition of glyclysarcosine uptake by vacv. The uptake of 0.02 m*M* glycylsarcosine was measured at room temperature in the presence of various concentrations of vacv. The reported uptake rate was calculated by subtracting the uptake rate in water-injected oocytes from PepT1-injected oocytes. Each point represents the mean ± SEM of 6–10 oocytes.

should be combined with DNA within 30 min. Longer incubation may decrease the transfection activity. This dilution can be prepared in bulk for multiple wells.

4. Combine the diluted PepT1 cDNA with diluted lipofectamine and incubate at room temperature for 20 min to let the PepT1/lipofectamine complex form.
5. Remove the cell growth medium from the wells, and wash the cells with 1X PBS twice. Add 0.5 mL of Opti-MEM I medium to each well. Then add 100 µL of the PepT1/lipofectamine complex directly to one well. For the mock-transfected cells that are used as a control, add 100 µL of the pcDNA3/lipofectamine complex to one well (*see* **Note 7**).
6. Incubate the cells at 37°C in a CO_2 incubator for 5 h, and then remove the complex and replace the medium with 0.5 mL of normal growth medium.

3.2.2. Uptake of vacv Using PepT1-Transfected CHO Cells

The uptake procedures, such as time-course, concentration dependence, and inhibition studies, are similar to those described for the cRNA-injected oocytes. Therefore, these will not be described again, and the reader is referred to the previous sections. In this section, only the time dependence of vacv uptake is described.

1. PepT1 or mock-transfected cells were used for uptake studies 24 h after the initiation of transfection.

2. Prepare the test compound. vacv was diluted in Hank's balanced salt solution (HBSS) as a concentration of 20 m*M* spiked with [^{3}H]vacv.
3. The cells are then washed with 37°C HBSS three times.
4. The uptake is initiated by adding 0.5 mL of 20 m*M* vacv to each well.
5. The uptake is stopped at the indicated time points (1, 3, 5, 10, and 30 min) by the immediate removal of the drug solutions.
6. Wash the cells three times by using ice-cold HBSS (*see* **Note 8**).
7. After washing, add 200 µL of 0.2 *N* NaOH solution and lyse the cells by pipetting up and down several times.
8. Add 200 µL of 0.2 *N* HCl to each well to neutralize the cell lysate.
9. Put 350 mL of the cell lysate into each scintillation count vial, add 4 mL of scintillation fluid, and vortex. Measure the radioactivity using the scintillation counter.
10. Take 20 µL of the cell lysate and measure the protein concentration using the BCA protein assay reagent.
11. Normalize the vacv uptake in each well to the protein concentration, and express the uptake as vacv pmol/mg protein.

4. Notes

1. Depending on the quality of oocytes, the DMSO concentration can be as high as 5%.
2. Sometimes, the oocytes cannot freely roll in the well; in that case, the plate can be coated by Barth's media overnight before culturing oocytes.
3. This is a radioactive solution, so an appropriate safety procedure should be used.
4. Try to transfer only one drop of buffer that includes the oocytes.
5. The oocytes have to be lysed completely until no obvious cell debris can be observed.
6. An equal amount of cells should be seeded across the wells.
7. The preparation of the pcDNA3/lipofectamine complex is similar to the PepT1/ lipofecatime complex described in **steps 3** and **4**.
8. This is a radioactive solution, so an appropriate safety procedure should be used.

References

1. Balimane, P. V., Tamai, I., Guo, A., Nakanishi, T., Kitada, H., Leibach, F. H., Tsuji, A., and Sinko, P. J. (1998) Direct evidence for peptide transporter (PepT1)-mediated uptake of a nonpeptide prodrug, valacyclovir. *Biochem. Biophys. Res. Commun.* **250,** 246–251.
2. Guo, A., Hu, P., Balimane, P. V., Leibach, F. H., and Sinko, P. J. (1999) Interactions of a nonpeptidic drug, valacyclovir, with the human intestinal peptide transporter (hPEPT1) expressed in a mammalian cell line. *J. Pharmacol. Exp. Ther.* **289,** 448–454.

8

Plasma Protein-Binding Methods in Drug Discovery

Lucinda H. Cohen

Summary

This chapter focuses on the three most widely used in vitro protein binding techniques in pharmaceutical research, which each reflect a diversity of speed, data quality, and complexity. Chromatographic separation using a human serum albumin-immobilized column to allow relative ranking by percent binding is described. Also, 96-well ultrafiltration, perhaps the most widely used in the pharmaceutical industry is discussed. Ultrafiltration allows automation and rapid determinations for multiple compounds in a batch. However, the quality of data from this technique is notoriously dependent on the extent of nonspecific binding of the analyte to the plastic housing or ultrafiltration membrane surface. In addition, 96-well equilibrium dialysis, long considered the definitive or "gold-standard" means of protein binding determinations, is described. Commercial devices have only recently been introduced to allow automation of this technique in a 96-well format.

Key Words: Plasma protein binding; equilibrium dialysis; ultrafiltration; ADME screening.

1. Introduction

The use of in vitro absorption, distribution, metabolism, and excretion (ADME) tools offers the exciting prospect of better understanding a new chemical entity's (NCE's) mechanism of action while potentially reducing costly attrition during drug development. Over the past two decades, enormous investment and interest has blossomed in high-throughput ADME screens for permeability and metabolic stability, liability, and drug–drug interaction potential. From a hierarchical perspective, in vitro methods of plasma protein binding for NCEs are less preferred and less frequently used than other ADME

From: *Methods in Pharmacology and Toxicology*
Optimization in Drug Discovery: In Vitro Methods
Edited by: Z. Yan and G. W. Caldwell © Humana Press Inc., Totowa, NJ

screens. However, plasma protein-binding experiments advance our understanding of ADME properties to aid in candidate selection and development by determining the unbound drug blood concentrations as well as (potentially) drug concentration at the site of action. Unbound drug levels should also be closely related to the pharmacological effects of a compound as the principal determinant of tissue distribution, cell entry, receptor interactions, and availability for elimination. Plasma protein binding may contribute to a wide variety of phenomena such as drug–drug interaction potential, nonlinear or stereoselective pharmacokinetics, or interindividual variability. Therefore, the potential exists to identify and differentiate drug candidates based on plasma protein binding values ***(1,2)***. Ideally, plasma protein-binding data help guide both structure-activity relationships and promising chemical series' mechanism of action against a specific target.

Prior to the past 5 yr, a significant stumbling block of plasma protein-binding methods has been lack of automation. Plasma protein binding is traditionally performed by equilibrium dialysis during drug development using ^{14}C-labeled compounds. The timing of these experiments is largely determined by the effort and expense to obtain radiolabeled material. In addition, traditional methods consume a significant amount of material, are very labor-intensive, and not easily automated. Significant effort has been invested to search for high-throughput screening methods that reliably and accurately determine protein binding in early drug discovery. Possible techniques include biosensors ***(3,4)***, turbulent flow chromatography ***(5)***, 96-well fluorescence plate readers ***(6)***, 96-well equilibrium dialysis ***(7,8)***, capillary electrophoresis, 96-well ultrafiltration, and high-performance liquid chromatography (HPLC) using a column containing immobilized plasma proteins ***(9–12)***. **Table 1** describes the relative advantages, issues, and equipment requirements for the most commonly used in vitro plasma protein-binding techniques.

The 96-well fluorescence approach relies on the detection of intrinsic fluorescence of the tryptophan resides of human serum albumin (HSA) and α-glycoprotein (α-GP), the primary plasma protein constituents. As drugs bind to the protein, the fluorescence signal is quenched as a function of analyte concentration. The analyte's dissociation constant, K_D, can then be calculated. Although this method is readily automated, its universality is questionable because tryptophan residues reflect only a portion of the potential binding sites to both α-GP and HSA.

Another high-throughput technique for plasma protein binding uses the Biacore™ surface plasmon resonance (SPR) technology to determine both percent binding and dissociation constants. The rigor of the experiments can be tailored to the users' needs, with more rapid methods providing comparative data to known compounds to allow low, medium, or high percent binding rank-

Table 1
Comparison of In Vitro Methods for Protein Binding

Technique	Advantages	Issues	Equipment required
Chromatographic methods (HSA, α-GP columns)	Easy setup; low cost; relatively low sample consumption; minimal hands-on preparation or intervention	Binning/relative ranking not absolute percent binding	HPLC with detector (UV, radiometric, mass spectrometric, or circular dichroism)
96-Well fluorescence	Rapid; automated; easy setup; K_D	Monitoring binding only to tryptophan residue of HSA and α-GP; may miss other binding interactions	Fluorescence plate reader
Biosensor	Semiautomated; percent binding and K_D	Higher time commitment for setup; more sample needed; skilled operator	Biacore; albumin and α-GP biosensor chips
96-Well ultrafiltration	Percent binding; commercially available plates; automated	Nonspecific binding; must correct for volume shifts; not true equilibrium experiment	Millipore 96-well device; centrifuge; HPLC with detector (UV, radiometric, mass spectrometric, or circular dichroism)
96-Well equilibrium dialysis	Percent binding; automated; "gold standard"; flexible	May require long equilibration times; long-term plasma stability of analyte at 37°C may be problematic; devices not widely available	96-Well equilibrium device; HPLC with detector (UV, radiometric, mass spectrometric, or circular dichroism)

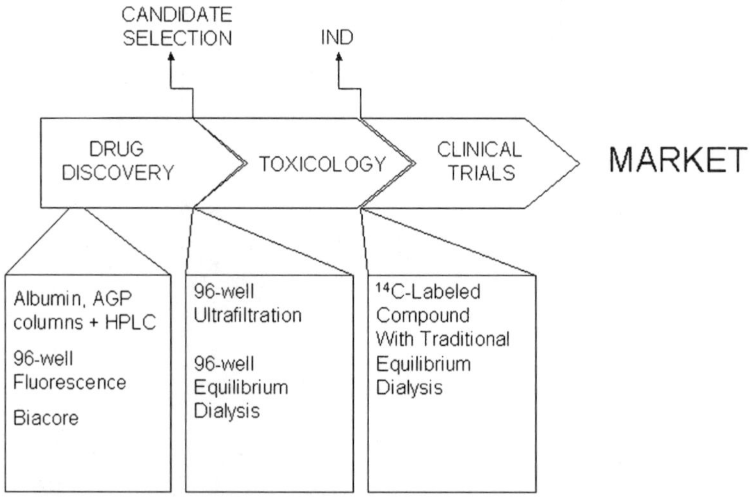

Fig. 1. Conduct of plasma protein-binding experiments during drug discovery and development.

ing. This "binning" process can swiftly be applied to large numbers and classes of compounds for evaluation purposes. When additional rigor is desired and sufficient compound is available, definitive K_D constants can be obtained. The need to purchase Biacore™ SPR instrumentation, as well as instrument and chip synthesis proficiency, can be potential limitations.

The purpose of this chapter is to focus on the three most widely used in vitro protein-binding techniques in pharmaceutical research, which each reflect a diversity of speed, data quality, and complexity. First, chromatographic separation using an HSA-immobilized column to allow relative ranking of percent binding will be described. Next, 96-well ultrafiltration, perhaps the most widely used in industry, will be discussed. Ultrafiltration allows automation and rapid determination for multiple compounds in a batch. However, the quality of data from this technique is notoriously dependent on the extent of nonspecific binding of the analyte to the plastic housing or ultrafiltration membrane surface. Third, 96-well equilibrium dialysis, long considered the definitive or "gold-standard" means of protein-binding determinations, will be described. Commercial devices have only recently been introduced to allow automation in a 96-well format.

The normal timings of the previously discussed techniques are shown in **Fig. 1**. Early in drug discovery, rapid screening techniques that allow binning into low, medium, and high binding categories are used. As a given NCE progresses forward in the drug discovery process and more of it is synthesized, more definitive approaches such as ultrafiltration and equilibrium dialysis are

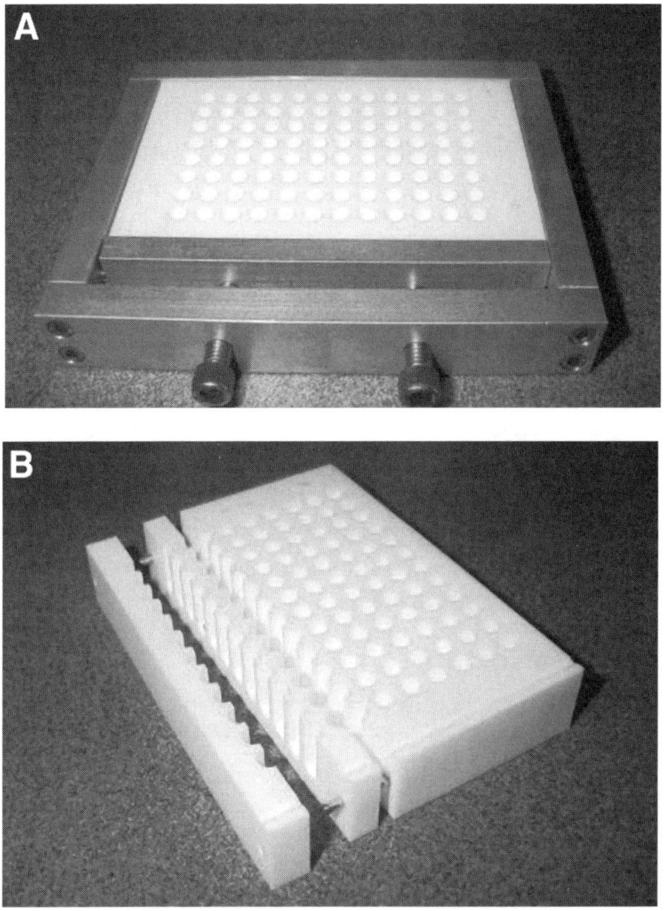

Fig. 2. 96-Well equilibrium dialysis apparatus. Reprinted with permission from Banker, M. J., Clark, T. H., and Williams, J. A. (2003) *J. Pharm. Sci.* **92,** 967–974. Copyright 2003 John Wiley & Sons.

applied. Once an NCE's likelihood of success seems greater, traditional equilibrium dialysis using radiometric detection is usually performed. This experiment is considered sufficiently rigorous to permit its inclusion in regulatory submissions. However, as 96-well techniques are validated, the need for the final low-throughput "definitive" radiometric experiment is becoming less and less compelling. Two different views of a recently described 96-well device are shown in **Fig. 2A** (front) and **2B** (side). In this apparatus, eight dialysis membranes are vertically mounted between Teflon spacers that comprise the individual wells. As a result of the vertical design, 96-well liquid-handling devices can be used for automated buffer and plasma transfers. The 96-well

Dispo-Equilibrium Dialyzer proposed by Kariv et al. *(8)* uses a single horizontally mounted dialysis membrane.

Recently, the clinical relevance of plasma protein binding has been challenged by Benet and Hoener *(13)*, who demonstrated through careful study that protein binding is relevant primarily for iv-administered drugs with a high extraction ratio, as well as oral drugs with a high extraction ratio and a nonhepatic clearance mechanism. Examination of data for 456 currently marketed drugs showed that protein binding influenced exposure for 25, which fell into the two categories described previously. If the therapeutic index is considered, protein-binding influences even fewer compounds. However, the clear need for protein binding in the discovery and preclinical development stages to conduct allometric scaling and understand species-different behavior is well understood. Protein-binding behavior of a drug candidate may not be in and of itself decision making but has a profound influence on a variety of in vivo and in vitro properties during ADME experiments. Thus, its determination early in drug discovery can provide significant input into understanding tissue distribution, mechanism of action, and potentially the much desired drug concentrations at the pharmacological site of action.

2. Reagents and Method

Analysis equipment for all three methods: high-performance liquid chromatography (HPLC) system, containing pump, autosampler, and detector (UV-Vis or mass spectrometric) from numerous vendors, including Waters, Agilent, AB/Sciex, Perkin-Elmer, and Shimadzu.

2.1. Chromatographic Methods

1. 37°C Temperature-regulating jacket or column heater: may be integral to HPLC or purchased separately.
2. 4.6 × 50-mm HSA column (Hypersil, Runcorn, UK).
3. Mobile phase: potassium phosphate dibasic–potassium phosphate monobasic buffer (50 m*M*, pH 7.4), modified with 5% (v/v) *n*-propanol (UV detection) or 94% 50 m*M* ammonium acetate, pH 7.4, and 6% *n*-propanol (mass-spectrometric detection). The mobile phases should be filtered (0.45 μm) and degassed with helium prior to use.
4. Injection volume: 10 μL.
5. Flow rate: 0.8 mL/min.

2.2. Ultrafiltration

1. 96-Well device: Microcon YM-10 for 10,000 Daton molecular weight cutoff (Millipore, Billerica, MA).
2. 37°C Centrifuge: capable of 3000*g* at fixed-angle rotation.
3. pH meter.

4. 37°C Water bath for plasma stability experiment.
5. Blank plasma in desired species, which is also used to generate blank ultrafiltrate for analytical standard preparation.

2.3. Equilibrium Dialysis

1. Dialysis Membrane (Spectra/Por) membranes: typical pore sizes for protein-binding studies are 12,000 to 14,000 mol wt cutoff.
2. 96-Well device such as 96-well Dispo-Equilibrium Dialyzer (Harvard Apparatus, Holliston, MA).
3. Phosphate-buffered saline (PBS), pH 7.4.
4. Blank plasma in desired species.
5. 37°C Water bath.

3. Experimental Procedures

3.1. Chromatographic methods Using Human Serum Albumin and α-Glycoprotein Columns

1. A series of compounds with known plasma protein-binding values should be chromatographically analyzed using an HSA column. The recommended analyte concentration is 5 μg/mL. In addition, an α-GP column may be used in serial or parallel. The degree of plasma protein binding can either be found in the literature ***(14,15)*** or obtained by comparative ultrafiltration or equilibrium dialysis methods.
2. The capacity factor (k') of each compound is calculated based on its retention time, using the following formula:

$$k = \frac{t_r - t_m}{t_m}$$

   where t_r is the retention time of the analyte, and t_m is the retention time of an unretained compound, also known as the column void volume. t_m can be assessed using glucose, cesium iodide, or ammonium nitrate. From the k' values, ($k'/k'+1$) is calculated.
3. As shown in **Fig. 3**, ($k'/k'+ 1$) is plotted as a function of the known plasma protein binding. After the correlation plot is generated, the plasma protein binding of unknown compounds can be calculated based on their retention time on the albumin or α-GP column. In general, the factor $k'/k'+ 1$, rather than k', shows better linear correlation with plasma protein-binding values. As shown in the figure, compounds can be binned into low-, medium-, and high-protein binding categories to aid in screening.

3.2. 96-Well Ultrafiltration

The overall workflow process for 96-well ultrafiltration and equilibrium dialysis is shown in **Fig. 4**.

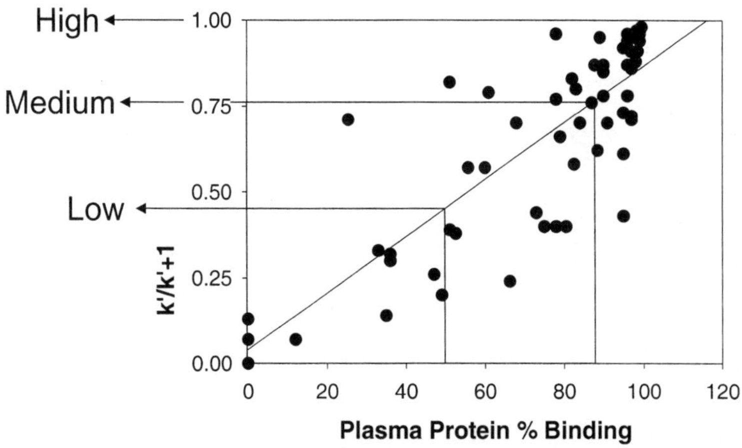

Fig. 3. Binning of low, medium, and high binding by chromatographic retention.

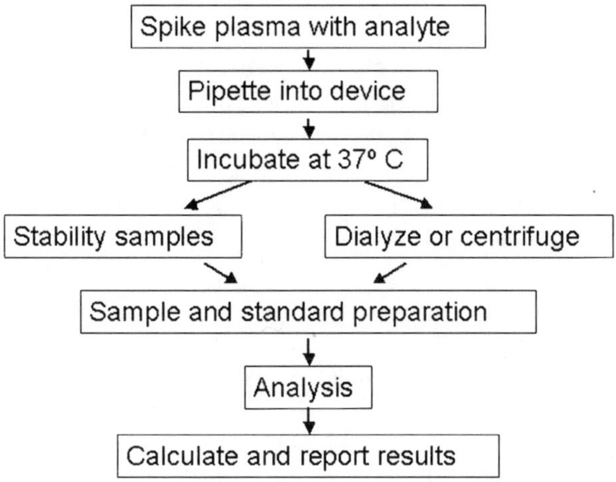

Fig. 4. Process flow for 96-well equilibrium dialysis or ultrafiltration.

1. The pH of plasma samples must be checked after the plasma has thawed. Adjust to pH 7.4 ± 0.1 by bubbling CO_2 gas through the plasma to lower the pH or by vigorous shaking to raise the pH.
2. Pipet 250 µL of analyte-spiked plasma (5 µg/mL recommended concentration) into each well. Three replicates for each plasma type and analyte are recommended. Usually, at least human plasma and plasma from one preclinical species, such as rat, are determined. Spiked ultrafiltrate may be used to assess nonspecific binding.

3. Spin the plate in a fixed-angle rotation at 37°C centrifuge for approx 1–4 h. Use the maximum allowable speed for centrifuge to obtain enough volume of ultrafiltrate in a reasonable time frame.
4. Simultaneously incubate spiked plasma at 37°C for the duration of the ultrafiltration experiment to assess plasma stability. Compare the determined concentration of initial and incubated plasma stability samples to determine if the analyte (NCE) is stable at 37°C over the course of the experiment. Usually no more than a 20% decrease in concentration is considered acceptable for plasma stability.
5. Prepare calibration standards for an appropriate dynamic range in the desired blank matrix, such as ultrafiltrate and plasma.
6. Analyze the samples and standards using an appropriate method such as liquid chromatography/tandem mass spectrometry (LC/MS/MS).
7. Calculate the percent bound using the following formula:

$$\textit{Percent bound} = \left(1 - \frac{[\textit{Post-centrifuged spiked plasma}]}{[\textit{Post-centrifuged ultrafiltrate}]}\right) \times 100$$

3.3. 96-Well Equilibrium Dialysis

1. Soak the membrane strips in buffer solution for at least 30 min prior to the experiment.
2. With an appropriate single-channel or multichannel pipet, add 150 to 200 µL of buffer solution to one side of the membrane in each well and an equal volume of analyte-spiked plasma (recommended concentration 5 µg/mL) to the other side.
3. Cover the plate with adhesive sealing film to prevent evaporation.
4. Incubate the device in a horizontally rotating 37°C incubator for the required equilibrium time (typically 2, 4, 6, or 24 h).
5. At the end of incubation, transfer 100 µL from the buffer and plasma halves of the dialysis cells into a sample container.
6. Prepare calibration standards for an appropriate dynamic range in the desired blank matrix, such as buffer and plasma.
7. Analyze the samples and standards using an appropriate method such as LC/MS/MS.
8. The analyte free fraction at the end of the incubation period is calculated using the following equation. This equation assumes that error added as a result of a volume shift is within the error of the assay method and therefore negligible. As a result of the small size of the 96-well apparatus, potential error is minimized.

$$f_u = \frac{C_{buffer}}{C_{plasma}}$$

where C_{buffer} is the unbound compound concentration in buffer after dialysis, and C_{plasma} is the postdialysis plasma concentration. The percentages of drug unbound (free) and bound to protein are calculated as follows:

$$\% \text{ Free} = f_u \cdot 100 \qquad \% \text{ Bound} = (1 - f_u) \cdot 100$$

4. Notes

1. HSA and α-GP columns should be used without exposure to acetonitrile, which can cause stationary phase collapse. The immobilized α-GP column is reputedly not as predictive or representative of in vivo plasma protein-binding behavior as its HSA counterpart ***(16,17)***.
2. The choice of which preclinical species to examine should be dictated by the purpose of the protein-binding experiment, such as pharmacokinetic calculations or allometric scaling.
3. The 96-well equilibrium dialysis or ultrafiltration studies should be designed such that protein binding is evaluated over an anticipated therapeutically and/or toxicologically relevant concentration range for the compound of interest. In addition, these methods can be used to investigate individual binding proteins (i.e., human serum albumin and α_1-acid glycoprotein [α-GP], preclinical species' albumin).
4. Plasma harvested using ethylenediaminetetraacetic acid (EDTA) as an anticoagulant is recommended. Frozen plasma can be used for these studies. Concerns have been raised that the anticoagulant heparin may interfere with protein binding, and it should thus be avoided. During preparation of initial analyte-spiked plasma, maintain minimal organic content (<2% by volume). Spiking using a larger percentage of organic solvents such as dimethylsulfoxide (DMSO) can adversely interfere with protein binding.
5. The stability of the compound in all species and matrices, including buffer solutions, should be assessed over the time period used for equilibration. This is accomplished by incubating an aliquot of the matrix standard and spiked buffer at the lowest concentration under the same conditions as the equilibrium dialysis apparatus. Samples taken at time zero and at the end of experiment should be assessed to determine percent analyte remaining.
6. A potential problem and source of high variability with equilibrium dialysis is protein breakthrough from the protein-rich plasma side to the aqueous side of the dialysis cell, causing false elevation in the buffer compound concentrations. This can be monitored by taking an aliquot of any remaining buffer, adding acetonitrile to precipitate the protein, and checking the solution for visible particulates. Use of a membrane with an appropriate molecular weight cutoff (10 kDa minimum) will help prevent this problem.
7. During equilibrium dialysis, an equilibration time of 24 h is recommended for the sake of efficiency. However, scientific judgment can be used to reduce this time to 4, 6, or 8 h.
8. Analytes can be lost during equilibrium dialysis by nonspecific binding to the membrane and apparatus, by decomposition of the compound, or as a result of solubility issues. Assessment of this loss can be performed in a separate experiment or during determination of equilibration time. To assess nonspecific compound loss, pre- and postdialysis plasma and buffer concentrations are measured in each half of the cell. These measurements are used to calculate the amount of drug lost by comparing the amount of drug added to the dialysis system to the amount recovered at the end of the experiment.

References

1. Oravcova, J., Boehs, B., and Lindner, W. (1996) Drug-protein binding studies: new trends in analytical and experimental methodology. *J. Chromatogr. B* **677,** 1–28.
2. Vallner, J. J. (1977) Binding of drugs by albumin and plasma protein. *J. Pharm. Sci.* **66,** 447–465.
3. Danelian, E., Karlen, A., Karlsson, R., Winiwarter, S., Hansson, A., Lofas, S. et al. (2000) SPR biosensor studies of the direct interaction between 27 drugs and a liposome surface: correlation with fraction absorbed in humans. *J. Med. Chem.* **43,** 2083–2086.
4. Frostell-Karlsson, A., Remaeus, A., Roos, H., Andersson, K., Borg, P., Hamalainen, M., et al. (2000) Biosensor analysis of the interaction between immobilized human serum albumin and drug compounds for prediction of human serum albumin binding levels. *J. Med. Chem.* **43,** 1986–1992.
5. Yang, E., Kartz, J., McSurdy-Freed, J., and Spooner, N. (1999) The study of drug-plasma protein binding by turbulent flow LC/MS and its application in screening mode. Paper presented at the national meeting of the American Association of Pharmaceutical Scientists.
6. Parikh, H. H., McElwain, K., Balasubramanian, V., Leung, W., Wong, D., Morris, M. E., et al. (2000) A rapid spectrofluorimetric technique for determining drug-serum protein binding suitable for high-throughput screening. *Pharm. Res.* **17(5),** 632–637.
7. Banker, M. J., Clark, T. H., and Williams, J. A. (2003) Development and Validation of a 96-well equilibrium dialysis apparatus for measuring plasma protein binding. *J. Pharm. Sci.* **92,** 967–974.
8. Kariv, I., Cao, H., and Oldenburg, K. R. (2001) Development of a high throughput equilibrium dialysis method. *J. Pharm. Sci.* **90,** 580–587.
9. Tiller, P. R., Mutton, I. M., Lane, S. J., and Bevan, C. D. (1995) Immobilized human serum albumin: liquid chromatography/mass spectrometry as a method of determining drug-protein binding. *Rapid Commun. Mass. Spectrom.* **9,** 261–263.
10. Noctor, T. A. G., Diaz-Perez, M. J., and Wainer, I. W. (1993) Use of a human serum albumin-based stationary phase for high-performance liquid chromatography as a tool for the rapid determination of drug-plasma protein binding. *J. Pharm. Sci.* **82,** 675–676.
11. Buchholz, L., Cai, C. H., Andress, L., Cleton, A., Brodfuehrer, J., and Cohen, L. (2002) Evaluation of the human serum albumin column as a discovery screening tool for plasma protein binding. *Eur. J. Pharm. Sci.* **15,** 209–215.
12. Beaudry, F., Coutu, M., and Brown, N. K. (1999) Determination of drug-plasma protein binding using human serum albumin chromatographic column and multiple linear regression model. *Biomed. Chromatogr.* **13,** 401–406.
13. Benet, L. Z. and Hoener, B. (2002) Changes in plasma protein binding have little clinical relevance. *Clin. Pharm. Ther.* **71,** 115–121.
14. Obach, R. S. (1999) Prediction of human clearance of twenty-nine drugs from hepatic microsomal intrinsic clearance data: an examination of in vitro half-life approach and nonspecific binding to microsomes. *Drug Metab. Disp.* **27,** 1350–1359.

15. Gilman, A. G., Goodman, L. S., Rall, T. W., and Murad, F., eds. (1996) *The Pharmacological Basis of Therapeutics*, 7th ed. Macmillan, New York.
16. Jewell, R. C., Brouwer, K. L. R., and McNamara, P. J. (1989) α_1-Acid glycoprotein high-performance liquid chromatography column (Enantiopac) as a screening tool for protein binding. *J. Chromatogr.* **487,** 257–264.
17. Schill, G., Wainer, I. W., and Barkan, S. A. (1986) Chiral separations of cationic and anionic drugs on an α_1-acid glycoprotein-bonded stationary phase (Enantiopac®): II. Influence of mobile phase additives and pH on chiral resolution and retention. *J. Chromatogr.* **365,** 73–88.

9

Isothermal Titration Calorimetry Characterization of Drug-Binding Energetics to Blood Proteins

Gary W. Caldwell and Zhengyin Yan

Summary

Techniques such as calorimetry, spectroscopy, and hydrodynamic methods can be used to investigate the binding energetics of drugs bound to macromolecules. In this chapter, the authors describe the use of isothermal titration calorimetry (ITC) to measure the binding energetics of drugs bound to blood proteins (i.e., human serum albumin [HSA] and α-acid glycoprotein [AGP]). The stoichiometry (n), the association-binding constant (K_a), and the enthalpy (ΔH^0) of binding can be rapidly, directly, and precisely measured using ITC. Because the free energy (ΔG^0) and the entropy (ΔS^0) are readily calculated from K_a and ΔH^0, a complete thermodynamic characterization of binding can be acquired in a single experiment.

Key Words: Isothermal titration calorimetry; protein binding.

1. Introduction

The binding of drugs to various blood proteins and tissues can significantly influence the pharmacokinetics of drugs and, therefore, the pharmacodynamic and toxicologic action of drugs *(1)*. For example, the extent of drug–protein binding may contribute to effects such as the volume of distribution of a drug and its interindividual variability. Drugs that are highly bound to blood proteins have a smaller volume of distributions compared to drugs with low binding to blood proteins. Drugs with high tissue affinities may also accumulate in lipid or adipose tissue. Premature displacement of drugs from blood proteins or tissues by other drugs or endogenous compounds may result in an increase in free drug in the systemic system that may diffuse to pharmacologic receptor sites, thus causing an unexpected intense or unwanted drug response. This situ-

From: *Methods in Pharmacology and Toxicology*
Optimization in Drug Discovery: In Vitro Methods
Edited by: Z. Yan and G. W. Caldwell © Humana Press Inc., Totowa, NJ

ation is particularly relevant for drugs with high extraction ratios and nonhepatic clearance mechanisms *(2)*. In addition, formation of reactive metabolites of drugs that irreversibly bind to proteins or tissues may cause certain types of toxicity *(3)*. Therefore, an understanding of the binding characteristics of drugs and metabolites to blood proteins, such as human serum albumin (HSA), α-acid glycoprotein (AGP), lipoproteins, and immunoglobulins, and to tissues such as lipid or adipose is useful information in the design and administration of therapeutic drugs. The energetics of drugs binding to both blood proteins and tissues can be studied by in vivo and in vitro methods. Here, we concentrate on drugs binding to blood proteins, using calorimetry methods.

Three types of in vitro methodologies can be used to investigate the binding energetics of drugs bound to macromolecules *(4)*. These methods can be broadly classified as calorimetry, spectroscopy, and hydrodynamic techniques. Calorimetry methods include isothermal titration *(5)* and differential scanning *(6)*. Spectroscopy methods include techniques such as optical and absorption (e.g., fluorescence) spectroscopy *(7)*, nuclear magnetic resonance *(8)*, electron spin resonance *(9)*, optical rotatory dispersion and difference circular dichroism *(10)*, and surface plasmon resonance *(11)*. The advantage of calorimetry and spectroscopy methods is that they allow the thermodynamics and/or kinetics of the interaction between drug molecules and macromolecules to be determined accurately, as well as the topography of the binding site to be investigated. Hydrodynamic methods are typically separation techniques such as equilibrium dialysis *(12)*, ultracentrifugation *(13)*, ultrafiltration *(14)*, gel filtration *(15)*, size-exclusion chromatography *(16)*, and capillary electrophoresis *(17)*. With these methods, the free drug, the free protein, and the bound drug–protein complex under equilibrium conditions are physically separated from each other, and the corresponding concentration of each is measured. Once the free (or bound) drug concentration is determined, the percent binding can be calculated. Other thermodynamic parameters can be determined by varying the concentrations of the drug or protein or the temperature of the system. The reliability of these methods depends on the accuracy of the free drug (or bound) concentration determination under equilibrium conditions.

Many in vitro methods are used to measure the binding energetics of drugs binding to blood proteins. In the present work, step-by-step experimental details are discussed on the use of isothermal titration calorimetry (ITC). ITC is powerful tool for the characterization of the thermodynamics and kinetics of drugs binding to macromolecules *(5,6,18,19)*. Substantial improvement in ITC instrumentation has occurred over the past two decades, and several easy-to-use commercial instruments are available. In most experiments, the rate of heat flow induced by changing the composition of a macromolecule solution by titration of a compound (or vice versa) is measured. These heat effects can be used to rapidly, directly, and precisely measure the stoichiometry (n), the association-binding constant (K_a), and the enthalpy (ΔH^0) of binding. The free energy (ΔG^0) and the entropy (ΔS^0) are readily calculated from K_a and ΔH^0. Thus, a complete thermodynamic characterization of binding can be acquired in a single experiment.

1.1. Terminology and Definitions of the Thermodynamics of Binding

Drug–protein complexes $[DP]$ are formed when drug molecules $[D]$ interact and bind to blood proteins $[P]$. This binding phenomenon is modeled in reaction **1**.

$$[D] + [P] = [DP] \tag{1}$$

The binding process can be classified as either irreversible or reversible. Irreversible drug–protein binding occurs when covalent bonds are formed between the drug and the protein or when the binding affinity between the drug and protein is so strong ($>10^{12}M^{-1}$) that the complex does not fall apart. For irreversible binding, no thermodynamic information can be obtained. Reversible drug–protein binding occurs when the drug binds to the protein with weak chemical bonds such as hydrogen bonds or van der Waals forces. Most drugs interact with blood proteins by a reversible process, and this binding event can be described by thermodynamic parameters such as the association binding constants (K_a) and the enthalpy (ΔH^0) of binding. For the reversible case, the free drug $[D]$, the free protein $[P]$, and the bound drug $[DP]$ in reaction **1** eventually come to equilibrium. Under equilibrium conditions, the concentrations of all chemical species are constant. It should be noted that equilibrium is a dynamic condition and not a static condition; that is, the concentrations of the chemical species are constant because the rate of association between the drug and the protein forming the bound complex $[PD]$ is equal to the rate of disassociation of $[PD]$ not because all activity has ceased. Using reaction **1** and assuming that this reaction is under equilibrium conditions, the association constant K_a is defined as the ratio of the bound drug to the free drug and protein concentrations.

$$K_a = \frac{[DP]}{[D][P]}. \tag{2}$$

If the chemical species are measured in moles per liter (M), then K_a has units of M^{-1}. The degree of drug–protein binding is controlled by the magnitude of K_a. In other words, if K_a is large ($>10^9$), the drug–protein complex is the dominant chemical species in the reaction. If K_a is small (10^3), then significant concentrations of all chemical species are present in the reaction mixture. The disassociation constant (K_d) of reaction **1** is simply the inverse of K_a (i.e., $K_d = 1/K_a$). The association constant K_a (or K_d) can be also related to the free energy (ΔG^0) using **Eq. 3**.

$$\Delta G^0 = -RT \ln K_a \tag{3}$$

In **Eq. 3**, R (1.986 cal/mol/K or 8.313 J/mol/K) is the gas constant, T is the absolute temperature expressed in Kelvin (K = °C ± 273.16), and K_a is the association constant in M^{-1} units. Note that to take the natural logarithm of any number, the number must be dimensionless. To create a dimensionless number, we simply divide K_a (M^{-1}) by a standard state concentration of 1 M^{-1}. The normalization procedure chosen here is not unique and can be accomplished by other means ***(20)***. The free energy can be dissected into enthalpy (ΔH^0) and entropy (ΔS^0) components using **Eq. 4**.

$$\Delta G^0 = \Delta H^0 - T\Delta S^0 \tag{4}$$

The interpretation of **Eq. 4** is not complicated. If ΔG^0 is negative, the reaction is spontaneous; that is, it releases energy (exergonic). If ΔG^0 is positive, the reaction is nonspontaneous; that is, it absorbs energy (endergonic). The energy we are referring to here is the amount of heat released or absorbed for reaction **1**. The most favorable circumstance for ΔG^0 to be negative is when ΔH^0 is negative and ΔS^0 is positive. When chemical bonds are broken, heat is released ($-\Delta H^0$). It requires heat ($+\Delta H^0$) to form chemical bonds. Therefore, the observed enthalpy (ΔH^0) for reaction **1** is a function of all the heats of formation of molecular bonds being formed or broken. The entropy (ΔS^0) is interpreted as a measure of the randomness or disorder of the reaction. Because a disordered state is more statistically probable than an ordered one, ΔS^0 is regarded as a probability function. If the reaction becomes more ordered when chemical bonds are created or broken, entropy becomes less probable ($-\Delta S^0$). If the reaction becomes less ordered when chemical bonds are created or broken, entropy becomes more probable ($+\Delta S^0$). Thus, **Eq. 4** simply represents the balance for chemical species in reactions to seek a minimum energy ($-\Delta H^0$) and a maximum randomness ($+\Delta S^0$). The heat capacity (ΔCp) of a reaction predicts the change of ΔH^0 and ΔS^0 with temperature. The heat capacity can be expressed as

$$\Delta C_p = \frac{\Delta H^{\circ}_{T2} - \Delta H^{\circ}_{T1}}{T_2 - T_1} \tag{5}$$

or

$$\Delta C_p = \frac{\Delta S^{\circ}_{T2} - \Delta S^{\circ}_{T1}}{\ln\left(\frac{T_2}{T_1}\right)} \tag{6}$$

The subscript p in **Eqs. 5** and **6** denotes that the system is at constant pressure. In some cases, ΔH^0 and ΔS^0 will be constant over some particular temperature range and $\Delta Cp = 0$. In other cases, ΔH^0 and ΔS^0 may change as the temperature of the reaction changes and $\Delta C_p \neq 0$. It is known that if ΔC_p is negative, then hydrophobic bonds are formed. If ΔC_p is positive, then hydrophobic bonds are broken. The value ΔC_p is itself temperature dependent in some cases, and this may complicate the interpretation of ΔC_p. Because there is no way to predict this temperature dependence, ΔC_p is usually determined to examine the change of ΔH^0 and ΔS^0 with temperature.

Protein macromolecules may have a single binding site or several binding sites. In addition, binding sites may accommodate a single drug molecule or more than one drug molecule. Thus, another important parameter is the stoichiometry or binding capacity number (n). The binding capacity number gives information on the different types of binding sites and the capacity of each in the protein. Typically, we assume that each binding site is independent, and thus each site has a unique n, K_a, and ΔH^0. In other words, if a drug (or drugs) binds at one site of a protein, it does not influence the binding characteristics at other sites. This independent site approximation is used to simplify the analysis and interpretation of the raw data. In reality, there is cooperativity in binding; therefore, binding at one site influences the successive binding of other drug molecules at other sites *(1)*. Therefore, some caution is warranted in the overinterpretation of these results. Binding sites are commonly referred to as being high affinity (large K_a) with a low capacity ($n = 1$) or as being low affinity (small K_a) with a high capacity ($n > 1$) or vice versa.

1.2. Terminology and Definitions for Human Blood

After introduction into the portal circulation system, most drugs can bind to various constituents such as blood proteins and tissues. Binding competition typically occurs between drugs bound to tissues and blood proteins. Drugs that are very lipophilic tend to be highly fat soluble and thus tend to accumulate in lipid or adipose (fat) tissue. Human blood consists of three major systems. The first system is the formed elements (i.e., erythrocytes, leukocytes, and blood platelets), the second is an aqueous portion, and the third is large amounts of various salts. The major cell body in the blood are the erythrocytes (i.e., red blood cells), which comprise approx 95% of the total cellular fraction in the blood. Four major components in the erythrocytes are capable of binding drugs—hemoglobin, carbonic anhydrase, and the cell membrane. If blood is allowed to naturally coagulate, a clear straw-colored fluid (i.e., serum) can be separated from the cellular fraction by centrifugation. In contrast, plasma is obtained by centrifugation of blood to which an anticoagulant was added immediately after removal from the body. Thus, serum contains water (90%–92%), all blood proteins (6%–8%), and various salts (e.g., 0.1 *M* NaCl), whereas plasma samples contain water, proteins minus the clotting factors, and salts. The approximate concentrations of proteins in serum (or plasma) are

Table 1
Properties of Selected Human Serum (or Plasma) Proteins

Fraction	Protein	Molecular weight (Daltons)	Amounts in normal serum (g/L)	Typical concentration (m*M*)
	Prealbumin61,000	0.28–0.35	5	
	Albumin (HSA)	69,000	35–45	580
α_1	Antitrypsin45,000	2.1–4.0	68	
	High-density lipoproteins	435,000	0.37–1.17	2
	α_1-Acid44,100 glycoprotein (AGP)	0.75–1.0	20	
α_2	α_2HS-Glycoprotein haptoglobin	49,000	0.30–0.90	12
	Type 1-1100,000	1.0–2.2	16	
	Type 2-1, 2-2	100,000	1.2–2.6	19
β_1	Low-density lipoproteins	3.2×10^6	2.8–4.4	1
γ	Globulins	$150{,}000–10^6$	7–15	11–73

listed in **Table 1** *(21)*. The concentration of various serum proteins can vary from person to person, as well as from day to day, by as much as 10% of the average value.

HSA, AGP, the high-density lipoproteins (HDL), and the low-density lipoproteins (LDL) are the more important proteins responsible for the binding of drugs in serum or plasma. HSA represents approx 73% of the total proteins, whereas AGP is 3%, HDL is 0.3%, and LDL is 0.1%. HSA is largely responsible for serum binding of acidic and neutral drugs, whereas AGP and lipoproteins bind mainly basic drugs. HSA is a single polypeptide chain containing 585 amino acid residues that is greatly stabilized by 17 disulfide bonds. HSA consists of three different albumin proteins (i.e., albumin, pre- and postalbumin) that differ in their amount of carbohydration. Albumin has at least six classes of high-specificity binding sites and an even larger number of low-affinity binding sites based on competitive binding results *(22)*. Of these, two major binding areas on albumin have been extensively investigated—namely, the warfarin site (I) that primarily interacts with cumarins, salicylates, and pyrazolidines and the indole site (II) that specifically binds benzodiazepines, arylpropionates, and L-tryptophan.

AGP is composed of a single polypeptide chain and five carbohydrate moieties. The polypeptide chain consists of 183 amino acid residues and two disulfide bonds *(23)*. The five carbohydrate moieties are located in the first half of the polypeptide chain and are linked to asparagine residues. The carbohydrate moieties consist of approx 11% sialic acid, 14% neutral hexoses, 14% hexosamine, and 1% fructose. The unusually low isoelectric point of 2.7 is caused by the high sialic acid content. From the results of drug displacement studies, it has been concluded that AGP has primarily one major specific binding site and several low-affinity binding sites.

Compared to HSA and AGP, very little is known about the binding sites of lipoproteins. There are three major groups of lipoproteins: very low-density lipoproteins (VLDL), LDL, and HDL. VLDL is the major carrier for triglycerides, whereas in LDL and HDL, cholesterol is the predominant lipid. Serum lipoproteins have distinct structural domains with which drugs can interact. These spherical pseudomicellar complexes (i.e., chylomicrons) have a hydrophobic core region surrounded by a phospholipid monolayer. Lipoprotein binding is generally considered a nonsaturable and reversible phenomenon. Little information concerning the number and types of binding sites is known about the other proteins listed in **Table 1**.

2. Isothermal Titration Calorimetry (ITC)

2.1. Instrumentation

The basic principle of ITC is simply to measure the heat released or absorbed in a liquid sample after the addition of another liquid sample. This heat is proportional to the total amount of binding that occurs within the calorimeter cell. The instrument has a pair of identical cells (1.4 mL), denoted as the reference and sample cells (**Fig. 1**). These cells, along with access stems, are enclosed in a temperature-controlled thermal jacket. The reference and sample cells (and stems) are filled with identical protein solutions. The injector syringe is filled with a known concentration of a drug and placed into the sample cell. Solutions injected into the sample cell are rapidly mixed using a stirring paddle that is attached to the syringe. After the addition of the drug solution to the protein solution, the temperature difference between the sample cell and the reference cell is measured. For our particular instrument (VP-ITC, Microcal, Inc.) the temperature difference is calibrated to power units (μcal/sec or μJ/s). This power is applied back (or restricted) to the sample cell so that the temperature between the sample cell and the reference cell remains the same. The power (or heat) difference between the sample and reference cells is used to determine n, K_a, and ΔH^0.

2.2. ITC Determination of n, K_a, *and* ΔH^0

The accuracy of the measured thermodynamic parameters (i.e., n, K_a, and ΔH^0) depends on correct experimental design and analysis. Experiments can be designed to measure all three parameters in a single experiment, or they can

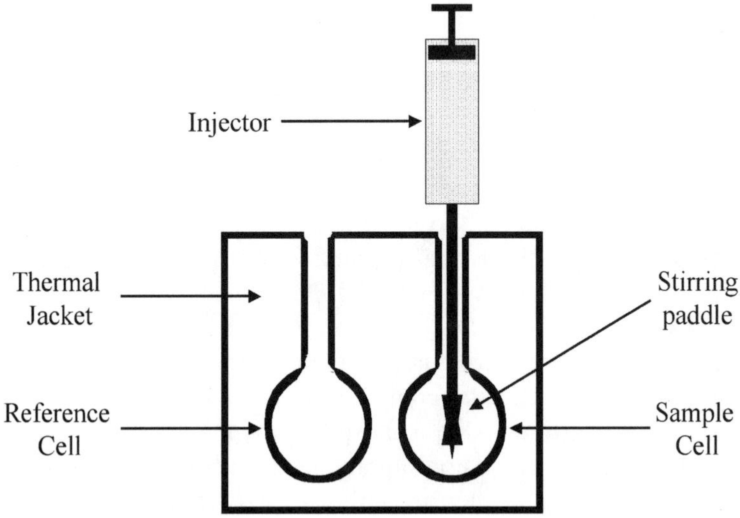

Fig. 1. Isothermal titration calorimeter.

be designed to measure them individually. Typically, the experiment is initiated by setting the thermal jacket to a known and constant temperature (i.e., isothermal). A precise amount of a drug solution is injected (i.e., titrated) into the sample cell (i.e., calorimeter) that contains a known protein concentration. The heat difference is measured, and the data are analyzed. It is important to remember that the correct choice of injection times and drug and protein concentrations is imperative for determining accurate parameters. In addition, the matrix (solution or buffer system) in the injector, the reference cell, and the sample cell must be nearly identical to eliminate heats of mixing effects. Establishing these conditions will be discussed in the next section.

An example of an ITC experiment is shown in **Fig. 2A** to illustrate raw data collection. The power required in maintaining the parity between the sample and reference cell for an exothermic binding reaction is measured for each injection. The initial injection of drug results in the binding of most of the drug molecules to the protein. This initial injection therefore requires the greatest power compensation and thus generates the greatest amount of heat. On subsequent injections of drug, there is less protein available for binding and, therefore, less heat of binding is generated. After approx 20 injections of drug, all the sites on the proteins are bound with drug molecules, and no further heat of binding is observed. The remaining heat generated at this point is as a result of the heat of diluting the drug solution into the protein solution. Typically, the drug concentration in the injector is at least 10 times more concentrated than in the sample cell. By integrating these deflections with respect to time and cor-

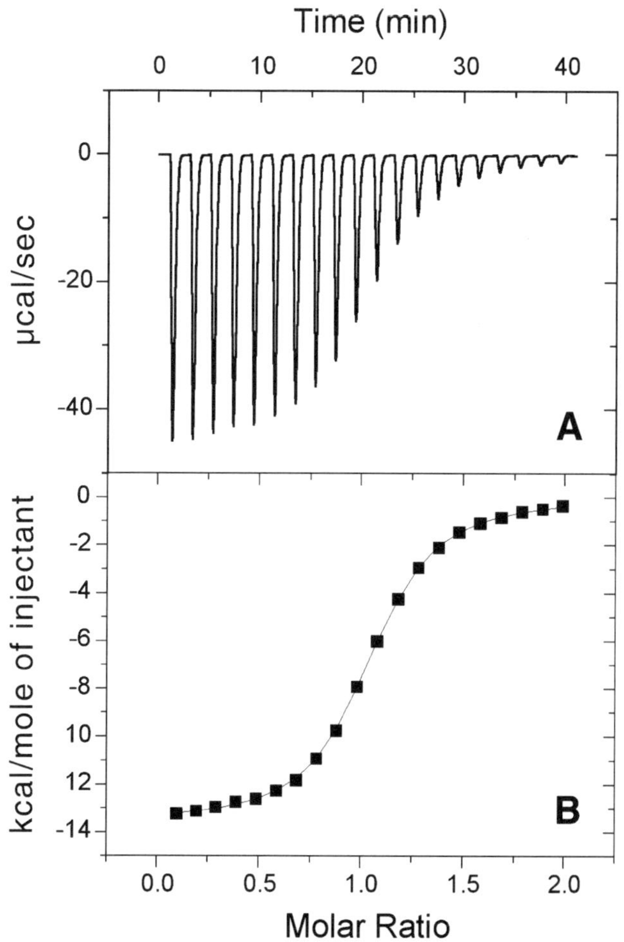

Fig. 2. Raw (**A**) and integrated (**B**) data from an ITC experiment.

recting for the heat of dilution, the heat of binding per injection (kcal/mol/injection) is calculated and plotted against the molar ratio of the drug to protein (**Fig. 2B**). The association constant (K_a) is related to the shape of the curve, and the binding capacity (n) is determined from the ratio of the drug to protein at the equivalence point of the curve. The enthalpy (ΔH^0) for the reaction is approximately the intercept at a zero molar ratio. To extract thermodynamic data from this plot (**Fig. 2B**), we must fit the data to a binding model. More on binding site model selection is given in the next section. For this particular example using a single binding site model, $\Delta H^0 = -13.6$ kcal/mol, $K_a = 5543\ M^{-1}$ ($K_d = 180\ \mu M$), and $n = 1$.

2.3. ITC Analysis of the Raw Data

It should be recognized that the data generated in **Fig. 2B** and the thermodynamic data (n, K_a, and ΔH^0) derived from these data are actually apparent (or observed) values because the measured heat of binding per injection can arise from any linked equilibria *(24)*. In other words, it is the total heat released or absorbed in the sample cell on each addition of the drug. The heat released or absorbed may arise from other sources other than the binding of the drug to the protein (reaction **1**). For drug-blood protein studies, these additional sources of heat are summarized as follows:

$$\Delta H^0 \approx \Delta H_{bind} + \Delta H_{dilution} + \Delta H_{matrix} + \Delta H_{ion} \qquad (7)$$

where ΔH_{bind} denotes the heat of binding of the drug to the protein (i.e., the parameter we are interested in measuring), $\Delta H_{dilution}$ represents the heat of dilution of the drug into the matrix of the protein, ΔH_{matrix} arises from mixing the drug and protein matrixes, and ΔH_{ion} denotes a change in pH in the sample cell upon addition of drug. By setting up the experiment under correct conditions, some of these enthalpies (ΔH_{matrix} and ΔH_{ion}) can be eliminated or diminished such that they can be neglected. For example, if the drug and the protein solutions are prepared in the same buffering solution, then ΔH_{matrix} and ΔH_{ion} will be approximately zero. For $\Delta H_{dilution}$, it must be measured in a separate experiment or approximated using the last few heat of binding per injection data points (**Fig. 2B**) and then subtracted from ΔH^0 to determine ΔH_{bind}. This procedure will become clear in the next few sections.

Once the binding data are corrected for contributions arising from nonspecific enthalpies, a model is chosen to fit the data such that the parameters—n, K_a, and ΔH^0—can be determined. To do this correctly, one must know the type of binding that is generating the heat of binding per injection (**Fig. 2B**). This molecular binding information is typically obtained from other experimental techniques. The fact that this information must be obtained from other sources is a serious disadvantage of the ITC technique. Fortunately, many drug–protein binding interactions in isolated systems are described reasonably well using a single binding site model. For experiments that use HSA, we will use a single or a two-binding site independent model; for AGP, a single-binding site model will be used.

3. Single and Multiple Independent-Binding Site Models for Fitting ITC-Binding Data

After the raw ITC has been corrected for nonspecific heat contribution, the data are fitted to a binding model. The simplest model is a single site model. If we define the quantity r as the moles of drug bound per mole of total protein and use the association constant definition $[PD] = K_a [P] [D]$ from **Eq. 2**, then

$$r = \frac{\text{moles drug bound}}{\text{total moles protein}} = \frac{[PD]}{[P] + [PD]} = \frac{K_a[P][D]}{[P] + K_a [P][D]} = \frac{K_a[D]}{1 + K_a[D]} \tag{8}$$

Therefore, the quantity r is the fraction of sites occupied by the drug (D) with an association constant K_a. Rearranging **Eq. 8** leads to **Eq. 9**.

$$K_a = \frac{r}{(1 - \mathrm{r})\,[D]} \tag{9}$$

The total concentration of drug $[D]_T$ is also known and can be represented by **Eq. 10**, in which $[P]_T$ represents the total concentration of protein and n denotes the capacity number.

$$[D]_T = [D] + nr[P]_T \tag{10}$$

It is clear from **Eq. 10** that $nr[P]_T = [PD]$. Combining **Eqs. 9** and **10** gives quadratic **Eq. 11**:

$$r^2 - r\left[\frac{[D]_T}{n[P]_T} + \frac{1}{nK_a[P]_T} + 1\right] + \frac{[D]_T}{n[P]_T} = 0 \tag{11}$$

Solving **Eq. 11** for r leads to **Eq. 12**:

$$r = \frac{1}{2}\left[\left(\frac{[D]_T}{n[P]_T} + \frac{1}{n[K]_a[P]_T} + 1\right) - \sqrt{\left(\frac{[D]_T}{n[P]_T} + \frac{1}{n[K]_a[P]_T}\right)^2 - \frac{4\,[D]_T}{n[P]_T}}\,\right] \tag{12}$$

The total heat content (Q) contained in the sample cell at volume (V) can be defined as

$$Q = nr[P]_T\,\Delta H^0 V \tag{13}$$

where ΔH^0 is the heat of binding of the drug to the protein, and $nr[P]_T = [PD]$. Substituting **Eq. 12** into **Eq. 13** gives the following equation:

$$Q = \frac{n[P]_T\,\Delta H^0 V}{2}\left[\left(\frac{[D]_T}{n[P]_T} + \frac{1}{n[K]_a\,[P]_T} + 1\right) - \sqrt{\left(\frac{[D]_T}{n[P]_T} + \frac{1}{n[K]_a\,[P]_T} + 1\right)^2 - \frac{4\,[D]_T}{n[P]_T}}\,\right] \tag{14}$$

Therefore, the total heat content (Q) in the sample cell is a function of n, K_a, and ΔH^0 because $[P]_T$, $[D]_T$, and V are known for each experiment.

The heat content measured in **Fig. 2B** represents the change in heat content with the injection of a known volume of drug solution into the sample cell containing a known volume of protein solution (V). Therefore, after completing the injection of drug, the volume of the sample cell changes by a known amount (ΔV_i). The change in the heat content is defined by **Eq. 15**.

$$\Delta Q(i) = Q(i) + \frac{\Delta V_i}{V}\left[\frac{Q(i) + Q(i-1)}{2}\right] - Q(i-1) \tag{15}$$

Fitting the raw data in **Fig. 2B** to **Eq. 15** involves the following steps:

1. Input the starting drug and protein concentrations ($[D]_T$ and $[P]_T$).
2. Input the initial volume of the sample cell (V).
3. Guess the initial values of n, K_a, and ΔH^0 and calculate Q.
4. Calculate $\Delta Q(i)$ for all injections and compare to experimental data.
5. Change the values of n, K_a, and ΔH^0 and recalculate $\Delta Q(i)$.
6. Repeat **steps 2–4** until there is no significant improvement in the fit between calculated and experimental results.

For two independent sites, **Eq. 8** can be rewritten as a linear combination of these sites:

$$r_1 + r_2 = \frac{K_{a1}[D]}{1 + K_{a1}[D]} + \frac{K_{a2}[D]}{1 + K_{a2}[D]} \tag{16}$$

The total concentration of drug $[D]_T$ is rewritten as

$$[D]_T = [D] + (n_1 r_1 + n_2 r_2)[P]_T \tag{17}$$

Eq. 17 can be inserted into **Eq. 16** to yield a cubic equation. The same procedure is followed as outlined above, except in this case, the cubic equation has to be solved numerically.

4. Materials

4.1. Instrument

1. VP-ITC MicroCalorimeter (MicroCal, Inc., Northampton, MA).
2. Origin Analysis Software (Origin Lab., Northampton, MA).
3. Hewlett Packard 8453 UV/vis spectrophotometer (HP, CA).
4. Benchtop pH Meter Corning Model 245 (VWR, NJ).

4.2. Chemicals

1. Barium chloride dihydrate, 99%, cat. no. B-6394 (Sigma, St. Louis, MO).
2. 1,4,7,10,13,16-Hexaoxacyclooctadecane (18-Crown-6), 99%, cat. no. C-5515 (Sigma, St. Louis, MO).
3. Cytidine 2'-monophosphate (2'CMP), 98%, cat. no. C-7137 (Sigma, St. Louis, MO).
4. Ribonuclease A from bovine pancreas (RNase A), 90%, cat. no. R-5500 (Sigma, St. Louis, MO).
5. (±)Propranolol hydrochloride, 99%, cat. no. P-0884 (Sigma, St. Louis, MO).
6. AGP, 99%, purified from Cohn Fraction VI, cat. no. G-9885 (Sigma, St. Louis, MO).
7. 3-(α-Acetonylbenzyl)-4-hydroxycoumarin (warfarin), 98%, cat. no. A-2250 (Sigma, St. Louis, MO).
8. HSA, 99%, lyophilized powder essentially fatty acid free, cat. no. A-3782 (Sigma, St. Louis, MO).

4.3. Reagents

1. Purified water (less than 5 ppb total organics and 18 Mohms/cm electrical resistance) (Millipore Milli-Q Gradient System, Bedford, MA).
2. Phosphate-buffered saline without calcium or magnesium (PBS; pH 7.4) (Mediatech Cellgro, VA): 8 g NaCl (58.44 g/mol); 0.2 g KH_2PO_4 (136.1 g/mol); 2.8 g of Na_2HPO_4 $7H_2O$ (268.1 g/mol); 0.2 g of KCl (74.55 g/mol). Dissolve in purified water to 1 L.
3. 0.2 *M* KCl and 0.2 *M* CH_3COOK buffer (acetate buffer, pH 5.5): 14.9 g of KCl (74.55 g/mol); 19.6 g of CH_3COOK (98.14 g/mol). Dissolve in purified water to 1 L adjusted with HCl.

4.4. Equipment

3500 MWCO dialysis tubing (VWR, NJ).

5. Calibrations

Calorimeters can be calibrated electrically or chemically. Electric calibrations are simple and fast. Briefly, an electric heater is positioned near or on the sample cell. Over a known period of time, a precise quantity of heat is released from the electric heater, and the amount of heat required maintaining an isothermal system is measured. The procedure is repeated several times using different amounts of heat, and the results are recorded. Action can be taken if serious deviations from the norm are observed. Chemical calibrations are used to calibrate ITC instruments or to examine systematic errors with a system that is closely related to the chemical process that is under investigation ***(25,26)***. The ITC technique is vulnerable to systematic errors such as unidentified chemical side reactions, evaporation during degassing, and condensation of protein or drug at high concentrations. Therefore, attempts should be made to minimize these errors. In this case, we are interested in chemical binding processes. Two common binding studies can be used to establish confidence in using an ITC system (barium chloride/18-crown-6 and 2'-CMP/RNase A). Although these systems are not universally accepted as calibration procedures for binding phenomena, they are easy to analyze and have been measured many times in the literature.

5.1. Barium Chloride and 18-Crown-6 Ether

The following equilibrium is established upon the addition of barium chloride to 18-crown-6 ether in water. We will now determine *n*, *Ka*, and ΔH^0.

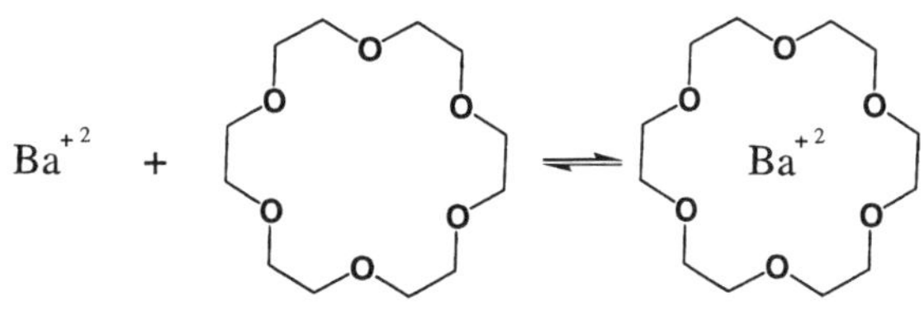

(18)

5.1.1. Preparation of Samples

$BaCL_2$ $2H_2O$: 244.3 g/mol. A 0.1 *M* stock solution was prepared by weighting out 488.6 mg and dissolving it into 20 mL of purified water. This stock solution was used for several days. The 10-mL working solution (0.03 *M*) was prepared by pipetting 3 mL of the 0.1 *M* stock solution and adding it to 7 mL of purified water. This 0.03 *M* solution of $BaCL_2$ was degassed and loaded into a 300-µL injection syringe.

18-Crown-6: 264.3 g/mol. A 0.01 *M* stock solution was prepared by weighting out 105.72 mg and dissolving it into 40 mL of purified water. This stock solution was used for several days. The 50-mL working solution (0.002 *M*) was prepared by pipetting 10 mL of the 0.01 *M* stock solution and adding it to 40 mL of purified water. This 0.002 *M* solution of 18-crown-6 was degassed and loaded into the reference and sample cells (i.e., approx 4 mL total).

5.1.2. Data Collection

The following experimental parameters were set:

Number of injections:	49
Run temperature:	25°C
Reference power:	30 mcal/s
Initial delay:	300 s
Syringe concentration:	30 m*M*
Cell concentration:	2 m*M*
Stirring speed:	300 rpm
Injection volume:	3 mL
Duration:	2 s
Spacing:	200 s
Filter period:	2 s

Because the reference and sample cells contain the same matrix—in this case, water—the heat of solvent mixing (ΔH_{matrix}) that arises from mismatched solvents is zero. Because there is no pH dependence for this reaction system, the heat of ionization (ΔH_{ion}) will be zero. Thus, the observed heat of interaction (ΔH^0) is

$$\Delta H^0 \approx \Delta H_{bind} + \Delta H_{dilution} \tag{19}$$

where ΔH_{bind} denotes the heat of binding of Ba^{+2} to 18-crown-6 (i.e., the parameter we are interested in measuring), and $\Delta H_{dilution}$ represents the heat of dilution of $BaCL_2$ into water. To obtain ΔH_{bind}, we must subtract $\Delta H_{dilution}$ from ΔH^0.

$$\Delta H_{bind} \approx \Delta H^0 - \Delta H_{dilution} \tag{20}$$

Therefore, we must measure $\Delta H_{dilution}$ in a separate experiment or approximate it using the last few heat of binding data points where the reaction

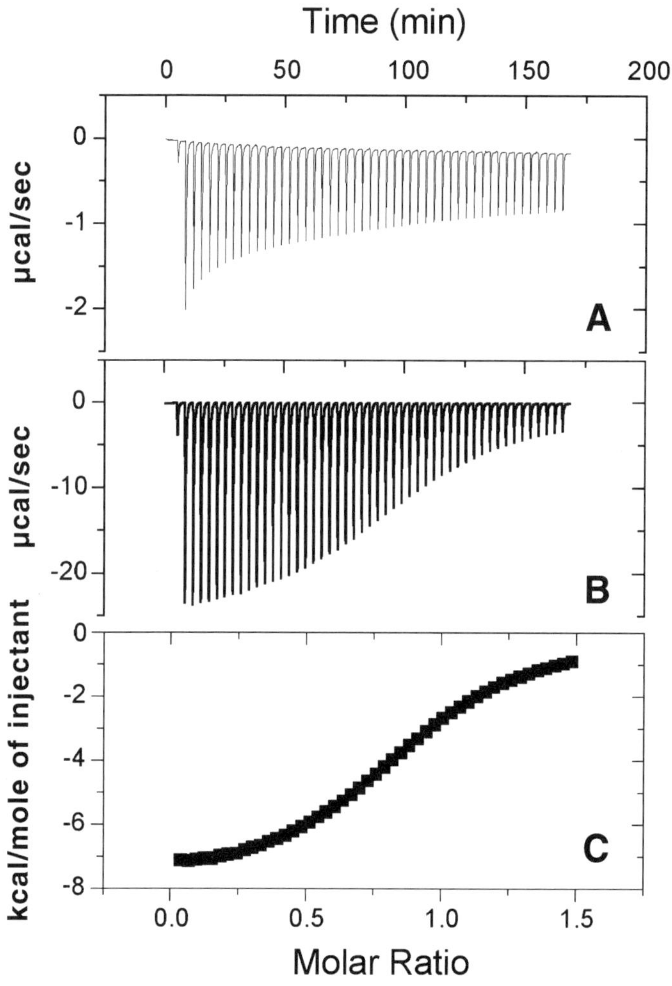

Fig. 3. The results obtained from $BaCL_2$ (0.03 *M* in 3-μL injections) and 18-crown-6 (0.002 *M* in the sample cell) at 25°C (298 K) in H_2O as the solvent. (**A**) Raw data of $BaCL_2$ injected into H_2O. (**B**) Raw data of $BaCL_2$ injected into 18-crown-6. (**C**) After subtracting **B** – **C**, enthalpy data are fitted with a single binding site model. For this particular example, $\Delta H^0 = -7.87 \pm 0.01$ kcal/mol, $K_a = 6194 \pm 62\ M^{-1}$ (161 μ*M*), and $n = 0.9032 \pm 0.0011$.

has become saturated. In **Fig. 3A**, we have measured the heat of dilution for $BaCL_2$ (30 m*M*) being mixed into water. The experiment resulted in producing a maximum power of approx –2 μcal/s. When $BaCL_2$ (30 m*M*) was mixed with a solution of 18-crown-6 (2 m*M*), the experiment resulted in producing a maximum power of approx –24 μcal/s (**Fig. 3B**). These two data sets were inte-

Table 2
Thermodynamic Data for the Binding of $BaCL_2$ to 18-Crown-6

Reference	ΔG^0 (kcal/mol)	ΔH^0 (kcal/mol)	ΔS^0 (cal/mol/K)	K_a (M^{-1})	ΔC_p (cal/mol/K)	Temperature (°C)
27	–5.3	–7.58 ± 0.01	–7.9	7413 ± 1		25
28	–5.0			4800		
29	–5.14 ± 0.02	–7.51 ± 0.05	–7.9	5900 ± 200	30.1	25
30	–5.1	–7.51 ± 0.01	–8.2	5140 ± 40	33.3	25
24	–5.1	–8.0 ± 0.1	–9.9	5100 ± 750	30.3 ± 2.4	25
Average	–5.1	–7.7	–8.4	5671	31.2	25
Standard deviation	0.1	0.2	1.0	1055	1.8	
%CV	2	3	12	19	6	
Figure 3	–5.2	–7.9	–9.2	6194	32	25

grated and subtracted, which resulted in the binding curve shown in **Fig. 3C**. Using **Eq. 14**, the best fit for n, K_a, and ΔH^0 was determined, and the results are shown in **Fig. 3** and **Table 2**.

By repeating the experiment at a different temperature, ΔC_p can be calculated using **Eq. 5**. The results obtained from $BaCL_2$ (0.03 M in 3-µL injections) and 18-crown-6 (0.002 M in the sample cell) at 37°C (310 K) in H_2O was $\Delta H^0 = -7.49 \pm 0.01$ kcal/mol, $K_a = 3767 \pm 65\ M^{-1}$ (265 µM), and $n = 0.9884 \pm 0.0032$. Therefore, ΔC_p equals approx 32 cal/mol/K:

$$\Delta C_p = \frac{\Delta H^0_{T2} - \Delta H^0_{T1}}{T_2 - T_1} = \frac{-7490 + 7870}{310 - 298} = 31.7 \text{ cal / mol / K} \qquad (21)$$

Depending on the experiment, the ITC system may require a few minutes or up to an hour to equilibrate. During this equilibration time, the $BaCL_2$ solution contained in the syringe can diffuse into the sample cell. Thus, the first injection may not be accurate. To correct for this situation, the first injection is typically set to 1 µL, and this data point is then discarded during data fitting.

5.1.3. Data Analysis

The $BaCL_2$/18-crown-6 equilibrium has been measured many times by several different groups. In **Table 2**, the literature data for this reaction are given along with the average value, standard deviation, and the coefficient of variation (%CV) for each thermodynamic parameter. Note that our data in **Fig. 3** are in agreement with the average data.

5.2. 2'CMP and RNase A

Bovine pancreatic ribonuclease A (RNase A) is a 124-residue protein (enzyme) that contains four interweaving disulfide bonds (Cys-26-Cys-84, Cys-40-Cys-95, Cys-58-Cys-110, and Cys-65-Cys-72). Based on its amino acid sequence, its molecular weight is 13,699 g/mol ***(31)***. This digestive enzyme mediates the hydrolysis (acid and base) of ribonucleic acid (RNA) to its component nucleotides. This digestive reaction exhibits a pH profile in which the

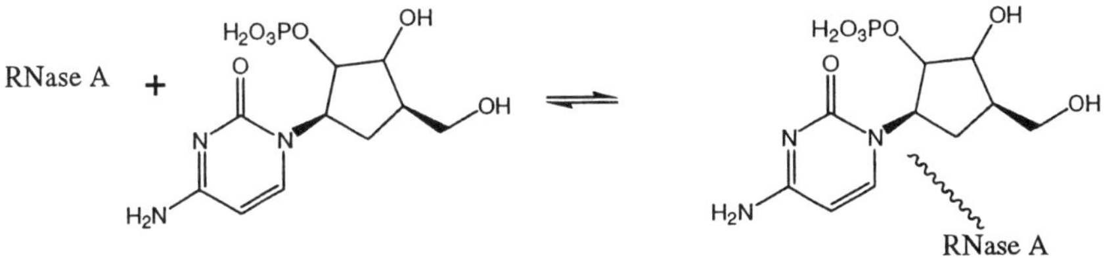

(22)

maximum rate of hydrolysis occurs near pH 6.0. It has been determined that His-12 and His-119 are the main amino acids (one acting as a proton acceptor and the other as a proton donor) responsible for its digestive properties ***(32)***. The binding of the nucleotide cytidine 2'-monophosphate (2'-CMP) to RNase A has been extensively studied by calorimetry. Depending on concentrations of the drug and the protein, the temperature, the pH of the buffer, the ionic strength, and the type of salt used, the association constant can vary from 10^4 to 10^6 M^{-1}, whereas the enthalpy can range from –8 to –25 kcal/mol.

5.2.1. Preparation of Samples

2'-CMP: 323.2 g/mol. The 2'-CMP working solution was prepared from the acetate buffer. A 2.5-m*M* working solution was prepared by weighting out 16.16 mg and dissolving it into 20 mL of acetate buffer at pH 5.5. This working solution was used for several days. This 2.5-m*M* solution of 2'-CMP was degassed and loaded into a 300-μL injection syringe.

RNase A: 13,699 g/mol. The RNase A working solution was prepared from the acetate buffer. A 0.1-m*M* working solution was prepared by weighting out 27.40 mg and dissolving it into 20 mL of acetate buffer at pH 5.5. The working solution was allowed to equilibrate for 24 h at 4°C and was used for several days. This 0.1-m*M* solution of RNase A was degassed and loaded into the reference and sample cells (i.e., approx 4 mL total).

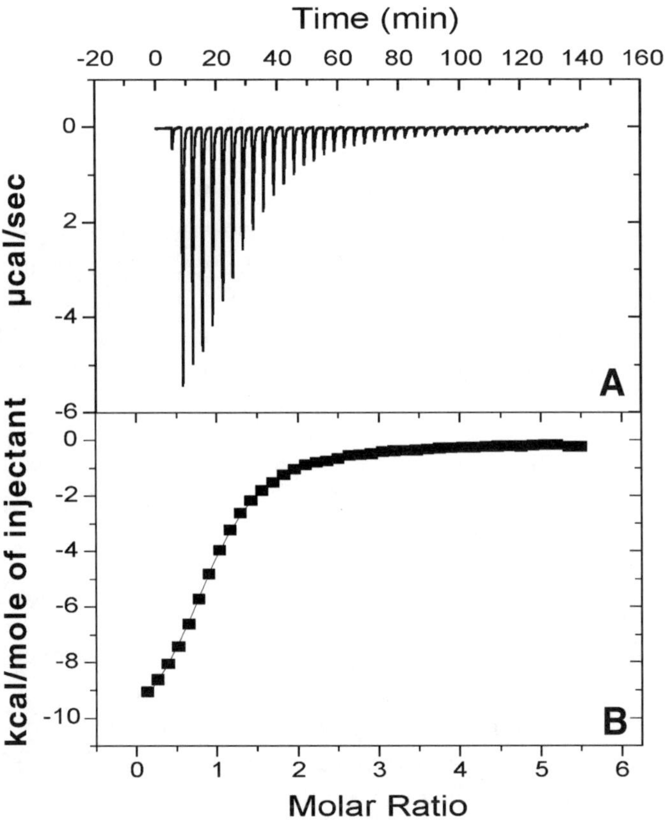

Fig. 4. The results obtained from 2'-CMP (2.57 m*M* in 7-μL injections) and RNase A (0.1 m*M* in the sample cell) at 28°C (301 K) in acetate buffer. (**A**) Raw data of 2'-CMP injected into RNase A. (**B**) After subtracting $\Delta H_{dilution}$, enthalpy data were fitted with a single binding site model. For this particular example, $\Delta H^0 = -11.48 \pm 0.15$ kcal/mol, $K_a = 50{,}470 \pm 1863\ M^{-1}$ (20 μ*M*), and $n = 0.9120 \pm 0.0088$.

5.2.2. Data Collection

The following experimental parameters were set:

Number of injections:	40
Run temperature:	25°C, 28°C, 37°C
Reference power:	30 mcal/s
Initial delay:	300 s
Syringe concentration:	2.5 m*M*
Cell concentration:	0.1 m*M*
Stirring speed:	300 rpm
Injection volume:	7 mL

Table 3
Thermodynamic Data for the Binding of 2'-CMP to RNase A

Reference	ΔG^0 (kcal/mol)	ΔH^0 (kcal/mol)	ΔS^0 (cal/mol/K)	K_a (M^{-1})	ΔC_p (cal/mol/K)	Temperature (°C)
33	–6.9	–10.67 ± 0.12	–12.7	112,000 ± 3000		25
Conditions	Buffer: 0.2 *M* KCl/0.2 *M* KAc/pH 5.5 Concentrations: 2'-CMP (0.177 m*M*) and RNase A (0.177 m*M*)					
Our data	–6.6	–10.66 ± 0.09	–13.7	65,580 ± 1905		25
34	–6.9	–12.3 ± 0.3	–18.0	98,000 ± 2200		28
Conditions	Buffer: 0.2 *M* KCl/0.2 *M* KAc/pH 5.5 Concentrations: 2'-CMP (4.2 m*M*) and RNase A (0.17 m*M*)					
Our data	–6.5	–11.48 ± 0.15	–16.6	50,470 ± 1863		28
35	–6.3	–13.7	–23.9	27,400		37
Conditions	Buffer: 0.2 *M* KCl/0.2 *M* KAc/pH 5.5 Concentrations: 2'-CMP (0.6 m*M*) and RNase A (0.6 m*M*)					
Our data	–6.4	–13.03 ± 0.15	–21.4	31,700 ± 598	–800	37

Duration:	2 s
Spacing:	200 s
Filter period:	2 s

When 2'-CMP (2.5 m*M*) was mixed with a solution of RNase A (0.1 m*M*), the experiment resulted in producing a maximum power of approx –6 μcal/s (**Fig. 4A**). The $\Delta H_{dilution}$ was approximated by using the last few heat of binding data points (–0.2 μcal/s) in which the reaction was saturated. The heat of dilution was integrated and subtracted, which resulted in the binding curve shown in **Fig. 4B**. Using **Eq. 14**, the best fit for n, K_a, and ΔH^0 were determined, and the results are shown in **Fig. 4** and **Table 3**.

5.2.3. Data Analysis

The 2'-CMP/RNase A equilibrium has been measured many times under a variety of conditions by several different groups. In **Table 3**, the literature data for this reaction are compared to our data over three different temperatures.

6. AGP

AGP is composed of 183 amino acid residues and five carbohydrate moieties *(11)*. AGP is a blood carrier protein that transports molecules throughout the body. It has one major specific binding site and favors cationic drugs over anionic drugs.

6.1. Preparation of Samples

(±)**Propranolol HCl: 295.8 g/mol**. The propranolol working solution was prepared from the PBS buffer. A 3.0-m*M* working solution by weighting out 17.75 mg and dissolving it into 20 mL of PBS buffer at pH 7.4. This working solution was used for several days. This 3.0-m*M* solution of propranolol was degassed and loaded into a 300-µL injection syringe.

AGP: 44,100 g/mol. The AGP working solution was prepared from the PBS buffer. A 0.3-m*M* working solution by weighting out 264.6 mg and dissolving it into 20 mL of PBS buffer at pH 7.4. The working solution was allowed to equilibrate for 24 h at 4°C and was used for several days. This 0.3-m*M* solution of AGP was degassed and loaded into the reference and sample cells (i.e., approx 4 mL total).

6.2. Data Collection

The following experimental parameters were set:

Number of injections:	40
Run temperature:	37°C
Reference power:	30 mcal/s
Initial delay:	300 s
Syringe concentration:	3.0 m*M*
Cell concentration:	0.3 m*M*
Stirring speed:	300 rpm
Injection volume:	5 mL
Duration:	2 s
Spacing:	200 s
Filter period:	2 s

When propranolol (3.0 m*M*) was mixed with a solution of AGP (0.3 m*M*), the experiment resulted in producing a maximum power of approx –6 µcal/s (**Fig. 5A**). The $\Delta H_{dilution}$ was measured (–0.05 kcal/mol) and subtracted from the binding curve shown in **Fig. 5B**. Using **Eq. 14**, the best fit for n, K_a, and ΔH^0 was determined, and the results are shown in **Fig. 5**.

6.3. Data Analysis

Propranolol binding to AGP has been measured several times using a variety of techniques *(17)*. The association constants range from 1×10^5 to 4×10^5 M^{-1}. As shown in **Table 4**, our data are consistent with these data.

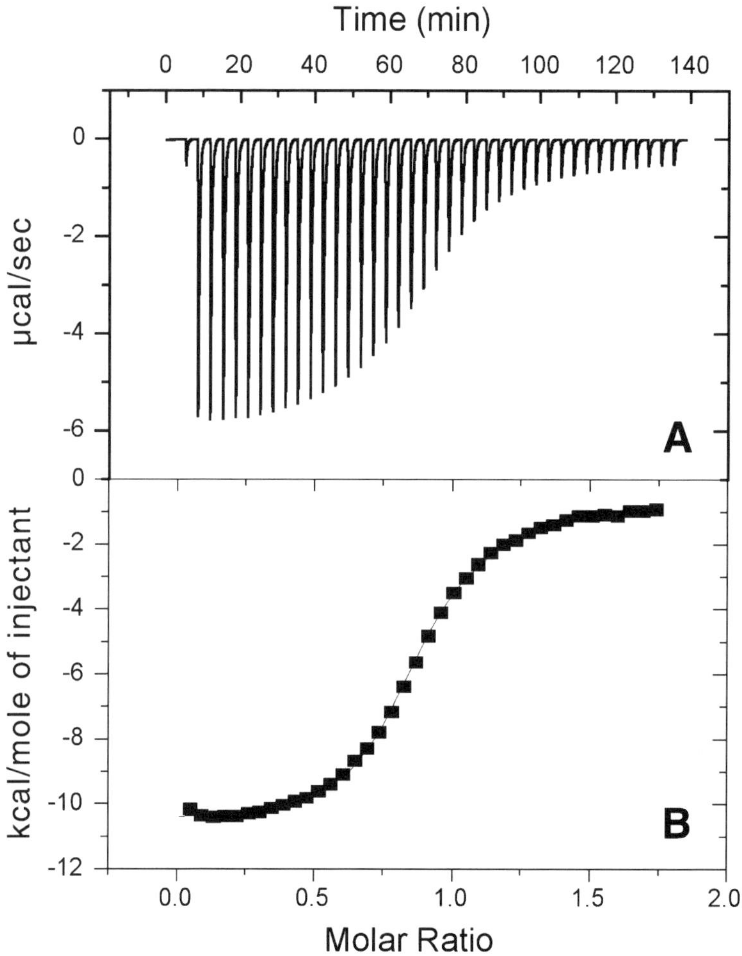

Fig. 5. The results obtained from propranolol (3.0 m*M* in 5-μL injections) and AGP (0.3 m*M* in the sample cell) at 37°C (310 K) in PBS buffer. (**A**) Raw data of propranolol injected into AGP. (**B**) After subtracting $\Delta H_{dilution}$, enthalpy data were fitted with a single binding site model. For this particular example, $\Delta H^0 = -11.10 \pm 0.12$ kcal/mol, $K_a = 110{,}400 \pm 8713\ M^{-1}$ (9 μ*M*), and $n = 0.9043 \pm 0.0071$.

7. HSA

HSA is composed of 585 amino acid residues with 17 disulfide bonds. HSA is a blood carrier protein that transports molecules throughout the body. It has two major specific binding sites and favors acidic and neutral drugs: the warfarin site (I), which primarily interacts with cumarins, salicylates, and pyrazolidines, and the indole site (II), which specifically binds benzodiazepines, arylpropionates, and L-tryptophan.

Table 4
Thermodynamic Data for the Binding of Propranolol to AGP

Reference	ΔG^0 (kcal/mol)	ΔH^0 (kcal/mol)	ΔS^0 (cal/mol/K)	K_a (M^{-1})	ΔC_p (cal/mol/K)	Temperature (°C)
Our data	–6.9	–10.10 ± 0.10	–10.8	111,900 ± 18,450		25
Our data	–7.2	–11.10 ± 0.12	–12.7	110,400 ± 8713		37

7.1. Preparation of Samples

Warfarin: 308.3 g/mol. The warfarin working solution was prepared from the PBS buffer. A 1.0-m*M* working solution was prepared by weighting out 12.34 mg and dissolving it into 40 mL of PBS buffer at pH 7.4. Vigorous shaking and heating of the solution was required to dissolve the warfarin sample. This working solution was made up fresh before each experiment. This 1.0-m*M* solution of warfarin was degassed, and the pH was checked, and the solution was loaded into a 300-μL injection syringe.

HSA: 69,000 g/mol. The HSA working solution was prepared from the PBS buffer. A 1.0-m*M* working solution was prepared by weighting out 276.0 mg and dissolving it into 40 mL of PBS buffer at pH 7.4. The working solution was allowed to equilibrate for 24 h at 4°C and was used for several days. This 0.1-m*M* solution of HSA was degassed, the pH was measured, and the solution was loaded into the reference and sample cells (i.e., approx 4 mL total).

7.2. Data Collection

The following experimental parameters were set:

Number of injections:	40
Run temperature:	37°C
Reference power:	30 mcal/s
Initial delay:	300 s
Syringe concentration:	1.0 m*M*
Cell concentration:	0.1 m*M*
Stirring speed:	300 rpm
Injection volume:	7 mL
Duration:	2 s
Spacing:	200 s
Filter period:	2 s

When warfarin (1.0 m*M*) was mixed with a solution of HSA (0.1 m*M*), the experiment resulted in producing a maximum power of approx –1.5 μcal/s

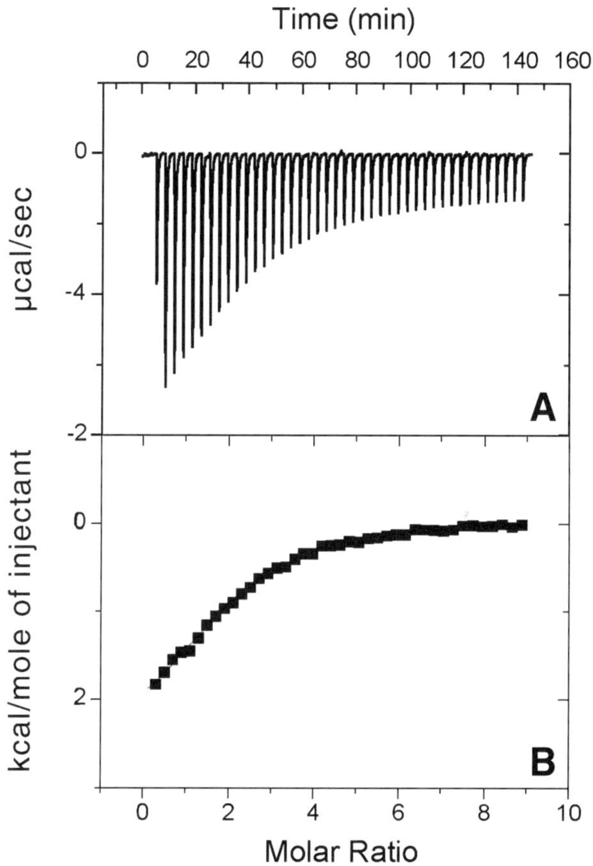

Fig. 6. The results obtained from warfarin (1.0 m*M* in 7-µL injections) and HSA (0.1 m*M* in the sample cell) at 37°C (310 K) in PBS buffer. (**A**) Raw data of warfarin injected into HSAP. (**B**) After subtracting $\Delta H_{dilution}$, enthalpy data were fitted with a single binding site model. For this particular example, $\Delta H^0 = -2.44 \pm 0.07$ kcal/mol, $K_a = 205{,}400 \pm 1369\ M^{-1}$ (5 µ*M*), and $n = 2.054 \pm 0.046$.

(**Fig. 6A**). The $\Delta H_{dilution}$ was measured (–0.3 kcal/mol) and subtracted from the binding curve shown in **Fig. 6B**. Using **Eq. 14**, the best fit for n, K_a, and ΔH^0 was determined, and the results are shown in **Fig. 6**.

7.3. Data Analysis

Warfarin binding to HSA has been measured several times using a variety of techniques *(36)*. The association constant for site (I) has been estimated to be on the order of $10^5\ M^{-1}$, whereas site (II) is on the order of $10^3 M^{-1}$. As shown in **Table 5**, our data are consistent with these data.

Table 5
Thermodynamic Data for the Binding of Warfarin to HSA

Reference	ΔG^0 (kcal/mol)	ΔH^0 (kcal/mol)	ΔS^0 (cal/mol/K)	K_a (M^{-1})	ΔC_p (cal/mol/K)	Temperature (°C)
36	–7.1			140,000 ± 31,000		37
Our data	–7.5	–2.44 ± 0.07	16.4	205,400 ± 1369		37

8. Notes

1. Experiments can be preformed at any temperature between 2°C and 80°C. A good starting point is 25°C.
2. The starting concentrations of the drug and protein are important for accurate results because they determine the shape of the binding curve (**Fig. 2B**), which describes n, K_a, and ΔH^0. The values of K_a and ΔH^0 only depend on the accuracy of the drug concentration, whereas n depends on the accuracy (and activity) of the protein concentration.
3. For a 300-µL injector syringe and a sample cell volume of 1.4 mL, the concentration in the syringe should be 5 to 30 times greater than the concentration in the sample cell. The starting protein concentration in the sample cell $[P]_T$ in molar (M) units can be estimated by guessing the association constant K_a (M^{-1}) and the binding capacity n and by using the following relationship: $n \cdot K_a \cdot [P]_T = 10$ to 100. ***(34)***. For HSA and AGP, $n = 1$ or 2, and $K_a = 10^3$ to 10^5. A good starting point is $[P]_T = 0.0001\ M$ and $[D]_T = 0.001\ M$.
4. The same matrix (solvent or buffering system) must be used to prepare the drug and protein solutions. This procedure minimizes any additional heat effect caused by matrix dilutions. In many cases, it is best that the protein be extensively dialyzed against the matrix. In addition, this dialyzed matrix solution can be used to prepare the drug solution. The molar concentration of the protein and drug solution must be accurately known. For purified small organic compounds and small stable proteins, this is not a problem because they can be accurately weighed out on an analytical balance. However, in some cases, the molar concentration of protein solutions may have to be determined by spectroscopic methods such as UV/vis absorbance, provided molar extinction coefficients are available ***(37,38)***.
5. In some cases, the measurement of the protein concentration may be very accurate. However, the average number of binding sites (n) may be less than 1 or greater than 1. When $n < 1$, this situation may indicate that the protein is not correctly folded. This is a common problem with recombinant proteins.
6. Most organic solvents, buffers, and detergents are compatible with ITC cells. However, dithiothreitol (DTT) should be avoided or used at very low concentrations because it causes baseline problems. The reference and the sample cell solutions/buffers should be degassed before loading into the instrument. Bubble

formation in the cell during the titration will produce artifacts. Care should be taken to load the solution in a manner that avoids air bubbles. Volatile additives are a problem, and the weight of the solution should be taken before and after degassing.

7. The rotation spin of the syringe can be set from 0 to 580 revolutions per minute (rpm). A good speed is 310 rpm.
8. The injection parameters are used to set up the volume, duration, spacing between injections, and the total number of injections. Remember that the titration syringe is 300 µL. It is a good idea to discard the first injection because the instrument can take several minutes to possibly an hour to equilibrate. A good starting point is as follows:

Volume:	5 mL
Duration:	10 s
Spacing:	200 s
Number of injections:	60

References

1. Shargel, L. and Yu, A. B. C. (1993) *Applied Biopharmaceutical and Pharmacokinetics.* 3rd ed. Appleton & Lange, Stamford, CT.
2. Benet, L. Z. and Hoener, B. (2002) Changes in plasma protein binding have little clinical relevance. *Clin. Pharm. Ther.* **71,** 115–121.
3. Uetrecht, J. P. (1997) Current trends in drug-induced autoimmunity. *Toxicology* **119,** 37–43.
4. Harding, S. E. and Chowdhry, B. Z. (2001) *Protein-Ligand Interactions: Hydrodynamics and Calorimetry.* Oxford University Press, Oxford, UK.
5. Leavitt, S. and Freire, E. (2001) Direct measurement of protein binding energetics by isothermal titration calorimetry. *Curr. Opin. Struct. Bio.* **11,** 560–566.
6. Cooper, A. (2000) Microcalorimetry of protein-DNA interactions, in *DNA-Protein Interactions*, (Travers, A. and Buckle, M., eds.), Oxford University Press, Oxford, UK, pp. 125–139.
7. Alexander, K. A. and Phelps, W. C. (1996) A fluorescence anisotropy study of DNA binding by HPV-11 E2C protein: a hierarchy of E2-binding sites. *Biochemistry* **35,** 9864–9872.
8. Tanaka, M., Asahi, Y., Masuda, S., and Ota, T. (1991) Interaction between drugs and water-soluble polymers: IV. Binding position of azathioprine with bovine serum albumin determined by measuring nuclear magnetic resonance relaxation time. *Chem. Pharm. Bull.* **39,** 2771–2774.
9. Neuhofen, S., Theyssen, H., Reinstein, J., Trommer, W. E., and Vogel, P. D. (1996) Nucleotide binding to the heat-shock protein DnaK as studied by ESR spectroscopy. *Eur. J. Biochem.* **240,** 78–82.
10. Ascoli, G., Bertucci, C., and Salvadori, P. (1995) Stereospecific and competitive binding of drugs to human serum albumin: a difference circular dichroism approach. *J. Pharm. Sci.* **84,** 737–741.
11. Frostell-Karlsson, A., Remaeus, A., Roos, H., Andersson, K., Borg, P.,

Haemaelaeinen, M., et al. (2000) Biosensor analysis of the interaction between immobilized human serum albumin and drug compounds for prediction of human serum albumin binding levels. *J. Med. Chem.* **43,** 1986–1992.
12. Banker, M. J., Clark, T. H., and Williams, J. A. (2003) Development and validation of a 96-well equilibrium dialysis apparatus for measuring plasma protein binding. *J. Pharm. Sci.* **92,** 967–974.
13. Lebowitz, J., Lewis, M. S., and Schuck, P. (2002) Modern analytical ultracentrifugation in protein science: a tutorial review. *Protein Sci.* **11,** 2067–2079.
14. Lee, K.-J., Mower, R., Hollenbeck, T., Castelo, J., Johnson, N., Gordon, P., et al. (2003). Modulation of nonspecific binding in ultrafiltration protein binding studies. *Pharm. Res.* **20,** 1015–1021.
15. Gell, D., Kong, Y., Eaton, S. A., Weiss, M. J., and Mackay, J. P. (2002) Biophysical characterization of the α-globin binding protein α-hemoglobin stabilizing protein. *J. Bio. Chem.* **277,** 40,602–40,609.
16. Blom, K. F., Larsen, B. S., and McEwen, C. N. (1999) Determining affinity-selected ligands and estimating binding affinities by online size exclusion chromatography/liquid chromatography-mass spectrometry. *J. Combin. Chem.* **1,** 82–90.
17. McDonnell, P. A., Caldwell, G. W., and Masucci, J. A. (1998) Using capillary electrophoresis/frontal analysis to screen drugs interacting with human serum proteins. *Electrophoresis* **19,** 448–454.
18. O'Brien, R., Ladbury, J. E., and Chowdhry, B. Z. (2001) Isothermal titration calorimetry of biomolecules, in *Protein-Ligand Interactions: Hydrodynamics and Calorimetry* (Harding, S. E. and Chowdhry, B. Z., eds.), Oxford University Press, Oxford, UK, pp. 263–286.
19. Todd, M. J. and Gomez, J. (2001) Enzyme kinetics determined using calorimetry: a general assay for enzyme activity? *Anal. Biochem.* **296,** 179–187.
20. Voet, D. and Voet, J. G. (1995) Biochemistry. 2nd ed. John Wiley, New York.
21. Schulze, A. and Heremans, C. (1966) *Molecular Biology of Human Proteins with Special Reference to Plasma Proteins.* Elsevier, Amsterdam, 1966.
22. Kragh-Hansen, U. (1981) Molecular aspects of ligand binding to serum albumin. *Pharmacol. Rev.* **33,** 17–53.
23. Fournier, T., Medjoubi-N, N., and Porquet, D. (2000) Alpha-1-acid glycoprotein. *Biochimica et Biophysica Acta* **1482,** 157–171.
24. Horn, J. R., Brandts, J. F., and Murphy, K. P. (2002) van't Hoff and calorimetric enthalpies: II. Effects of linked equilibria. *Biochem.* **41,** 7501–7507.
25. Wadso, I. (2000) Needs for standards in isothermal microcalorimetry. Thermochimica Acta **347,** 73–77.
26. Olofsson, G., Berling, D., Markova, N., and Molund, M. (2000) The dissolution of propan-1-ol and dilution of 10wt. % propan-1-ol solution in water as calibration and test reactions in solution chemistry. *Thermochimica Acta* **347,** 31–36.
27. Izatt, R. M., Terry, R. E., Nelson, D. P., Chan, Y., Eatough, D. J., Bradshaw, J. S., et al. (1976) Calorimetric titration study of the interaction of some uni- and bivalent cations with benzo-15-crown-5, 18-crown-6, dibenzo-24-crown-8, and

dibenzo-27-crown-9 in methanol-water solvents, at 25°C and $\mu = 0.1$. *J. Am. Chem. Soc.* **98,** 7626–7630.

28. Hasegawa, Y. and Date, H. (1988) Stability of strontium(II) and barium(II) complexes with 18-crown-6 in aqueous solution and their extractability as picrates. Sol. *Extra Ion Exchange* **6,** 431–437.
29. Briggner, L. E. and Wadsoe, I. (1991) Test and calibration processes for microcalorimeters, with special reference to heat conduction instruments used with aqueous systems. *J. Biochem. Biophys. Methods* **22,** 101–118.
30. Liu, Y. and Sturtevant, J. M. (1995) Significant discrepancies between van't Hoff and calorimetric enthalpies: II. Protein Sci. **4,** 2559–61. *See also* Horn, J. R., Russell, D., Lewis, E. A., and Murphy, K. P. (2001) van't Hoff and calorimetric enthalpies from isothermal titration calorimetry: are there significant discrepancies? *Biochemistry* **40,** 1774–1778.
31. Gutte, B. and Merrifeild, R. B. (1969) The total synthesis of an enzyme with ribonuclease A activity. *J. Am. Chem. Soc.* **91,** 501–502.
32. Zegers, I., Maes, D., Dao-Thi, M. H., Poortmans, F., Palmer, R., and Wyns, L. (1994) The structures of RNase A complexed with 3'-CMP and d(CpA): active site conformation and conserved water molecules. *Protein Sci.* **3,** 2322–2339.
33. Garcia-Fuentes, L., Baron, C., and Mayorga, O. L. (1998) Influence of dynamic power compensation in an isothermal titration microcalorimeter. *Anal. Chem.* **70,** 4615–4623.
34. Wiseman, T., Williston, S., Brandts, J. F., and Lin, L.-N. (1989) Rapid measurement of binding constants and heats of binding using a new titration calorimeter. *Anal. Biochem.* **179,** 131–137.
35. Kotelnikov, G. V., Moiseyeva, S. P., Mezhburd, E. V., and Krayev, V. P. (2002) New isothermal titration calorimeter for investigation on very small samples: theoretical and experimental results. *J. Therm. Anal. Calor.* **68,** 8003–8018.
36. Aki, H. and Yamamoto, M. (1994) Thermodynamic characterization of drug binding to human serum albumin by isothermal titration microcalorimetry. *J. Pharm. Sci.* **83,** 1712–1716.
37. Anders, J. C., Parten, B. F., Petrie, G. E., Marlowe, R. L., and McEntire, J. E. (2003) Using amino acid analysis to determine absorptivity constants: a validation case study using bovine serum albumin. *Biopharm. Intern.* **16,** 30–32, 34–37.
38. Pace, C. N., Vajdos, F., Fee, L., Grimsley, G., and Gray, T. (1995) How to measure and predict the molar absorption coefficient of a protein. *Protein Sci.* **4,** 2411–2423.

10

Metabolic Stability Assessed by Liver Microsomes and Hepatocytes

David C. Ackley, Kevin T. Rockich, and Timothy R. Baker

Summary

Metabolic stability is defined as the percentage of parent compound lost over time in the presence of a metabolically active test system. For metabolic stability assays, the typical test systems are liver microsomes, liver S9, or hepatocytes (plated or suspended), depending on the goal of the assay. To determine the metabolic stability of a new chemical entity, quantification of the drug candidate from incubate supernatants is required and usually accomplished by high-performance liquid chromatography (HPLC) with mass spectrometry. This analytical approach incorporates specificity, increased sensitivity, and higher throughput via decreased method development and analysis runtime. By understanding the metabolic stability of compounds early in discovery, compounds can be ranked for further studies, and the potential for a drug candidate to fail in development as a result of pharmacokinetic reasons may be reduced. This chapter details the procedures for performing a standard metabolic stability assay and the subsequent analysis of generated incubate samples.

Key Words: In vitro; hepatocytes; microsomes; LC/MS; metabolic stability.

1. Introduction

Various in vitro approaches are incorporated into the drug discovery process. With regards to optimizing pharmacokinetic parameters (e.g., bioavailability and clearance), the metabolic stability of new chemical entities (NCEs) can be determined from in vitro incubations with hepatocytes, S9 fractions (not discussed in this chapter), or microsomes. Metabolic stability has been defined as the percentage of parent compound lost over time in the presence of the test system *(1)*. These test systems, which will be discussed sepa-

From: *Methods in Pharmacology and Toxicology*
Optimization in Drug Discovery: In Vitro Methods
Edited by: Z. Yan and G. W. Caldwell © Humana Press Inc., Totowa, NJ

rately, are widely used throughout the pharmaceutical industry to assist with the identification of likely candidates to be further evaluated using in vivo models.

1.1. Test Systems Commonly Used in Determining Metabolic Stability

Because a majority of drug metabolism occurs in the liver, several in vitro liver preparations have been established to evaluate metabolic stability. The primary systems used are either hepatocytes (plated or suspended) or microsomes. Microsomes are prepared from liver homogenates, with the goal to isolate the endoplasmic reticulum. The cytochrome P450 (CYP) metabolizing enzymes are located within the endoplasmic reticulum. These enzymes are responsible for the majority of drug metabolism. However, microsomes do not contain other cytosolic or organelle-associated metabolizing enzymes (e.g., monoamine oxidase) or cytosolic conjugating enzymes (e.g., glutathione transferase). Microsomes must also be fortified with either nicotinamide adenine dinucleotide phosphate (NADPH) or an NADPH-regenerating system to function.

Besides microsomes, hepatocytes are obtained from the liver following a two-step collagenase digestion (***2***, with various modifications, ***3***). The primary cells can then be plated for long-term usage (1 wk or more), cyropreserved for future use, or used immediately in suspension (viability of 2–6 h). The advantage of using hepatocytes is that they contain the full complement of drug-metabolizing enzymes and need no supplementation to function properly.

The decision to use microsomes or hepatocytes depends on the goal of the evaluation. If the goal is to screen compounds in a high-throughput manner, microsomes may be more applicable because of the low volumes used in these assays. For more definitive work, hepatocytes may be more applicable because they contain the full complement of hepatic metabolizing enzymes (phases I and II).

1.2. Overview of Metabolic Stability Assay

Typically, metabolic stability assays are designed to follow the loss of the NCE over time in the presence of the test system (**Fig. 1**). For microsomes, the NCE is added at a low micromolar concentration to a buffer system, usually phosphate or Tris buffer, containing 0.1 to 1 mg/mL microsomal protein and either NADPH or an NADPH-regenerating system. The incubation is maintained at 37°C either in a shaking or static water bath and the reaction stopped by the addition of methanol, acetonitrile, or an acid, such as trichloroacetic, resulting in precipitation of the proteins. The samples are then centrifuged and prepared for analysis via high-performance liquid chromatography (HPLC) with tandem mass spectrometry (LC/MS/MS). Appropriate controls (inactivated microsomes and benchmark compound) are typically added to the assay to assist with the interpretation of the results.

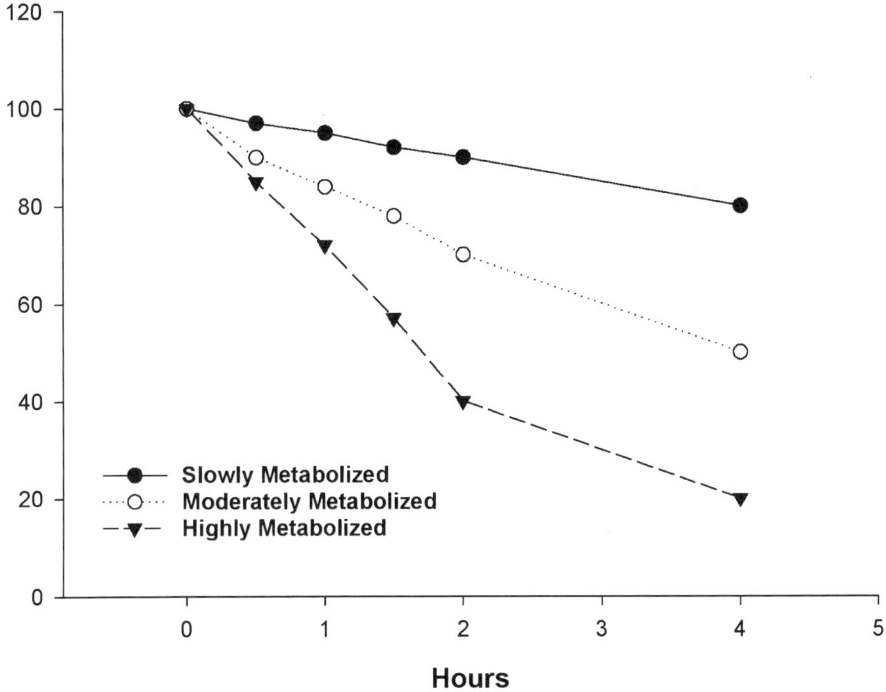

Fig. 1. Theoretical stability of three compounds in the presence of suspended hepatocytes. The disappearance of the compounds at different rates allows the compounds to be assigned rankings, such as slowly metabolized, moderately metabolized, and highly metabolized.

For hepatocytes in suspension, either fresh or cryopreserved cells can be used for metabolic stability studies. Hepatocytes are suspended in media with a final concentration in the range of 1.0×10^6 to 2.0×10^6 cells/mL *(4)*. The NCE is dissolved in an organic solvent and diluted with the same hepatocyte media such that the organic content is below the recommended concentration (dimethylsulfoxide [DMSO] < 0.2%, methanol and acetonitrile < 1%; *see* **Note 1**; ***5***). To a 48-well plate, 75 μL of the hepatocytes in suspension are added to each well, plus 75 μL of the NCE in media. The plate is placed in a 37°C incubator with 95% relative humidity and 5% CO_2. At appropriate time-points, aliquots are removed from the wells and placed in a microcentrifuge tube. Following centrifugation, the supernatant is removed for further LC/MS/MS analysis.

Briefly, plated hepatocytes, which will not be discussed in detail, are used somewhat similarly to suspended hepatocytes, except they are on a collagen or matrigel matrix. Briefly, primary hepatocytes are plated onto an extracellular matrix and allowed to adapt for 24 to 48 h. Compound in media is then added, and aliquots of media are removed for subsequent LC/MS/MS analysis.

1.3. Overview of LC/MS/MS Analysis of Samples From Metabolic Stability Incubations

The determination of metabolic stability requires the quantitation of the drug candidate from incubate supernatants. The level of the compound in the supernatants can be compared to a metabolically inactive control to determine the compound loss as a function of time. Initially, analyses of drug candidates in support of metabolic stability assays were performed via HPLC with ultraviolet (UV) detection (HPLC/UV). Those assays required adjustments to the chromatography to elute the analyte of interest in an interference-free portion of the chromatogram. Successful analysis included consideration of coeluting matrix components and metabolites. Generally, analytical considerations required incubations at levels above those analogous to therapeutic relevance (i.e., 10–50 μ*M*). Analysis was problematic in cases in which the drug candidate lacked a chromophore and was therefore not amenable to UV detection.

More recently, analysis of incubates has been conducted with HPLC coupled with mass spectrometry ***(6)***. The use of tandem mass spectrometry (MS/MS), in particular, has considerable advantages over HPLC/UV methodology. These advantages include speed, throughput, and sensitivity. The specificity of MS/MS detection allows abbreviated chromatography, with total analysis times of several minutes as opposed to the 20 to 30 min usually required by HPLC/UV, with a higher degree of assurance that similar compounds (metabolites) are differentiated. The sensitivity of LC/MS/MS permits the utilization of lower level incubations (easily down to 0.1 μ*M*), consuming less material and more closely approximating therapeutic levels. In practice, LC/MS/MS assays to determine multiple compounds can be readily developed to greatly increase throughput.

An LC/MS/MS determination of a single candidate from a metabolic stability incubate can usually be performed in a couple of minutes. Alternatively, a group of drug candidates (typically 2–10) can be incubated individually. Then, supernatants of like time-points can be combined into a single sample (i.e., the controls combined into one sample, the 30-min sample supernatants comprise another sample, and so on). Then, the combined samples are analyzed with an LC/MS/MS assay that determines each compound within less than 10 min. Within a compound class, generic HPLC gradients are possible as a result of the specificity of MS/MS. The various MS/MS detection schemes for individual analytes can be readily determined for each sample set. In this manner, the overall throughput for metabolic stability determinations is greatly increased, relative to single-candidate analysis via HPLC/UV.

A related strategy is the utilization of single-stage mass spectrometry with HPLC separation (LC/MS). LC/MS is used because of the two obvious advantages over LC/MS/MS: lower cost of instrumentation and slightly easier optimization of the mass-spectrometric detection. However, the lower specificity of the single-stage MS analysis often requires more development of compound-specific chromatography and longer elution times. It also provides less specificity (i.e., certainty) and makes the multiple-compound assay, described above, more difficult, if not impractical.

2. Materials

2.1. Metabolic Stability Using Microsome Incubations

*2.1.1. Generation of NADPH-Regenerating System (*see **Note 2***)*

1. Glucose 6-phosphate (Sigma, St. Louis, MO).
2. β-Nicotinamide adenine dinucleotide phosphate (NADP; Sigma, St. Louis, MO).
3. Glucose 6-phosphate dehydrogenase (Sigma, St. Louis, MO).
4. $MgCl_2 \cdot 6H_2O$ (J. T. Baker, Phillipsburg, NJ).

*2.1.2. NCE Stock Solution Preparation (*see **Note 3***)*

1. NCE with known molecular weight (P&GP, Mason, OH).
2. HPLC grade methanol or acetonitrile (Sigma, St. Louis, MO; *see* **Note 4**).

2.1.3. Materials for Microsome Incubation

1. 100 m*M* Potassium phosphate buffer, pH 7.4 (*see* **Note 5**).
2. Reaction tubes, polypropylene, 1.5 mL.
3. NADPH-regenerating system (*see* **Subheading 2.1.1.**).
4. Water bath, 37°C.
5. Crushed ice.
6. Diluted pooled rat or human liver microsomes, ~0.5 mg/mL final concentration (Xenotech LLC, Lenexa, KS; *see* **Note 6**).
7. NCE stock solution, 100 μ*M* (*see* **Subheading 2.1.2.**).
8. HPLC grade methanol (Sigma, St. Louis, MO).

2.1.4. Preparation of Samples for LC/MS/MS Analysis

1. Refrigerated centrifuge capable of 10,000*g*.
2. LC/MS/MS autosampler vials or deep-well blocks.
3. Appropriate internal standard.

2.2. Metabolic Stability Assessed by Suspended Hepatocytes

2.2.1. Preparation of 30% Isotonic Percoll

1. Percoll (Sigma).
2. 10X Phosphate-buffered saline (Invitrogen, Carlsbad, CA).
3. Hepatocyte thawing media (In Vitro Technology [IVT], Baltimore, MD).

2.2.2. Thawing of Cryopreserved Hepatoctyes

1. 1.5-mL Vial rat cryopreserved hepatocytes (Xenotech, LLC Lenexa, KS).
2. Cedra Complete Media (CEDRA Corporation, Austin, TX).
3. Shaking water bath 37°C.
4. Centrifuge capable of generating 40–60*g* and holding 50-mL tubes.
5. Incubator 37°C relative humidity (95%) and CO_2 (5%).
6. Trypan blue (Sigma Chemical Co., St. Louis, MO).
7. Hemacytometer.
8. 48-Well plates.
9. Liquid nitrogen storage.

2.3. Materials for the Analysis of Samples Generated in Metabolic Stability Assays

2.3.1. LC/MS/MS Materials

1. API 3000 LC/MS/MS system (ABS-Sciex, Toronto, Canada).
2. Shimadzu LC-10AD pumps and SCL-10A controller (Columbia, MD).
3. Autosampler (LEAP PAL, Carrboro, NC).
4. HPLC and mass spectrometry interfaced with a TurboIonSpray (ABS-Sciex; heated gas-assisted electrospray).
5. C18 or C8 columns with 2.0-mm internal diameter (i.d.) (various vendors).

3. Methods

3.1. Metabolic Stability Using Liver Microsomes

Typically, a standard metabolic stability assay using microsomes can be performed on either the bench-top or with an adapted liquid-handling system (e.g., TECAN Genesis Workstation 200 [Durham, NC]). The procedure described here will be for a bench-top metabolic stability assay. Briefly, metabolic stability, equated with parent loss of the NCEs, is evaluated in either pooled rat or pooled human liver microsomes. The NCEs (1 μ*M*) are incubated in three (triplicate) individual tubes, and samples are collected at specified time-points. Compound stock solutions are prepared in 100% HPLC grade methanol and are diluted in the incubation mixture containing 0.1 *M* potassium phosphate buffer, pH 7.4, and an NADPH-regenerating system. The final organic concentration in each incubate is ~1%.

3.1.1. Phosphate Buffer Preparation

Typically, phosphate buffer (~100 m*M*) is used to maintain the pH of the reaction at ~7.4. The strength of the buffer will dictate the ability of the suspension to maintain proper pH. To make 500 mL of 100 m*M* potassium phosphate buffer, the following must be done:

1. Dissolve 8.71 g of dibasic potassium phosphate into 500 mL of water (dibasic stock).
2. Dissolve 2.05 g of monobasic potassium phosphate into 150 mL of water (monobasic stock).
3. Combine 405 mL of the dibasic stock with 95 mL of the monobasic stock.
4. To adjust the pH, add monobasic stock to lower the pH or dibasic stock to increase the pH.
5. Filter the buffer using a 0.2-mm Nalgene filter flask unit and store at 4°C.

3.1.2. NADPH-Regenerating System

NADPH is a required cofactor for functional CYPs within microsomes. NADPH supplies the necessary electrons to the CYP enzymes through NADPH-cytochrome P450 reductase, which is located in the endoplasmic reticulum *(7)*. In the current method, NADPH is regenerated from NADP with the use of the enzyme glucose-6-phosphate dehydrogenase. To prepare the NADPH regenerating system, consisting of 1.3 m*M* NADP, 3.3 m*M* glucose-6-phosophate, 0.4 U/mL glucose-6-phosphate dehydrogenase, and 3.3 m*M* magnesium chloride, perform the following:

1. Dissolve 37.2 mg glucose-6-phosphate into 1 mL of 100 m*M* potassium phosphate buffer.
2. Dissolve 39.8 mg NADP into 1 mL of 100 m*M* potassium phosphate buffer.
3. Dissolve 11.5 U glucose-6-phosphate dehydrogenase into 1 mL of 100 m*M* potassium phosphate buffer.
4. Dissolve 26.8 mg $MgCl_2 \cdot 6H_2O$ into 1 mL of water.
5. Combine the prepared solutions and store on crushed ice for immediate use (*see* **Note 7**).

3.1.3. NCE Stock Solution Preparation

The solubility of the NCEs is usually not known at the time of the metabolic stability assay. Therefore, NCEs are dissolved in either acetonitrile or methanol because these compounds have been shown to be weak inhibitors of CYPs when compared with other organic solvents, such as DMSO *(8,9)*. Typically, a 100-μ*M* stock solution of the NCEs is prepared before the initiation of the study because the stability of the compounds is unknown (*see* **Note 8**).

3.1.4. Microsomal Incubation Procedure

Once the stock solutions are prepared (*see* previous sections), the reagents can be placed on crushed (wet) ice. The following procedure details a bench-top stability incubation using pooled human liver microsomes. The volumes quoted below are for an incubation study with the final volume of 300 μL.

1. Add 271 µL buffer to reaction tubes.
2. Add 18 µL of the NADPH-regenerating system.
3. Immediately prior to use, thaw pooled human or rat liver microsomes in a 37°C water bath for 2 min.
4. Add 8 µL of pooled human or rat liver microsomes (20 mg/mL with final concentration of 0.53 mg/mL; *see* **Note 9**).
5. Remove incubation tubes from ice and place in a 37°C water bath.
6. Add 3 µL of NCE stock (*see* **Subheading 3.1.3.**) prepared in methanol to reaction tubes.
7. Quench reaction tubes at selected time-points—typically 15, 30, and 45 min—by the addition of 150 µL methanol.
8. Remove samples from water bath, close tube lids, vortex briefly, and centrifuge samples at 14,000*g* for 10 min.
9. A 200-µL aliquot of the supernatant is removed, spiked with an appropriate internal standard, and analyzed by LC/MS/MS.

3.2. Metabolic Stability Assessed With Hepatocytes in Suspension

3.2.1. Preparation of 30% Isotonic Percoll Gradient

1. Prepare isotonic percoll by adding 22.5 mL of percoll and 2.5 mL of 10X PBS to a 50-mL conical centrifuge tube.
2. A 30% isotonic percoll solution is prepared by the addition of 14.4 mL of the isotonic percoll solution (from **step 1**) to 33.6 mL of hepatocyte thawing media in another 50-mL centrifuge tube. Invert the tube several times for proper mixing.
3. Place tube containing 30% isotonic percoll (from **step 2**) and another tube that contains 48 mL of hepatocyte thawing media in to a 37°C incubator at 95% relative humidity and 5% CO_2.

3.2.2. Thawing Cryopreserved Hepatocytes

1. Follow procedure specified by the manufacturer for thawing cryopreserved hepatocytes. Typically, this involves placing the vial of cryopreserved hepatocytes in a 37°C water bath and shaking it vigorously either automatically or manually. This is done for 1 to 1.5 min or until the pellet just lifts off the bottom of the tube.
2. In a biological safety cabinet, the pellet containing the hepatocytes is slowly transferred to the 30% isotonic percoll solution. Invert the tube horizontally and gently mix the pellet until it is completely suspended in the solution (*see* **Note 10**).
3. Centrifuge the tube at 50*g* for 5 min at room temperature. Remove the supernatant and gently pour the 48 mL of hepatocyte thawing media down the side of the tube. Centrifuge the tube at 50*g* for 3 min at room temperature.
4. Remove the supernatant and add 2 mL of Cedra Complete Nutrient media to the pellet that has been allowed to reach 37°C. Agitate tube by hand (do not vortex) until the cells are suspended.

3.2.3. Trypan Blue Exclusion Method to Measure Cell Viability and Concentration

1. Dilute Trypan blue by adding 50 µL of Trypan blue solution to 400 µL of 1X PBS in a microcentrifuge tube.
2. Pipet 50 µL of the suspended hepatocytes (*see* **Subheading 3.2.2.**) into the Trypan blue solution and mix by tapping the bottom of the vial several times.
3. After 1 min, pipet 10 µL to each side of a hemacytometer. Count two squares that contain 16 compartments on each side of the hemacytometer. Total the number of live (clear) and dead (purple-stained) cells that were counted in the four squares (A, B, C, and D).
4. Determine cell viability by dividing the number of live cells by the total number of cells. For the cell concentration, take the average of the live cells (A + B + C + D/4) and multiply by the dilution factor of 10 and then by 10,000 (hemacytometer factor). This results in the number of cells per milliliter, with the target being 1.0×10^6 cells/mL.

3.2.4. Metabolic Stability Study for NCE

Hepatocytes in suspension for metabolic stability studies can be from either freshly isolated or cryopreserved hepatocytes. In the case of cryopreserved hepatocytes, these can be obtained from several different vendors (e.g., Xenotech, In Vitro Technologies, BD Biosciences) with various species available. Once the hepatocytes are in suspension (*see* **Subheading 3.2.3.**), they can be used in experiments for up to 6 h.

1. Prepare a 200 to 2000X stock of the NCE (depending on which solvent the NCE is soluble in; *see* **Note 11**).
2. Dilute the NCE stock (**step 1**) with media, such that the NCE concentration is twice the desired final concentration (*see* **Note 12**).
3. To a 48-well plate, add 75 µL of the NCE in media to the wells. The hepatocytes are removed from the 37°C incubator, and 75 µL is transferred into the appropriate wells, with the number of cells being $0.75–1.5 \times 10^5$ cells/well.
4. The plate is placed into a 37°C nonshaking incubator, which is set at 95% relative humidity and 5% CO_2. At appropriate times, the sample is removed from the well and placed into a microcentrifuge tube. The tube is centrifuged at 13,000 rpm for 2 min. The supernatant is removed, and internal standard is added and analyzed via LC/MS/MS.

3.3. LC/MS/MS Analysis of Metabolic Stability Samples

Supernatants are analyzed directly or combined (multiple analytes of the same time-point) without further sample preparation. A generic and rapid HPLC gradient using a 2.0-mm i.d. C18 or C8 column is used to perform a quick reverse-phase separation (e.g., 10%–90% organic in 1 min, with 0.1% formic acid overall). The total analysis time is typically less than 6 min. Analysis is performed by an API 3000 LC/MS/MS system with Shimadzu LC-10AD pumps and SCL-10A controller with a LEAP PAL autosampler. HPLC and mass spectrometry are interfaced using TurboIonSpray.

For each analyte, source conditions (orifice voltage, etc.) are optimized to produce the protonated molecular ion. These ions are then selected by the first quadrupole. Surviving ions are fragmented in the collision cell, and a single optimal product ion for each analyte is selected and allowed to pass through the second mass filter. This specific process, unique for each analyte, rejects the vast majority of interfering material that might obscure the signals of interest. In other words, only molecules that form an ion of a specific mass-to-charge ratio (*m/z*) in the source are allowed to pass the first mass filter. Only those ions that then fragment to another specific and selected *m/z* ion are allowed to pass through the second stage of mass spectrometry. The result is a specific and quantifiable trace that is unique to the analyte of interest and produces a peak at a specific chromatographic retention time. This specificity allows rapid and sensitive analysis.

3.4. Conclusion

The combination of improved cell culturing techniques for hepatocytes, liquid-handling systems, and LC/MS/MS has had a dramatic impact on the ability to conduct high-throughput screening of compounds for metabolic stability. By understanding the metabolic stability of compounds early in discovery, the potential for a drug candidate to fail in development as a result of pharmacokinetic reasons may be reduced. By adding in vitro absorption determinations with metabolic stability data, the likelihood of failure in development as a result of pharmacokinetic shortages should be reduced even further, which is one of the major goals in the pharmaceutical industry ***(10,11)***.

4. Notes

1. Organic solvent concentrations above those suggested have been demonstrated to decrease CYP activity.
2. The stability and functionality of the regenerating system have not been explored and should be prepared within 4 h of use.
3. The stability of NCEs is not usually known, and the stock solution is usually prepared the day of the study.
4. Methanol or acetonitrile is commonly used to dissolve NCEs because the solubility of these compounds is usually not known. However, if the NCE were soluble at a final concentration of 100 μ*M* in phosphate buffer, it would be advantageous to dissolve the compound in the aqueous matrix rather than the organic matrix.

5. The phosphate buffer is usually prepared in advance of the study and stored at 4°C until used. The pH of the buffer should be verified and adjusted prior to study initiation.
6. If a bench-top procedure is used instead of a liquid-handling system, the pooled microsomes, which are a suspension, should be vortexed prior to addition to each incubation tube. If a liquid-handling system is used, then the system should be evaluated to ensure proper transfer of the microsome suspension to result in equivalent protein concentration in each tube.
7. The stability of the combined regenerating system is unknown. Premade stock solutions are available from various vendors (e.g., BD Biosciences [Bedford, MA]).
8. Because NCEs are typically synthesized in batches of less than 100 mg, stock solutions are generally prepared using less than 5 mg of material.
9. Prior to each addition, the thawed microsomes are vortexed to maintain a homogeneous suspension.
10. The suspension should have no visible "clumps" of pellet remaining.
11. For example, an NCE dissolved in DMSO would have a 2000X stock prepared because it would need to be diluted with media to achieve a final organic concentration less than 0.2%.
12. The organic concentration in the diluted NCE stock should be less than or equal to 2%, except for DMSO, which should be less than or equal to 0.4%.

References

1. Li, A. (2001) Screening for human ADME/TOX drug properties in drug discovery. *Drug Discov. Today* **6,** 357–366.
2. Seglen, P. O. (1976) Preparation of isolated rat liver cells. *Methods Cell. Biol.* **13,** 29–83.
3. LeCluyse, E. L., Bullock, P. L., Parkinson, A., and Hochman, J. H. (1996) Cultured rat hepatocytes, in *Models for Assessing Drug Absorption and Metabolism,* (Borchardt, R. T., et al., eds.), Plenum, New York, pp. 121–159.
4. Li, A. P., Lu, C., Brent, J. A., Pham, C., Fackett, A., Ruegg, C. E., et al. (1999) Cyropreserved human hepatocytes: characterization of drug-metabolizing enzyme activities and applications in higher throughput screening assays for hepatotoxicity, metabolic stability and drug-drug interaction potential. *Chem. Biol. Interact.* **121,** 17–35.
5. Easterbrook, J., Lu, C., Sakai, Y., and Li, A. P. (2001) Effects of organic solvents on the activities of cytochrome P450 isoforms, UDP-dependent glucuronyl transferase, and phenol sulfotransferase in human hepatocytes. *Drug Metab. Dispos.* **29,** 141–144.
6. Baker, T. R., Foltz, D. J., Bornes, D. M., Peng, S. X., Hu, J. K., and Grace, J. M. (1999) Multiple-compound HPLC/MS/MS assays to obtain high-throughput metabolic stability data. Paper presented at the 47th ASMS Conference on Mass Spectrometry and Allied Topics, June, Dallas, TX.
7. deBethizy, J. D. and Hayes, J. R. (2001) Metabolism: a determinant in toxicity, in

Principles and Methods of Toxicology, 4th ed., (Hayes, A. W., ed.), Taylor & Francis, Philadelphia, pp. 77–136.

8. Hickman, D., Wang, J.-P., Wang, Y., and Unadkat, J. D. (1998) Evaluation of the selectivity of in-vitro probes and suitability of organic solvents for the measurements of human cytochrome P450 monooxygenase activities. *Drug Metab. Disp.* **26,** 207–215.
9. Chauret, N., Gauthier, A., and Nicoll-Griffith, D. A. (1998) Effect of common organic solvents on in vitro cytochrome P450-mediated metabolic activities in human liver microsomes. *Drug Metab. Disp.* **26,** 1–4.
10. Kariv, I., Rourick, R. A., Kassel, D. B., and Chung, T. D. (2002) Improvements of "hit-to-lead" optimization by integration of in vitro HTS experimental models for early determination of pharmacokinetic properties. *Comb. Chem. High Throughput Screen* **5,** 459–472.
11. Mandaagere, A. K., Thompson, T. N., and Hwang, K. K. (2002) Graphical model for estimating oral bioavailability of drugs in humans and other species from their Caco-2 permeability and in vitro liver enzyme metabolic stability rates. *J. Med. Chem.* **45,** 304–311.

11

In Vitro Drug Metabolite Profiling Using Hepatic S9 and Human Liver Microsomes

Wu-Nan Wu and Linda A. McKown

Summary

Following oral administration to animals and humans, drugs are absorbed, transported via portal circulation to the liver, and metabolized primarily via this organ. In general, drugs are predominantly metabolized by the oxidation of parent drug, which is typically mediated by cytochrome P450 (CYP450) enzymes. To a lesser degree, flavin monooxidation (FMO), as well as the reduction or cleavage of the parent drug via enzymatic (i.e., esterase and amidase) or nonenzymatic hydrolysis, forms other phase I metabolites. Subsequent conjugation (phase II reaction) of the phase I metabolites can produce glucuronide, sulfate, glutathione, glycine, and acetate conjugated metabolites. In many cases, hepatic in vitro metabolism studies can yield valuable preliminary information on the in vivo metabolism of a compound of interest by the liver. Experimental in vitro hepatic systems using hepatocytes, 9000*g* supernatant (S9), and microsomal fractions are presently used to characterize the in vitro metabolism of xenobiotics. Following the incubation of drugs with either of the systems above, solvent or solid-phase extraction, radio-TLC ($^{14}C/^{3}H$-labeled drugs), high-performance liquid chromatography (HPLC) (radiolabeled or unlabeled), liquid chromatography/mass spectrometry (LC/MS), nuclear magnetic resonance (NMR), and derivatization (phenolic, alcoholic, carboxylic, and/or amino metabolites) techniques are commonly used to analyze and evaluate the metabolic stability of drugs (percentage of parent remaining), as well as to quantify, characterize, and identify drug metabolites and their derivatives. In this chapter, valuable in vitro methods using animal and human hepatic S9, as well as human liver microsomal fractions, and unique techniques for estimating and understanding metabolic stability, as well as profiling and identifying metabolites,

From: *Methods in Pharmacology and Toxicology*
Optimization in Drug Discovery: In Vitro Methods
Edited by: Z. Yan and G. W. Caldwell © Humana Press Inc., Totowa, NJ

will be discussed for use in drug discovery and drug evaluation phases of a drug's development.

Key Words: In vitro drug metabolism; hepatic S9; liver microsomes; incubation; animals; human; metabolic stability; metabolite profiling and identification, phase I and phase II metabolism; metabolic pathways; thin-layer chromatography (TLC); HPLC; LC/MS and MS/MS; NMR; derivatization.

1. Introduction

Drugs that are orally administered to animals or humans and are absorbed to some degree from the gastrointestinal tract are subsequently transported through the portal-vein circulation to the liver. These absorbed drugs are readily subjected to potential hepatic metabolism, followed by biliary or renal elimination, and excreted in the feces or urine, respectively ***(1–3)***. In general, the predominant pathway for metabolite formation is via the oxidation of the parent drug and, in some cases, the reduction and cleavage of parent drug (phase I reaction), followed by the conjugation of phase I metabolites with highly polar molecules, such as glucuronic acid, sulfuric acid, glucose, acetic acid, glutathione, cysteine, glutamic acid, taurine, and so forth, to form phase II conjugated metabolites ***(1–4)***.

In the liver, the enzymes catalyzing drug metabolism reactions are located mainly in the endoplasm (microsomes) and soluble fraction of the cytoplasma (cytosol), along with small amounts in lysosomes, mitochondria, and nuclei ***(1–4)***. The important enzymes responsible for phase I oxidation are primarily the isoenzymes of the cytochrome P450 (CYP450) family ***(5–7)*** and, to a lesser degree, flavin monooxidase (FMO) ***(1–5,8)***, alcohol dehydrogenase, aldehyde dehydrogenase, and aldehyde oxidase ***(1–4)***. These enzymes are present in the microsomal fraction. The major human CYP450 enzymes mediating drug oxidation reactions consist of the following seven CYP450 isoforms: 1A2, 2A6, 2C9, 2C19, 2D6, 2E1, and 3A4 ***(5–7)***. Of these isoforms, the two most important ones are CYP3A4 and CYP2D6, which have been documented as being responsible for the formation of most oxygenated metabolites ***(5–7)***.

Enzymes mediating phase I reduction reactions such as azo, nitro, and quinone reduction are present in both microsomes and the cytosol ***(1–4)***. Likewise, enzymes responsible for hydrolysis reactions such as epoxide hydrolase are present in both microsomes and cytosol. However, carboxyesterase is present in microsomes only ***(1–4)***. The enzymes responsible for phase II reactions such as glucuronidation and glutathione conjugation are present primarily in microsomes, whereas the one responsible for sulfation conjugation is largely present in the cytosol ***(1–4,9–12)***. The major enzymes mediating phase II reactions are UDP-dependent glucuronyltransferase (UGT), sulfotransferase

(PST), and glutathione-*S*-transferase (GST), which are present as multiple isomers ***(9–12)***.

Drug metabolism has always been an important research area for drug discovery and drug development. From the new drug screening programs in drug discovery to drug evaluation and drug development, where identifying so-called "metabolically stable" drugs with better oral bioavailability is considered critical, drug metabolism is now one of the pivotal factors for further investigation of new therapeutic agents. Because the liver is the major target organ for drug metabolism and hepatic subcellular materials are readily available, high-throughput screening assays and preliminary in vitro metabolism data generated from hepatic S9, microsomes, and hepatocytes have become valuable in evaluating the metabolic stability of drugs and the acquisition of early structural information of drug metabolites ***(13,14)***. Presently, hepatic S9, liver microsomes, and hepatocytes are the experimental in vitro systems used for the metabolic investigation of novel drugs. The understanding of major metabolic pathways of xenobiotics via the identification and quantification of metabolites provides medicinal chemists and pharmacologists the information necessary to make chemical and structural modifications for increasing drug efficacy, decreasing drug toxicities, and implementing the synthesis of metabolites with increased biological activity ***(13–16)***. This chapter focuses on sharing the methodology used in determining the in vitro phase I metabolism of drugs using animal and human hepatic S9 and human liver microsomal incubations, thin-layer chromatography (TLC), high-performance liquid chromatography (HPLC) and liquid chromatography/mass-spectrometric (LC/MS) profiling, and unique techniques in the identification of metabolites.

2. Materials

2.1. Hepatic S9/Liver Microsomal Incubations

2.1.1. Generation of Small Animal Hepatic S9 (see **Note 1**)

1. Trishydroxymethylaminomethane hydrochloride (Tris-HCl) (Sigma Co., St. Louis, MO).
2. Potassium chloride (KCl) (Sigma Co., St. Louis, MO).
3. Hydrochloride (HCl) (Fisher Scientific, Fair Lawn, NJ).
4. Potassium hydroxide (KOH) (Fisher Scientific, Fair Lawn, NJ).
5. Mouse or rat (gender and strain of choice).
6. Decapitator.
7. Surgical scissors.
8. Top-loading balance.
9. Beakers, glass-stoppered graduated cylinder.
10. Homogenizer (Brinkman Polytron®).

11. Plastic sorval tubes.
12. High-speed refrigerated centrifuge with rotor (capable of generating 9000*g* at 4°C).

2.1.2. Generation of Rodent Microsomes

1. High-speed centrifuge tubes.
2. 4-(2-Hydroxyethyl)-1-piperazineethanesulfonic acid (HEPES) (Aldrich Chemical Co., Milwaukee, WI).
3. High-speed refrigerated centrifuge with type 40 rotor (capable of speeds >105,000*g* at 4°C).

2.1.3. Human Hepatic S9 and Microsomes (see **Note 2**)

1. Human hepatic S9 and microsomes (XenoTech, L.L.C., Kansas City, KS, or In Vitro Technologies, Baltimore, MD).

2.1.4. Incubation

1. Nicotinamide adenine dinucleotide phosphate (NADP) (Sigma Co., St. Louis, MO).
2. Reduced nicotinamide adenine dinucleotide phosphate (NADPH) (Sigma Co., St. Louis, MO).
3. Magnesium chloride ($MgCl_2$) (Sigma Co., St. Louis, MO).
4. Glucose-6-phosphate (G-6-P) (Sigma Co., St. Louis, MO).
5. Beakers.
6. Wide-mouth vials (Wheaton, 16 mL) or 25-mL Erlenmeyer flasks.
7. Dubnoff Metabolic Shaker Incubator (Precision Scientific, Chicago, IL).
8. Ethyl acetate (Burchick & Jackson Laboratories, Muskegon, MI).
9. Acetone (Burchick & Jackson Laboratories, Muskegon, MI).
10. Dry ice.

2.2. Sample Preparation

1. Extraction solvents: hexane, ether, dichloromethane, ethyl acetate, acetonitrile, methanol (Burdick & Jackson Laboratories, Muskegon, MI).
2. Acetic acid (EM Science, Gibbstown, NJ).
3. Ammonium hydroxide (EM Science, Gibbstown, NJ).
4. Solid-phase extraction cartridges: C_{18}, C_8, C_4, C_2 (Whatman Inc., Clifton, NJ).
5. Amberlite®-XAD2 resin (Rohm & Haas Co., Philadelphia, PA).
6. Compact II centrifuge (Becton Dickinson & Co., Sparks, MD).
7. Pipets (Wheaton, Millville, NJ).
8. Turbo Vap® evaporator (Zymark Corp., Hopkinton, MA).

2.3. Sample Derivatization Reagents

1. Acetylation: acetic anhydride and pyridine (EM Science, Gibbstown, NJ).
2. Methylation: *N*-methyl-*N*-nitroso-*p*-toluenesulfonamide (Diazald®) (Aldrich Chemical Co., Milwaukee, WI).

2.4. TLC and HPLC Chromatography

1. TLC and HPLC solvents: hexane, chloroform, dichloromethane, ethyl acetate, methanol, ethanol, acetonitrile, tetrahydrofuran, water (Burdick & Jackson Laboratories, Muskegon, MI).
2. Acetic acid (EM Science, Gibbstown, NJ).
3. Ammonium hydroxide (EM Science, Gibbstown, NJ).
4. Ammonium acetate (Aldrich Chemical Co., Milwaukee, WI).
5. Formic acid (Aldrich Chemical Co., Milwaukee, WI).
6. Trifluoroacetic acid (TFA) (Aldrich Chemical Co., Milwaukee, WI).
7. TLC plates: silica gel GF and neutral alumina (normal phase); C_{18}, C_8, C_2, phenyl (reverse phase) (Anatech, Inc., Newark, DE).
8. TLC development tank or jar.
9. TLC Radiochromatogram Imaging System (BID 100) (Bioscan, Inc., Washington, DC).
10. HPLC system (Beckman Instrument Co., Fullerton, CA).
11. HPLC Radioactive Monitor (RAM) (RAMONA, IN; US Service Corp., Fairfield, NJ).

2.5. LC/MS and MS/MS Application

1. PE Sciex API III-Plus and API 3000 Mass Spectrometers (Perkin-Elmer Sciex Instruments, Thornhill, Ontario, Canada).
2. HPLC system interfaced to MS-Hitachi HPLC solvent delivery system (L-6200A Intelligent pump) (Hitachi Co., Tokyo, Japan).
3. HPLC column: C_{18}, C_8, C_2, phenyl, cyano (Agilent Technologies, Fitchburg, MA); LiChorsorb RP-2 (C_2), RP-8 (C_8), and RP-18 (C_{18}) (Brownlee Laboratories, Inc., Santa Clara, CA).

3. Methods

3.1. Hepatic S9/Microsomal Generation

3.1.1. Small Animal Hepatic S9 Preparation

3.1.1.1. Buffer Preparation

The base buffer used in the preparation of any hepatic S9 is 1.15% KCl in 0.05 *M* Tris-HCl (pH 7.4) buffer. This may be prepared ahead of time as follows (*see* **Note 3**):

Tris-HCl:	6.055 g
KCl:	1.15 g
Water (distilled) q.s.:	1000 mL
Adjust pH to 7.4 with either HCl or KOH	

3.1.1.2. Hepatic S9 Preparation

A homogenate is prepared by first euthanizing a small rodent by decapitation. The liver is removed (wet weight determined), minced, and homogenized using a Brinkmann Polytron® in cold Tris-HCl buffer to a total volume of ~4 × the wet liver weight (*see* **Note 4**). The homogenate is divided into equal volumes into the sorval centrifuge tubes and spun at 9000*g* for 30 min. The supernatant (S9) is removed and should be used immediately or stored at –70°C to maintain viability for use at a later date. Typically, a male SD rat is used (*see* **Note 5**).

3.1.2. Microsomal Preparation

Microsomal suspensions are prepared by taking a measured volume of S9 and centrifuging again at 105,000*g* (type 40 rotor) in a high-speed centrifuge for 1 h. The subsequent supernatant is discarded, and the pellet is gently resuspended in cold 0.1 *M* HEPES/1.15% KCl buffer up to a volume one-half that of the original S9 (approx 12–16 mg of microsomal protein per milliliter with this method). The microsomal fraction should be used immediately or stored at –70°C or lower for use at a future time.

3.2. Hepatic S9/Microsomal Incubation

3.2.1. Hepatic S9 Incubation Preparation

Prior to an incubation, each of the following cofactors is prepared fresh daily in cold Tris-HCl buffer: (1) 5 m*M* $MgCl_2$ (i.e., 127 mg $MgCl_2 \times 6\ H_2O$ in 25 mL Tris-HCl), (2) 5 m*M* glucose-6-phosphate (i.e., 190 mg glucose-6-phosphate in 25 mL Tris-HCl), and (3) 0.5 m*M* NADP (i.e., 47.5 mg in 25 mL Tris-HCl).

To maintain a 5-mL volume in each 25-mL Erlenmeyer flask or suitable vial, 1 mL each of cold Tris-HCl buffer, $MgCl_2$, glucose-6-phosphate, and NADP solutions and the desired S9 (prepared in-house or purchased outside; ~20 mg/mL protein) are placed into each flask on ice in the order given (*see* **Note 6**). A flask containing drug but no S9 fraction, as well as one containing a compound with a documented in vitro metabolic profile (i.e., etoperidone or tramadol), is also incubated to serve as environmental and enzyme activity controls (*see* **Note 7**). Finally, the drug solution, typically 2.5 mg/mL, as well as reference standards can be spiked into each vial as a small volume (5–50) in methanol, ethanol, or dimethylsulfoxide (DMSO) or as an aqueous solution dissolved in Tris-HCl buffer (*see* **Note 8**) so that the spike (typically 20 µL) gives a final desired concentration of drug (1–10 µg/mL or 1–20 µ*M*/mL) (*see* **Note 9**). Each chilled flask is placed in the Dubnoff Metabolic Shaker Incubator and incubated in an open-air atmosphere for up to 120 min at 37°C. Aliquots (1 mL) may be removed and placed into prelabeled tubes at any time for analysis. Equal volumes of ethyl acetate or acetonitrile are added to aliquots to terminate the reaction (*see* **Note 10**). All samples are then immediately frozen in a dry ice/acetone bath and stored at –20°C or lower pending analysis *(17–27)*. When the incubation is complete, each remaining sample is transferred to a prelabeled storage vial, deactivated, and stored as described previously (*see* **Note 11**). This hepatic S9 system primarily generates phase I metabolites.

3.2.2. Hepatic Microsomal Incubation Preparation

Incubations with microsomes are prepared and carried out using the same methodology described for the S9 mixtures, substituting 1 mL of the microsomal suspension for the supernatant (*see* **Note 12**) and replacing 1 mL of NADPH solution for the NADP solution *(17,22,23)* (*see* **Note 13**). The hepatic microsomal incubation also chiefly produces phase I metabolites (*see* **Note 14**). The addition of uridine 5' diphosphoglucuronic acid (UDPGA) to the incubation mixture, as well as an increased incubation duration, may form glucuronide conjugates (phase II metabolites) because of the presence of UGT in the microsomal fraction *(28)*.

3.3. Sample Preparation for Metabolic Profiling

Acidified and or basified hepatic S9 and liver microsomal incubates can be extracted using organic solvents (i.e., ether, ethyl acetate, and dichloromethane for organic extractable drugs), or solid-phase extraction, such as C_{18}, C_8, or C_2 cartridges or Amberlite®-XAD2 resin, can be used for nonorganic extractable drugs. The extract is evaporated to dryness to yield a residue, which is reconstituted in methanol or acetonitrile and applied on the TLC plate or injected onto the HPLC system. For example, unchanged RWJ-34130 and its metabolites, generated from hepatic S9 and microsomal incubations, were profiled by HPLC, and then the drug-related peaks were individually collected from the HPLC effluents for subsequent MS analysis (**Fig. 1**) *(17,29)*.

3.4. Radio-TLC Metabolic Profiling and Isolation

This method only applies to radiolabeled drugs such as the two ^{14}C-labeled drugs, ^{14}C-fenoctimine and ^{14}C-fenobam, which has an in vitro metabolism that can be characterized by using a radio-TLC method that was previously reported *(18,19)*. In general, the organic extract residue from the incubate is reconstituted in a minimal amount of organic solvent, or the aqueous incubate (nonorganic extractable) is applied directly as a band or spot on a 20 × 20-cm TLC plate, along with reference samples (parent drug, synthetic metabolites), and developed in organic solvent systems (acidic, basic, and neutral). The developed plate is radioscanned to obtain the TLC metabolic profile, followed by visualization under a short-wavelength UV light to localize the drug-related

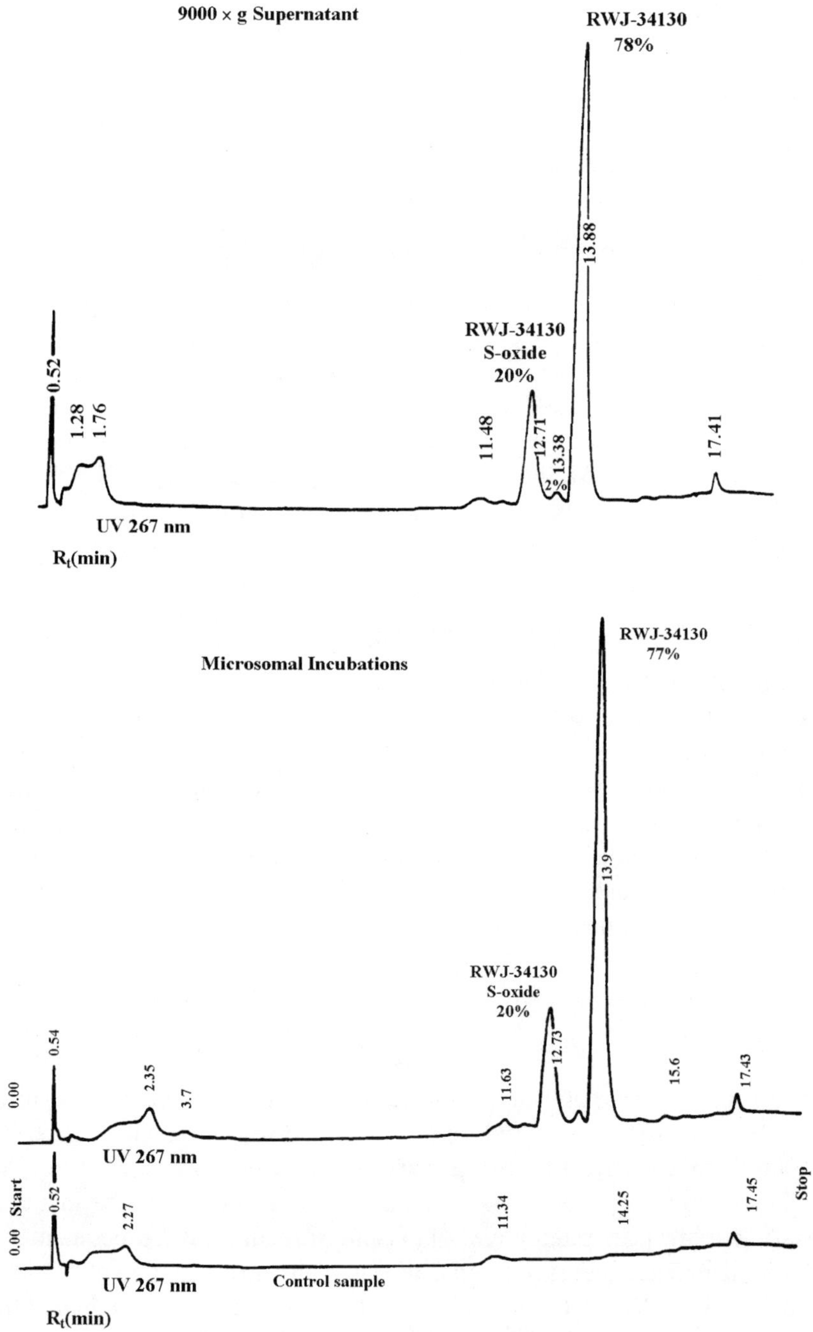

Fig. 1. HPLC profiles of the rat hepatic S9 and microsomal incubation of RWJ-34130.

zones or spots. These areas are removed by scraping and extracted with organic solvents (a mixture of methanol and dichloromethane or methanol and ethyl acetate). The extracts are filtered, followed by evaporation to yield dry residues, which are then analyzed using mass spectrometry (MS) and nuclear magnetic resonance (NMR) to gain structural information of metabolites. Derivatization using, for example, diazomethane for reacting with phenolic and carboxyl metabolites to form methyl ethers and methyl esters, respectively, or acetic anhydride/pyridine for reacting with the alcoholic, phenolic, and amino metabolites to form acetyl derivatives can be valuable for further structural confirmation of metabolites ***(19–22,25,27,30)***.

3.5. Radio-HPLC and HPLC Metabolic Profiling

The typical HPLC system used is a gradient liquid chromatograph with a UV detector. A LiChrosorb RP-2 (C_2) guard and analytical column (5 μm, 130 × 4.6 mm) are used for sample analysis at a flow rate of 2 mL min^{-1} for the mobile phase (*see* **Note 15**). The gradient elution is conducted from 2% to 100% B in 20 min, with water (mobile phase A) and methanol (mobile phase B) both containing 0.02% ammonium acetate. The in vitro metabolic profiling of RWJ-34130 from rat hepatic S9 fraction and liver microsomal incubations was conducted using the HPLC conditions described above (**Fig. 1**) ***(17,29)***. Unchanged drug and metabolites obtained from these samples were isolated by HPLC and analyzed by MS and NMR ***(17,19,21,30)***. An estimate of the relative percentages of unchanged drug and each metabolite in a given sample was made using the integrated peak intensity generated by the HPLC chromatogram for the unlabeled drugs and by using the integrated radioactive peaks from the RAM (radioactive monitor) for the radiolabeled drugs ***(17,30)***.

3.6. LC/MS and MS/MS Metabolic Profiling

Following organic solvent/solid-phase (C_2, C_8, C_{18}, Amberlite®-XAD2 resin) extraction of each acidified, basified, or neutral incubate (1 mL) (*see* **Note 16**), the residue is reconstituted in a 0.2- to 0.5-mL buffer (acetonitrile or methanol/water [50/50, v/v] with 5 m*M* ammonium acetate, pH 4.0), centrifuged, and then analyzed via a 20-μL flow-injection into a PE Sciex API III-Plus or PE Sciex API 3000. These are triple quadruple mass spectrometers, interfaced to a Hitachi HPLC (C_{18}, C_8, or C_2 column) solvent delivery system (L-6200 A Intelligent pump) via an ionsprayer using nitrogen as the curtain and nebulizing gas and argon (API III Plus) or nitrogen (API 3000) as the collision gas for MS/MS analysis. The isocratic mobile phase for this system is the same buffer as described for residue reconstitution, delivered at a flow rate of 0.5 to 0.1 mL min^{-1} (*see* **Note 17**). For each sample, the relative percentage of unchanged drug and its metabolites is estimated using the integrated chromatograms generated by the Sciex API-III Plus or API 3000 Q1 scan MS (total ion chromatogram). These data are not absolutely quantitative because of the potential differences in the degree of ionization of each analyte. However, they are reproducible ***(20–22,25,27)*** (*see* **Note 18**).

3.7. Metabolite Derivatization

3.7.1. Methyl Derivatization (see **Note 19**)

Each incubate (1 mL) extract residue is dissolved in 0.2 to 0.5 mL of methanol, an excess amount of ethereal diazomethane (generated from Diazald with 1 *N* methanolic KOH solution) is added, and the mixture is allowed to react at room temperature overnight. This mixture is subsequently evaporated to dryness to yield a methylated residue consisting of the phenolic and carboxylic metabolites derivatized to methyl ethers and methyl esters, respectively. Each residue is then further analyzed using LC/MS for the confirmation of metabolites ***(19,21,22,25,27,30)***.

3.7.2. Acetyl Derivatization

Each incubate (1 mL) extract residue is dissolved in 0.2 mL of acetic anhydride and 0.1 mL of pyridine and is allowed to react at room temperature for 4 h. Then, 5 mL of cold water is added to each sample followed by organic solvent extraction (ether, ethyl acetate, or dichloromethane). Each acetylated extract residue is further analyzed by LC/MS for the confirmation of metabolites ***(20)***. Phenolic, primary and secondary alcoholic, and primary and secondary amino metabolites can be derivatized as acetates.

3.8. Structural Elucidation of Unchanged Drugs, Metabolites, and Derivatives

The structures of unchanged drug, as well as its metabolites and derivatives, are characterized, quantified, and elucidated based on the generated MS, MS/MS, and NMR data and by comparison to synthetic samples, if available.

3.9. Proposed In Vitro Metabolic Pathways of Drugs

The proposed in vitro metabolic pathways for many investigational drugs have been established using the techniques already described. The in vitro metabolism of RWJ-34130 ***(17,29)***, RWJ-52763 ***(24,25)***, and RWJ-68025 ***(26,27)***, which have previously been published, are presented as examples of this methodology.

3.9.1. In Vitro Metabolism of RWJ-34130

RWJ-34130, 3-[2-(1-phenyl-2-pyrrolidinylideneamino)ethylthio]indole, is a potential antiarrhythmic drug. HPLC profiling was conducted for RWJ-34130

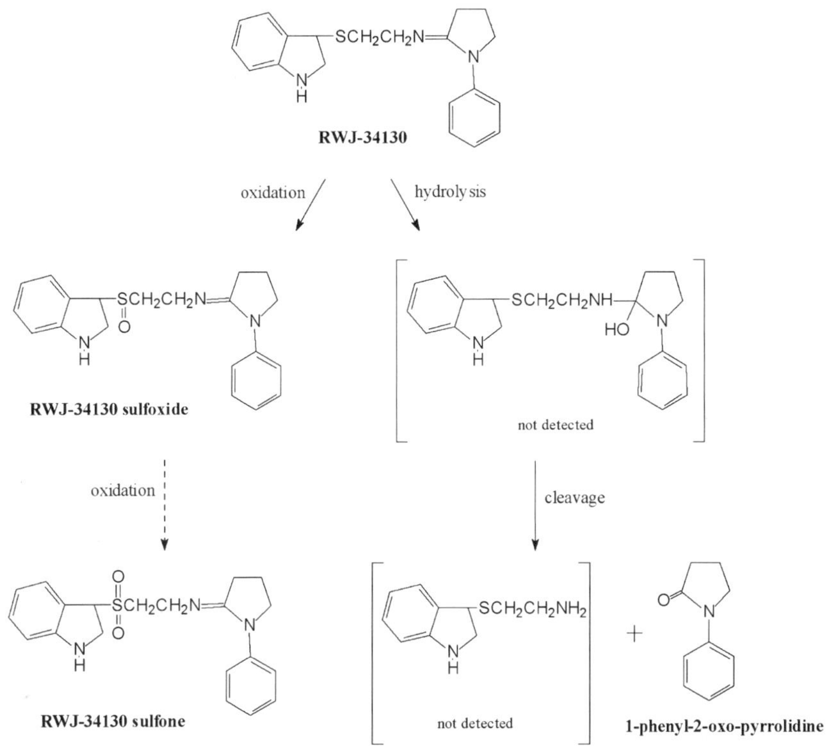

Fig. 2. In vitro metabolic pathways for RWJ-34130.

and four synthetic putative metabolites ***(17,29)***. Rat hepatic S9, liver microsomal, and control incubates (30 and 60 min) were profiled by HPLC, and they were all qualitatively and nearly quantitatively identical (**Fig. 1**). The profiles revealed unchanged RWJ-34130 (77% of the drug-related sample), one major metabolite, RWJ-34130 sulfoxide (20% of the drug-related sample), and one minor unidentified metabolite (2.5% of the drug-related sample). Unchanged RWJ-34130 and the major sulfoxide metabolite were subsequently isolated by HPLC and further confirmed by MS data in comparison with the synthetic standard. RWJ-34130 sulfoxide was synthesized by the oxidation of RWJ-34130 with *m*-chloro-peroxybenzoic acid. The in vitro metabolism of RWJ-34130 in rat hepatic S9 and microsomes appeared to form substantial amounts of the sulfoxide metabolite via oxidation at the sulfur atom of the molecule (**Fig. 2**) (*see* **Note 20**). Cimetidine is also largely metabolized to form cimetidine sulfoxide, which is an example of an *S*-oxidative metabolic pathway. Further oxidation of the sulfoxide could produce a sulfone that would also be synthesized, although it was not detected in these rat liver preparations.

3.9.2. In Vitro Metabolism of RWJ-52763

RWJ-52763, 6-*N*,*N*-dimethoxyethyl-1,2-dihydro-3-oxo-*N*-(2,6-difluorophenyl)pyrido[1,2-*a*]benzimidazole-4-carboxamide, is an anxiolytic agent. The in vitro metabolism of RWJ-52763 was conducted in the human hepatic S9 fraction ***(24,25)***. Unchanged RWJ-52763 (64% of the drug-related sample) and a total of six metabolites (M1 through M6) were profiled, quantified, and tentatively identified in 60-min incubates based on API ionspray-MS and MS/MS data in the positive mode. The representative MS metabolic profile for the 60-min human hepatic S9 incubate is shown in **Fig. 3**. The structures of RWJ-52763 and its metabolites, as well as their MS data, are also illustrated in **Fig. 4**. The MS and MS/MS data revealed protonated molecular ions and prominent as well as informative product ions for the structural elucidation of RWJ-52763 and its metabolites. The formation of RWJ-52763 metabolites in the human hepatic S9 fraction can be explained by two metabolic pathways: *N*/*O*-dealkylation and phenylhydroxylation. Pathway 1 appeared to be the most quantitatively important pathway, forming *N*-desmethyl-RWJ-52763 (M1; 22% of the drug-related sample) as a major metabolite, and *O*-desmethyl-RWJ-52763 (M2; 2% of the drug-related sample) and *N*,*N*-didesmethoxyethyl-RWJ-52763 (M3; 3% of the drug-related sample) were two minor metabolites. Pathway 2 produced two minor phenylhydroxylated metabolites, M4 and M5, and, in combination with pathway 1, formed a trace metabolite, hydroxy-M1. The proposed in vitro metabolic pathways for RWJ-52763 in human hepatic S9 fraction are depicted in **Fig. 5**. RWJ-52763 is substantially metabolized in this human hepatic in vitro system.

3.9.3. In Vitro Metabolism of RWJ-68025

RWJ-68025, 1-*R*-phenyl-2-*R*-(1-(3-methoxyphenyl)-*R*-ethylamino)methyl-cyclo-propane, is a calcium-mimetic agent. The in vitro metabolism of RWJ-68025 was investigated in rat and human hepatic S9 fractions ***(26,27)***. Following 60 min of incubation, unchanged RWJ-68025 (44%–48% of the sample) plus 12 metabolites were profiled, quantified, and tentatively identified from 30- and 60-min incubates based on API-MS and MS/MS data collected in positive mode and methyl derivatization. The representative MS metabolic profile and MS/MS spectrum of metabolite 1 from the 60-min incubate of human S9 are shown in **Fig. 6** and **Fig. 7**, respectively. Formation of the 12 RWJ-68025 metabolites from rat and human hepatic S9 can be explained by four metabolic pathways: (1) *O*-demethylation, (2) phenyl oxidation, (3) methyl oxidation, and (4) *N*-dealkylation. Pathway 1 appeared to be the most important pathway, forming a major metabolite, *O*-desmethyl-RWJ-68025 (M1; 26%–16% in rat and human). Pathway 2 produced one major metabolite,

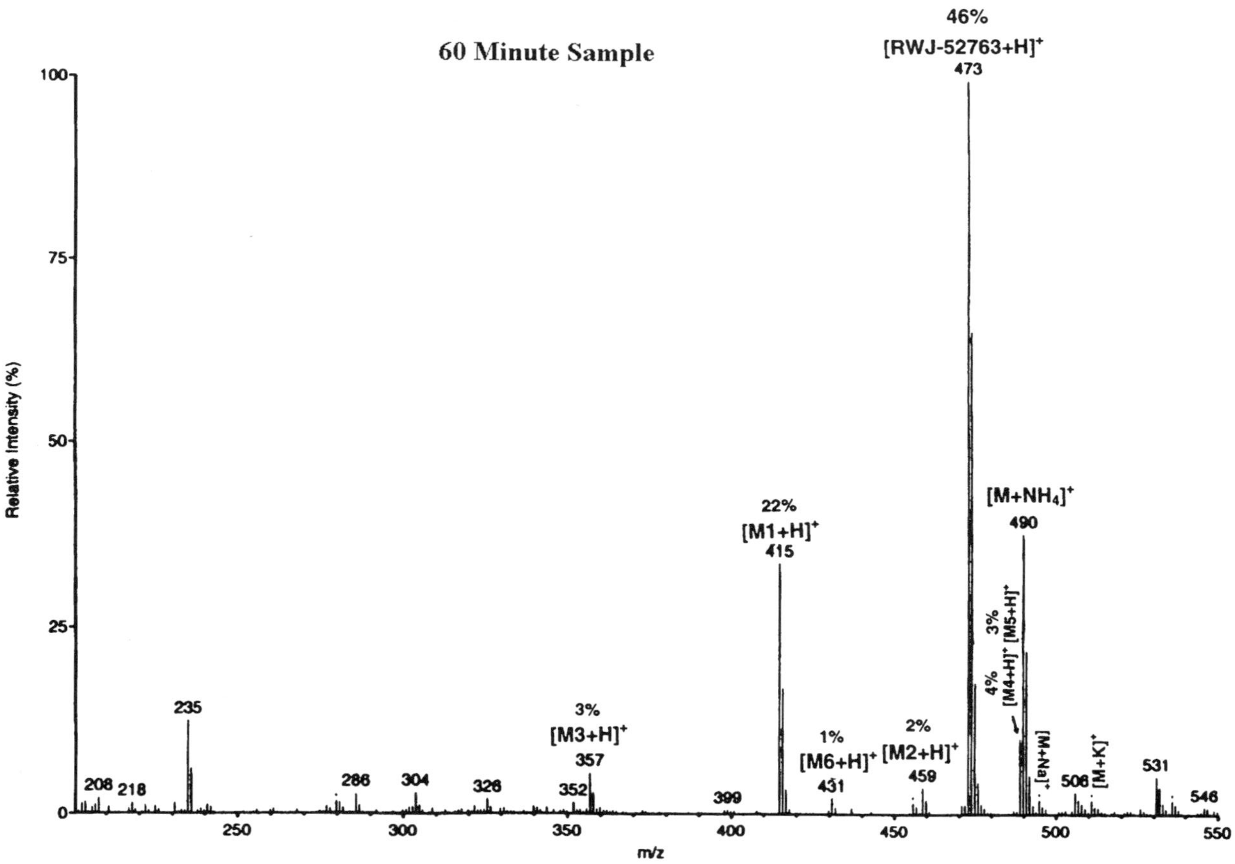

Fig. 3. API-MS profile of human hepatic S9 incubate of RWJ-52763 (60 min).

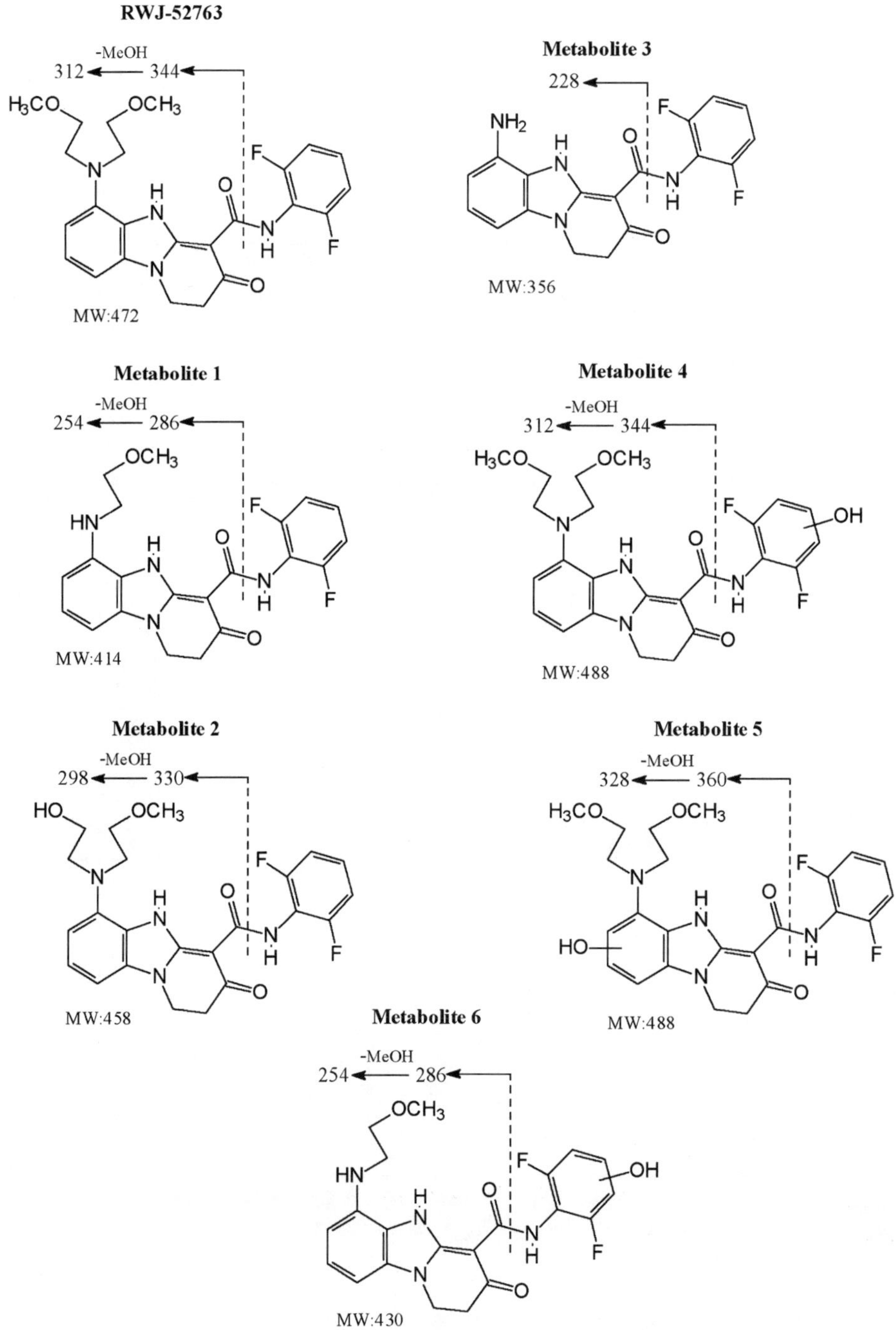

Fig. 4. Structures and MS/MS product ions for RWJ-52763 and metabolites.

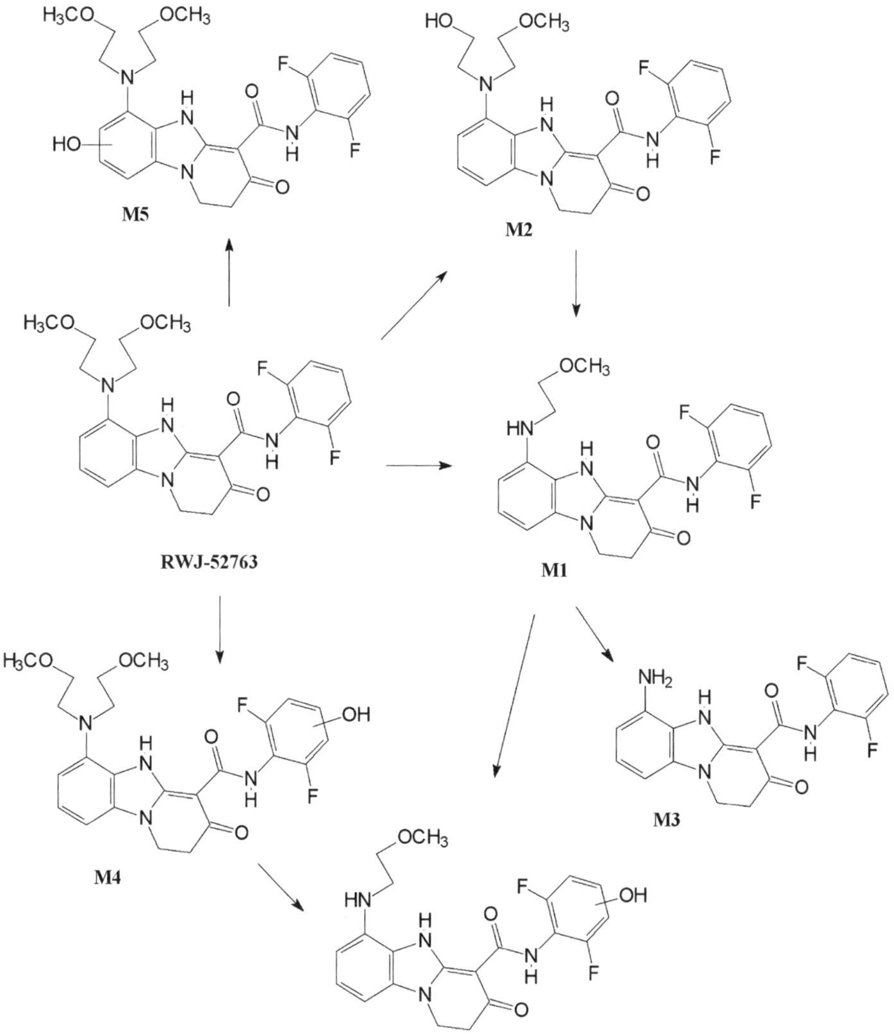

M6

Fig. 5. In vitro metabolic pathways for RWJ-52763 in human hepatic S9 fraction.

hydroxyphenyl-RWJ-68025 (M2; 12%–17% in both species), and two minor phenolic metabolites and, in conjunction with pathway 1, formed hydroxy-M1 (M3; 4%–5% in both species). Pathways 3 and 4 produced 7 minor methyl-oxidized and *N*-dealkylated/acetylated metabolites. The proposed in vitro metabolic pathways for RWJ-68025 in rat and human hepatic S9 fractions are depicted in **Fig. 8**. RWJ-68025 was rapidly and extensively metabolized in both rat and human hepatic S9 fractions.

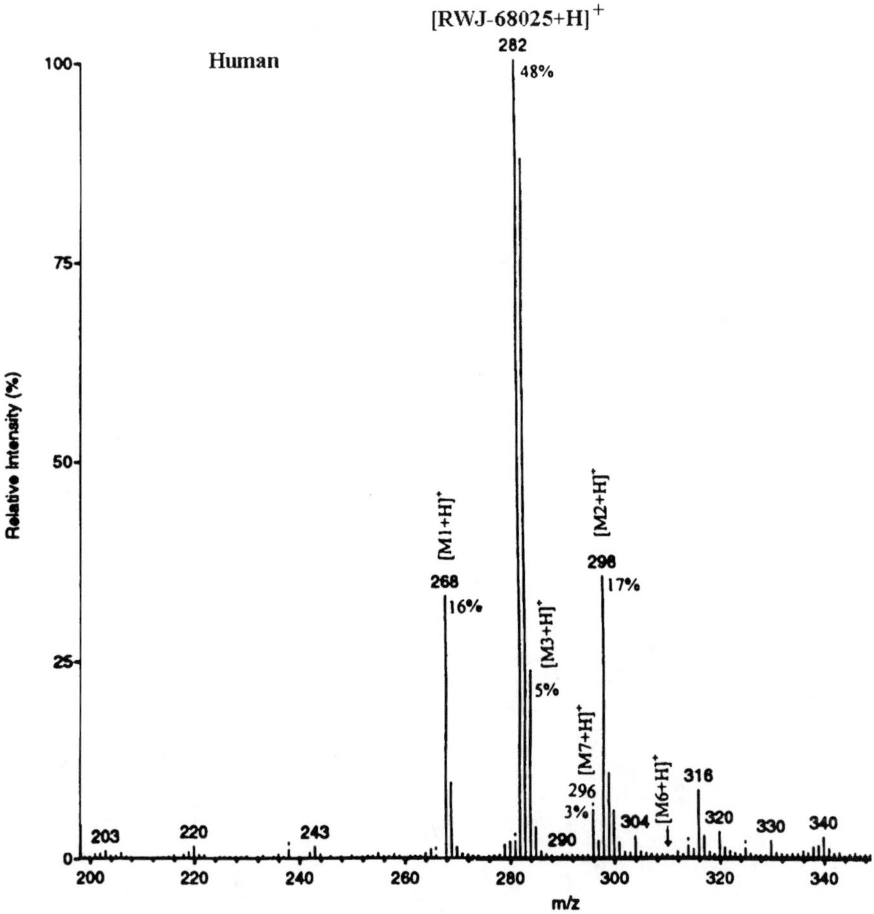

Fig. 6. API-MS profile of human hepatic S9 incubate of RWJ-68025 (60 min).

4. Notes

1. Hepatic S9 is also commercially available for a wide variety of animal species, strains, and genders. This material usually comes with a detailed characterization as well. A common source is In Vitro Technologies (Baltimore, MD).
2. Sources of human pooled liver preparations may vary in microsomal activity because of potential enzyme induction, for example, by those patients who may have been long-term drug users versus healthy subjects. One should try to maintain the same source of human S9/liver microsomes to obtain reproducible results *(1–3,6,7)*.
3. A total of 1.15% KCl in 0.05 *M* Tris-HCl buffer should be stored refrigerated after preparation and can then be used for up to ~4 mo. However, the remaining cofactors—5 m*M* $MgCl_2$, 0.5 m*M* NADP, 0.55 m*M* NADPH, and 5 m*M* glucose-

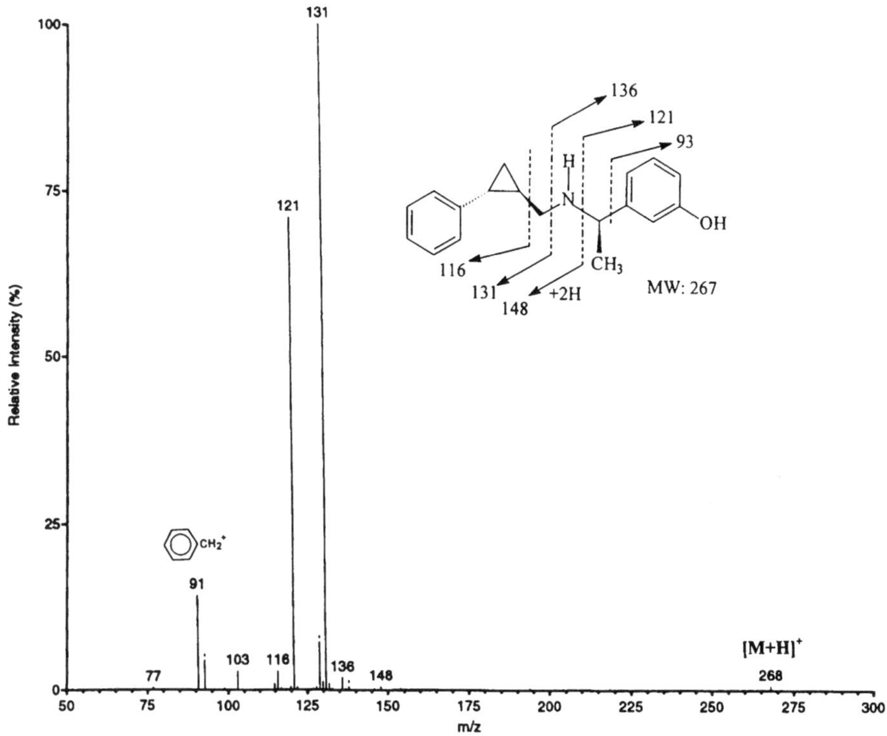

Fig. 7. API-ionspray MS/MS spectrum of metabolite 1 from RWJ-68025 incubate.

6-phosphate, all prepared in Tris-HCl buffer—must be prepared fresh daily just prior to preparing an incubation ***(1)***.

4. The preparation of hepatic S9 should be well planned out and done quickly. All materials should be chilled and procedures conducted on ice, if possible, to maintain the viability of the enzymes during processing.
5. The hepatic S9 and microsomal fractions of male rats have higher drug-oxidizing activity than that of females because of the higher level of CYP450 enzymes present in males ***(1–5)***.
6. It is possible to incubate a total volume less than 5 mL. To do so, one would just adjust volumes of all components equally. The larger volume that is used in these experiments allows for potential isolation of metabolites of interest.
7. It is important to test your incubation conditions and the activity of each specific lot of enzyme by incubating concurrently with a control drug whose in vitro metabolic profile is well documented (percent disappearance of parent drug, metabolites formed)—that is, etoperidone ***(23)*** and tramadol ***(22)***—used in these examples.
8. It is best to try to gain some solubility information about each drug or class prior to incubation. If no information is known, it is best to first try dissolving the neat

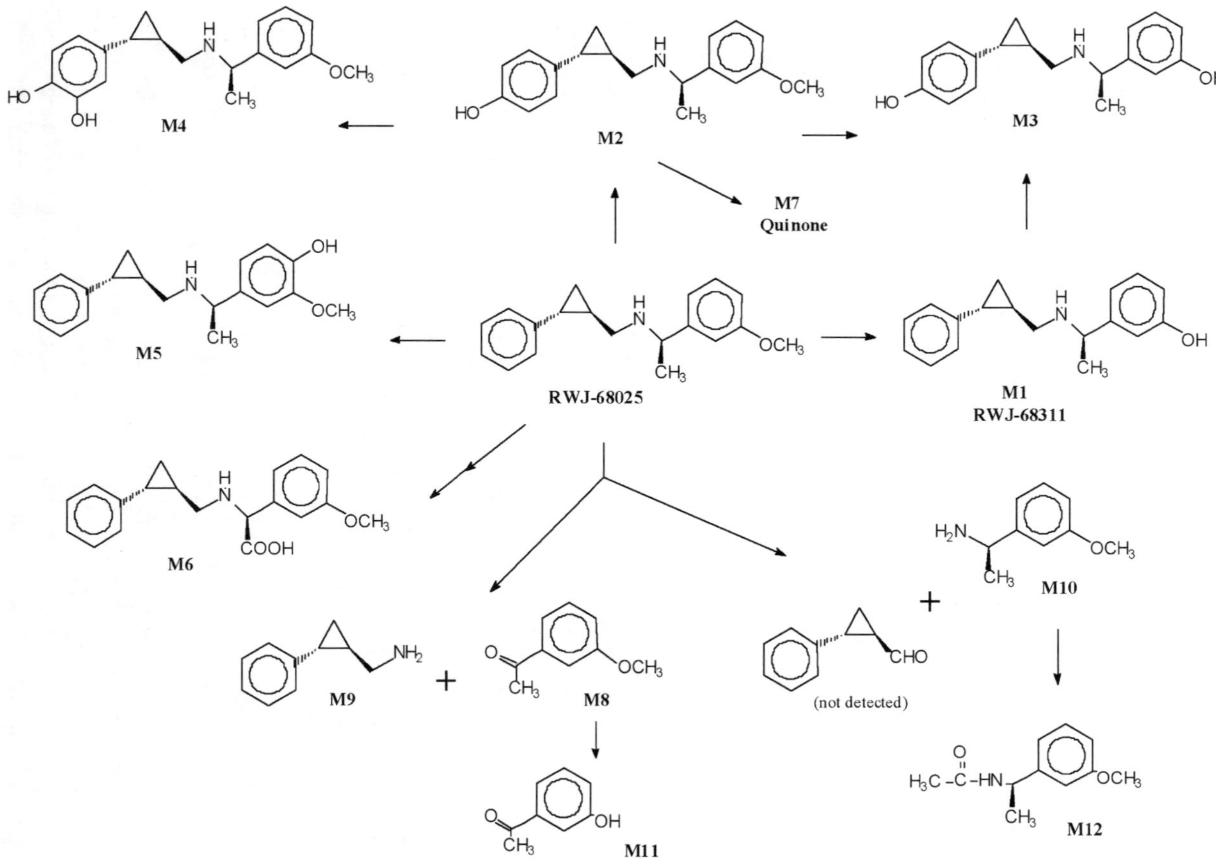

Fig. 8. In vitro metabolic pathways for RWJ-68025 in rat and human hepatic S9 fractions.

material in MeOH, which has a low impact on the biological system. If this is not successful, then it can be evaporated down and another solvent tested. DMSO is usually the last solvent tested and is typically successful ***(1)***.

9. In general, it can be said that the lower the drug concentration of the incubation mixture, the higher the percentage of metabolite generation will be ***(1–4,13, 20–22,25,27,30)***.
10. The enzymatic reactions of incubated samples need to be terminated quickly by the addition of organic solvents, such as acetonitrile, ethyl acetate, or dichloromethane, immediately following the removal of aliquots or incubates from the incubator. This should be followed by a quick freeze and storage at –20°C or lower pending analysis ***(1,17–19)***.
11. For light-sensitive drugs, lights should be kept low and amber glass used to avoid exposure to light during incubation, storage, sample preparation, and analysis ***(1,17–19)***.
12. In many cases, there are advantages to incubating drugs with the S9 fraction vs the microsomal fraction. The hepatic S9 is more convenient to prepare, the reaction is linear for a longer period of time, and the overall activity is better than that seen with microsomes ***(1–4,17)***.
13. It is unnecessary to add NADPH to the hepatic S9 (microsomes + cytosol) incubation because of the presence of endogenous isocitric and glucose-6-phosphate dehydrogenases in the cytosolic fraction, which, along with NADP, are used to generate NADPH. In contrast, NADPH is essential for the liver microsomal incubation ***(1)***.
14. Hepatic S9 and liver microsomal incubations primarily generate phase I metabolites only. However, in some cases, the formation of acetyl metabolites (phase II) has been documented following hepatic S9 incubation as a result of the presence of *N*-acetyltransferases in cytosol ***(26,27)***.
15. Sample proteins are removed by acetonitrile precipitation and centrifugation. The supernatant volume injected into the LC (~20 µL) is kept as small as possible for optimizing LC/MS separation and resolution ***(1–4,17,20–22,23,25,27,30)***.
16. Some drugs produce unstable metabolites (heat-labile, light-sensitive, and reactive) that need to be analyzed as quickly as possible after incubation and sample preparation. Avoid using CI and EI-MS for thermal-labile metabolites (i.e., *N*-oxides and conjugates) ***(1–5,8,9,17–19)***.
17. The formylation of a metabolite's amino group (addition of 28 am) could occur in LC/API-MS analysis if formic acid is used. A LC mobile phase containing ammonium acetate can remarkably enhance ionization efficiency in LC/MS analysis, but it can also produce ammonium-adduct molecular ions of unchanged drugs and its metabolites. The use of TFA to enhance ionization during LC/MS analysis might form TFA polymers in the MS ion source; therefore, one needs to periodically refresh the LC/MS system using methanol/water (50:50, v/v) ***(20–22,25,27)***.
18. The most commonly adducted molecular ions observed in LC/API/ES-MS analysis are ammonium adducts ($[M+18\ amu]^+$) if ammonium acetate or ammonium

carbonate is used, sodium adducts ([M+23 amu]$^+$), potassium adducts ([M+39 amu]$^+$), methanol adducts ([M+32 amu]$^+$), acetonitrile adducts ([M+41 amu]$^+$), acetic acid adducts ([M+60 amu]$^+$), and TFA adducts ([M+114 amu]$^+$). These adduct ions could form from the use of organic solvents, acids, and bases and from tubing and glassware. The methanol adduct of a drug may lead to the misinterpretation of the formation of a dioxidized metabolite, which will not derivatize with either diazomethane or acetic anhydride/pyridine but will fragment to form a protonated molecular ion of the parent drug via the loss of methanol, along with its product ions during MS/MS analysis ***(20–22,25,27)***.

19. Diazomethane derivatization reacts not only with phenolic and carboxylic metabolites but also with some heterocyclic nitrogens. However, it does not derivatize *N*-oxide, amino, and alcoholic metabolites. Acetic anhydride/pyridine acetylation derivatizes phenolic, alcoholic (primary and secondary), and amino (primary and secondary) metabolites but not amide and tertiary alcoholic metabolites ***(2,3,19–22,25,27,30)***.
20. *N*-oxide metabolites formed via cytochrome P450 or FMO may consist of two stereoisomers—for example, the *cis* and *trans* nicotine-*N*-oxides, which were formed via an in vitro system ***(8)***.

References

1. La Du, B. N., Mandel, H. G., and Way, E. L., eds. (1972) *Fundamentals of Drug Metabolism and Drug Disposition*. Williams & Wilkins, Baltimore.
2. Testa, B. and Jenner, P., eds. (1976) *Drug Metabolism: Chemical and Biochemical Aspects*. Marcel Dekker, New York.
3. Jenner, P. and Testa, B., eds. (1980–1981) *Concepts in Drug Metabolism Parts A and B*. Marcel Dekker, New York.
4. Parkinson, A. (1996) Biotransformation of xenobiotics, in *Casarett & Doull's Toxicology*, (Klaassen, C. D., ed.), pp. 113–186.
5. Ortiz de Montellano, P. R., ed. (1995) *Cytochrome P450: Structure, Mechanism and Biochemistry*. Plenum, New York.
6. Omura, T. (1999) Forty years of cytochrome P450. *Biochem. Biophys. Res. Commun.* **266,** 690–698.
7. Rendic, S. and Di Carlo, F. J. (1997) Human cytochrome P450 enzymes: a status report summarizing their reactions, substrates, inducers, and inhibitors. *Drug Metab. Rev.* **29,** 413–580.
8. Cashman, J. R. (2000) Human flavin-containing monooxygenase: substrate specificity and role in drug metabolism. *Curr. Drug Metab.* **1,** 181–191.
9. Mulder, G. J., ed. (1990) *Conjugation Reactions in Drug Metabolism*. Taylor & Francis, London.
10. Radominska-Pandya, A., Czernik, P. J., Little, J. M., Battaglia, and Mackenzie, E. (1999) Structural and functional studies of UDP-glucuronosyltransferase. *Drug Metab. Rev.* **31,** 817–899.

11. King, C. D., Rios, G. R., Green, M. D., and Tephly, T. R. (2000) UDP-glucuronosyltransferases. *Curr. Drug Metab.* **1,** 143–161.
12. Banoglu, E. (2000) Current status of the cytosolic sulfotransferases in the metabolic activation of promutagens and procarcinogens. *Curr. Drug Metab.* **1,** 1–30.
13. Li, A. P. (2001) Screening for human ADME/Tox drug properties in drug discovery. *DDT* **6,** 357–366.
14. White, R. E. (2000) High-throughput screening in drug metabolism and pharmacokinetic support of drug discovery. *Annu. Rev. Pharmacol. Toxicol.* **40,** 133–157.
15. Uetrecht, J. P. (2000) Is it possible to more accurately predict which drug candidates will cause idiosyncratic drug reactions? *Curr. Drug Metab.* **1,** 107–132.
16. Wu, W. N. and McKown, L. A. (2000) Recent advances in biotransformation of cns and cardiovascular agents. *Curr. Drug Metab.* **1,** 255–270.
17. Wu, W. N., McKown, L. A., Yorgey, K. A., and Pritchard, J. F. (1999) In vitro metabolic products of RWJ-34130, an antiarrhythmic agent, in rat liver preparations. *J. Pharm. Biomed. Anal.* **20,** 687–695.
18. McKown, L. A., Wu, W. N., and O'Neill, P. J. (1994) Characterization and identification of the metabolites of fenoctimine using in vitro drug metabolizing systems. *J. Pharm. Biomed. Anal.* **6,** 771–775.
19. Wu, W. N., McKown, L. A., and O'Neill, P. J. (1995) In vitro and in vivo metabolism of the antianxiolytic agent fenobam in the rat. *J. Pharm. Sci.* **84,** 185–189.
20. Wu, W. N., McKown, L. A., Moyer, M. D., Johannsen, T. B., and Takacs, A. R. (1999) In vitro metabolism of mifepristone (RU-486) in rat, monkey and human hepatic S9 fractions: identification of three new mifepristone metabolites. *Xenobiotica* **31,** 1089–1100.
21. Wu, W. N., McKown, L. A., Gauthier, A. D., Jones, W. J., and Raffa, R. B. (2001) Metabolism of the analgesic drug, tramadol hydrochloride, in rat and dog. *Xenobiotica* **31,** 423–441.
22. Wu, W. N., McKown, L. A., and Liao, S. (2002) Metabolism of the analgesic drug, ULTRAM® (tramadol hydrochloride) in humans: api-ms and ms/ms characterization of metabolites. *Xenobiotica* **32,** 411–425.
23. Yan, Z., Caldwell, G. W., Wu, W. N., McKown, L. A., Rafferty, B., Jones, W. J., et al. (2002) In vitro identification of metabolic pathways and cytochrome P450 enzymes involved in the metabolism of etoperidone. *Xenobiotica* **32,** 949–962.
24. Wu, W. N., McKown, L. A., and Reitz, A. B. (2001) In vitro metabolism of the anxiolytic agent, RWJ-52763 in human hepatic S9 fraction [abstract #243]. The 6th International ISSX Meeting. *Drug Metab. Rev.* **33,** 122.
25. Wu, W. N., McKown, L. A., and Reitz, A. B. (2003) In vitro metabolism of the new anxiolytic agent, RWJ-52763 in human hepatic S9 fraction—api-ms/ms identification of metabolites. *J. Pharm. Biomed. Anal.* **31,** 95–102.
26. Wu, W. N., McKown, L. A., and Rybczynski, P. J. (2000) In vitro metabolism of the endocrine agent, RWJ-68025, in rat and human hepatic S9 fraction [abstract #230]. The 10th North American ISSX Meeting. *Drug Metab. Rev.* **32,** 251.

27. Wu, W. N., McKown, L. A., Rybczynski, P. J., and Demarest, K. (2003) Hepatic biotransformation of the new calcium-mimetic agent, RWJ-68025, in the rat and in man—api-ms/ms identification of metabolites. *J. Pharm. Pharmacol.* **55,** 631–637.
28. Tang, C., Hochman, J. H., Ma, B., Subramanian, R., and Vyas, K. P. (2003) Acyl glucuronidation and glucosidation of a new and selective endothelin ETA receptor antagonist in human liver microsomes. *Drug Metab. Dispos.* **31,** 37–45.
29. McKown, L. A., Wu, W. N., and Pritchard, J. F. (1992) In vitro metabolism of McN-4130 (RWJ-34130) in the rat [abstract]. Presented at the AAPS Eastern Regional Meeting.
30. Wu, W. N., Masucci, J. A., Caldwell, G. W., and Carson, J. R. (1998) Excretion and metabolism of the antihypertensive agent, RWJ-26240 (McN-5691) in dogs. *Drug Metab. Dispos.* **26,** 115–125.

12

In Vitro Identification of UDP-Glucuronosyl-transferases (UGTs) Involved in Drug Metabolism

Michael H. Court

Summary

Glucuronidation catalyzed by the UDP-glucuronosyltransferases (UGTs) is a major pathway for drug metabolism and elimination in humans. Identification of the UGTs responsible for glucuronidation of existing and novel drugs will assist in the prediction of adverse reactions resulting from drug–drug interactions or genetic polymorphism. An integrated approach is proposed for UGT reaction phenotyping using recombinant enzymes and human liver microsomes. Described methods include screening of recombinant UGTs for activity, comparative enzyme kinetic analysis, correlations with isoform-selective marker activities, and chemical inhibition. The primary focus is on identification of the well-characterized hepatic UGTs, including UGTs 1A1, 1A4, 1A6, 1A9, 2B7, and 2B15, although a similar approach potentially could be used for the study of extrahepatic tissues, such as the kidney and gastrointestinal tract.

Key Words: UDP-glucuronosyltransferase; UGT; human liver microsomes; in vitro; glucuronide; glucuronidation; phenotype; glucuronidase.

1. Introduction

1.1. Role of Glucuronidation and the UGTs in Drug Metabolism

Glucuronidation represents one of the major pathways for drug metabolism in humans and other mammalian species (for review, *see* **ref. *1***). This reaction is catalyzed by the UDP-glucuronosyltransferases (UGTs) and involves transfer of the sugar group from UDP-glucuronic acid (UDPGA) to a small hydrophobic molecule (aglycone) that most commonly contains a carboxyl, hydroxyl, or nitrogen group. Substrates may include drugs that possess these functional groups or drug metabolites that have had these functional groups

From: *Methods in Pharmacology and Toxicology*
Optimization in Drug Discovery: In Vitro Methods
Edited by: Z. Yan and G. W. Caldwell © Humana Press Inc., Totowa, NJ

generated by other drug-metabolizing enzymes (most frequently by cytochrome P450 mono-oxygenase [CYP]). Although in most instances, glucuronidation results in inactivation of a drug, pharmacologic or toxicologic activation can occur. Examples include morphine-6-glucuronide, which is a more potent opioid agonist than morphine, and the acyl-glucuronides of various nonsteroidal anti-inflammatory and hypolipidemic drugs, which have the potential for adduct formation. **Table 1** compares substrates, possible enzyme-inducing agents, and tissue distribution for the 18 known human UGT isoforms.

1.2. In Vitro Phenotyping of Drug-Metabolizing Enzymes

In vitro reaction phenotyping is now routinely used to identify CYPs responsible for the oxidative metabolism of candidate compounds during the preclinical phase of drug development *(2,3)*. Such information has proven extremely useful in predicting drug–drug interactions as well as high interindividual variability in drug disposition resulting from genetic polymorphism. Drugs that could be problematic in clinical usage, such as compounds that induce or inhibit CYP3A4 or are metabolized exclusively by the highly polymorphic CYP2D6, can be identified relatively early in the development process. Accumulating evidence indicates that drug–drug interactions and genetic polymorphism may also complicate the clinical utility of drugs that are cleared primarily by glucuronidation *(1)*. For example, UGT1A1 has been identified as the principle isoform responsible for glucuronidation of SN-38, the active metabolite of irinotecan (Topotecan®), a novel and highly effective anticancer drug. However, persons with Gilbert's disease, caused by a common genetic polymorphism of UGT1A1 (7–10% of Caucasians), are more likely to show adverse effects of irinotecan, including severe diarrhea and hematologic toxicity *(4)*.

1.3. Strategy to Identify UGTs Relevant to In Vitro Glucuronidation of a Drug

The purpose of this chapter is to provide a methodology that can be used to identify UGT isoforms that are relevant to the metabolism of novel and existing drugs. The primary focus will be identification of the well-characterized hepatic UGTs (UGTs 1A1, 1A4, 1A6, 1A9, 2B7, and 2B15) because the liver is a major site of drug glucuronidation, and the research tools are better developed for these isoforms. However, it is clear that the gastrointestinal tract (contributing to first-pass metabolism) and the kidney are also major sites of glucuronidation for many drugs *(1)*. The strategy used here for UGT phenotyping is based on well-established procedures for the CYPs *(2,3)* with appropriate modifications. Although the available tools for this process are much less well developed, recent work in this and other laboratories have made

Table 1
Substrates, Inducers, and Tissue Distributions of UGT Isoforms in Humans

UGT	Substrates	Inducers	Liver	Kidney	Esophagus	Stomach	Intestine	Lung	Prostate	Testes	Mam. gland	Ovary	Nose	Brain
1A1[a]	Bilirubin, ethinylestradiol, buprenorphine, acetaminophen, SN-38, flavopiridol	Arylhydrocarbons, phenobarbital, rifampicin	+	–	–	–	+							
1A3[a]	Norbuprenorphine, nonsteroidal anti-inflammatory drugs (NSAIDs)		+	–	–	+								
1A4[a]	Tricyclic antidepressants, antipsychotics, antihistamines, Z-4OH-tamoxifen		+	–	–	–	+							
1A5	Not studied		–	–	–	–								
1A6[a]	Planar aromatic compounds, acetaminophen, serotonin	Arylhydrocarbons, antioxidants	+	+	–	+	+	+						+
1A7[a]	Benzo(α)pyrene		–	+	+	–								
1A8[a]	Benzo(α)pyrene, mycophenolic acid, raloxifene		–	–	+	–	+	–	–	–				–
1A9[a]	Bulky phenols, propofol, salicyclic acid, flavopiridol, mycophenolic acid, thyroid hormones	Arylhydrocarbons, antioxidants, PPAR agonists	+	+	+	–	+							
1A10[a]	Mycophenolic acid, raloxifene		–	–	+	+	+	–	–					–

(*Continued*)

Table 1 (*Continued*)
Substrates, Inducers, and Tissue Distributions of UGT Isoforms in Humans

UGT	Substrates	Inducers	Liver	Kidney	Esophagus	Stomach	Intestine	Lung	Prostate	Testes	Mam. gland	Ovary	Nose	Brain
2A1	Multiple, including odorants, menthol, citronellol		–					±					+	±
2B4[a]	Bile acids, hyodeoxycholic acid, codeine		+	±	–			+	+	+	+			
2B7[a]	Opioids, AZT, NSAIDs, epirubicin, catechol estrogens, retinoids, fatty acids	Phenobarbital	+	+	+	–	+	±	–	–	±			+
2B10	Arachidonate metabolites		+	+	+			+	+	+	+			
2B11	Arachidonate metabolites		+	+				+	+	±	+			
2B15[a]	Androgens, flavonoids, S-oxazepam, E-4OH-tamoxifen, 5OH-rofecoxib	Rifampicin	+	+	+	±	+	+	+	+	+			
2B17[a]	Androgens		+	+				+	+	+	+			
2B28	Steroids		+	+		+	+	±	+	+	+	+		

[a]Recombinant UGTs commercially available.

UGTs 1A2, 1A11, and 1A12 are pseudogenes in humans. +, detectable messenger ribonucleic acid (mRNA) (constitutively); –, no detectable mRNA (constitutively); ±, results differ between studies. Blank cells indicate no data.

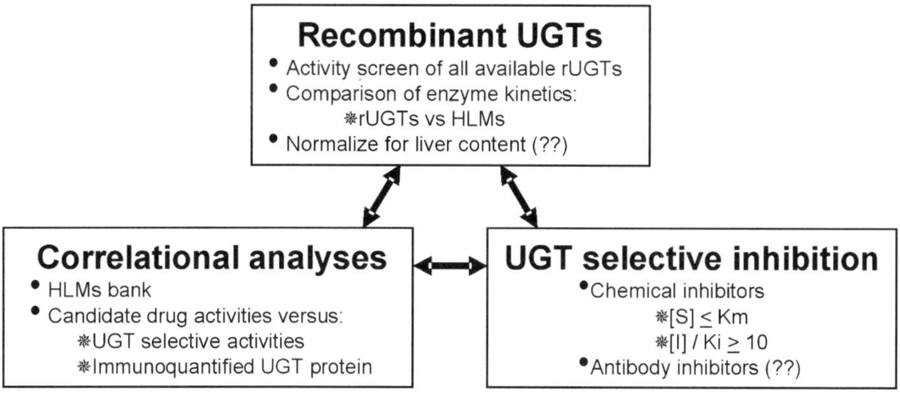

Fig. 1. An integrated approach to the identification of UDP-glucuronosyltransferases mediating glucuronidation of a drug in vitro. "(??)" in figure indicates that these particular methods are not yet practicable because of a lack of appropriate research tools.

substantial progress in this regard. There are essentially three components of this strategy, including the use of recombinant UGTs (rUGTs), correlation analyses, and isoform-selective inhibition, each of which provides complementary and supportive information (*see* **Fig. 1**).

2. Materials

2.1. In Vitro Glucuronidation Assay

1. Candidate drug and glucuronide.
2. Recombinant expressed UGTs (e.g., BD-Gentest, Woburn, MA).
3. Human liver microsomes: pooled and from individuals (e.g., BD-Gentest, Woburn, MA; CellzDirect, Tucson, AZ; Xenotech LLC, Lenexa, KS).
4. High-performance liquid chromatography (HPLC) system equipped with gradient capability, C18 reverse-phase column, and UV absorbance detector (*see* **Note 1**).
5. HPLC mobile phase reagents (*see* **Table 4**).
6. Incubation buffer, 50 m*M* phosphate, pH 7.5 (*see* **Note 2**).
7. UDP-glucuronic acid (cat. no. U6751, Sigma-Aldrich, St. Louis, MO).
8. Magnesium chloride solution (50 m*M* in water).
9. Alamethicin, 2.5 mg/mL of methanol (cat. no. A4665, Sigma-Aldrich, St. Louis, MO).
10. Saccharolactone, 50 m*M* in water (cat. no. S0375, Sigma-Aldrich, St. Louis, MO).
11. *Helix pomatia* β-glucuronidase solution, 100 U/μL (cat. no. G-0762, Sigma-Aldrich, St. Louis, MO).
12. Vacuum oven set at 45°C (*see* **Note 3**).
13. Water bath incubator set at 37°C (*see* **Note 4**).

2.2. UGT Marker Activities

2.2.1. Substrates

1. Estradiol (cat. no. E1024, Sigma-Aldrich, St. Louis, MO).
2. Trifluoperazine (cat. no. T6062, Sigma-Aldrich, St. Louis, MO).
3. Serotonin; 5-hydroxytryptamine (cat. no. H9523, Sigma-Aldrich, St. Louis, MO).
4. Propofol; 2,6-diisopropylphenol (cat. no. W50,510-2, Sigma-Aldrich, St. Louis, MO).
5. Azidothymidine (AZT); 3'-azido-3'-deoxythymidine (cat. no. A2169, Sigma-Aldrich, St. Louis, MO).
6. Oxazepam (cat. no. O5254, Sigma-Aldrich, St. Louis, MO).

2.2.2. Glucuronides

1. Estradiol-3-glucuronide (cat. no. E2127, Sigma-Aldrich, St. Louis, MO).
2. AZT-glucuronide (cat. no. A0679, Sigma-Aldrich, St. Louis, MO).
3. Serotonin glucoronide (NIMH code S-803, NIMH Chemical Synthesis and Drug Supply Program).

2.2.3. Internal Standards

1. Phenacetin (cat. no. A2375, Sigma-Aldrich, St. Louis, MO).
2. Acetaminophen (cat. no. A7085, Sigma-Aldrich, St. Louis, MO).
3. 3-Acetamidophenol (cat. no. A4911, Sigma-Aldrich, St. Louis, MO).
4. Thymol (cat. no. N8280, Sigma-Aldrich, St. Louis, MO).

2.3. Chemical Inhibition

1. Tangeretin; 5,6,7,8,4'-pentamethoxyflavone (Sequoia Research Products, Oxford, UK).
2. Hecogenin (cat. no. H2261, Sigma-Aldrich, St. Louis, MO).
3. 4-Nitrophenol (cat. no. 73560, Sigma-Aldrich, St. Louis, MO).
4. Propofol; 2,6-diisopropylphenol (cat. no. W50,510-2, Sigma-Aldrich, St. Louis, MO).
5. Naproxen (cat. no. N8280, Sigma-Aldrich, St. Louis, MO).

2.4. Data Analyses

1. Graphical computer program capable of nonlinear curve fitting and correlation analyses (e.g., GraphPad Prism v3.00 for Windows, GraphPad Software, San Diego, CA).

3. Methods

3.1. Development of an In Vitro Glucuronidation Assay for the Candidate Drug

The following is a general approach to developing an HPLC-based method to quantify the rate of formation of a glucuronide metabolite using tissue microsomes or recombinant enzyme. A literature search should be conducted prior to starting to determine whether previous assay methods for the substrate and glucuronide have been published and gathering any other useful information (such as UV absorbance wavelength maxima [λ max]). Although not essential, the process is simplified if a small quantity of glucuronide of the candidate drug is available to assist in identifying the appropriate peak on the HPLC chromatogram and enable accurate quantitation. If a glucuronide standard is not available, it can be identified using the methods described below and roughly quantified by reference to a standard curve using the parent compound, assuming similar UV absorbance. For accurate quantitation and identification, milligram amounts of the glucuronide can be synthesized biologically with this system and purified using methods previously described *(5)*.

3.1.1. Initial Assay Method Development

1. The following assumes a 100-μL incubation volume but can be scaled to other volumes.
2. Dissolve substrate and glucuronide in 50 to 100 mL methanol and store in a sealed glass container in a –20°C freezer (*see* **Note 5**).
3. Set up an HPLC apparatus and allow it to equilibrate with 1% solvent A (acetonitrile) and 99% solvent B (20 m*M* potassium phosphate, pH 2.2) at a 1 mL/min flow rate (*see* **Note 6**). Set the UV absorbance detector at the λ max for the glucuronide analyte (*see* **Note 7**).
4. Prepare the UDP-glucuronic acid (UDPGA) cofactor solution on ice in a microcentrifuge tube. For each 100-μL incubation volume, add the following:
   a. 0.645 mg UDPGA (5 m*M* final).
   b. 10 μL 50 m*M* magnesium chloride solution (5 m*M* final).
   c. 10 μL 50 m*M* saccharolactone (optional).
   d. 25 μL 100 m*M* potassium phosphate buffer, pH 7.5.
   e. Balance to 50 μL with water and vortex.
5. Add 100 μL of substrate dissolved in methanol to empty incubation tubes (0.5- or 1.5-mL polypropylene microcentrifuge) and dry down in the vacuum oven.
6. Place incubation tubes on ice and add 50 μg of pooled human liver microsomes (HLM) protein, 2.5 μg alamethicin (2.5 μg/ μL methanol; 50 μg alamethicin/mg microsomal protein) and balance to a volume of 50 μL with 50 m*M* potassium phosphate buffer, pH 7.5 (0.5 mg protein/mL final concentration).
7. Preincubate tubes at 37°C for 5 min.
8. Start reaction by adding 50 μL of UDPGA cofactor solution, mix by gently flicking the tube (do not vortex rUGTs), cap tube, and incubate for up to 6 h.
9. To aid in identifying the glucuronide metabolite peak, also include three negative controls that (1) contain no UDPGA, (2) contain no substrate, and (3) are not incubated, immediately treated with stop solution, vortexed, and centrifuged.
10. Stop reactions with 100 μL of ice-cold acetonitrile, vortex, and centrifuge at 14,000*g* for 10 min. For acyl-glucuronides, the acetonitrile stop solution should

also contain 5% glacial acetic acid to enhance stability.

11. Transfer 190 µL to glass HPLC vials, dry down in a vacuum oven, and reconstitute with 95 µL of water.
12. Analyze 10 to 50 µL of the incubate by HPLC using a solvent gradient program that increases solvent A from 1% to 50% over 20 mins and then to 90% solvent A over the next 5 min (balance with solvent B) (*see* **Note 8**).
13. Chromatogram peaks from the incubate are identified by comparison of peak retention times to reference standards (substrate and glucuronide if available) and negative controls. Glucuronide peaks will be absent in all negative controls (*see* **Note 9**).
14. If an authentic glucuronide standard is not available, the identity of the glucuronide peak should be confirmed by showing sensitivity to glucuronidase treatment or by mass determination (HPLC–mass spectroscopy). Treatment with acids or alkalis can also assist in identification in that acyl-glucuronides tend to hydrolyze under alkaline conditions, whereas some *N*-glucuronides (especially primary amines) tend to hydrolyze when treated with acids. If multiple potential conjugation sites are present on the substrate, determination of the exact site of conjugation will require purification and nuclear magnetic resonance (NMR) analysis.

3.1.2. Confirmation of Metabolite Identity by β-Glucuronidase Treatment

1. Generate glucuronide as in the previous section, but place on ice without adding the stop solution.
2. To 100 µL of incubate, add 10 µL of 100 m*M* potassium phosphate buffer (pH 4.0) to adjust the pH to about 5.0.
3. Add 5 µL (1000 U) of *Helix pomatia* β-glucuronidase solution.
4. Cap tube and incubate overnight.
5. Continue as per **step 10** in previous section and analyze for glucuronide content by HPLC.
6. Confirm glucuronide peak identity by comparison with an untreated matched sample (*see* **Note 10**).

3.1.3. Optimization of the In Vitro Glucuronidation Assay

Once an assay has been developed, it will then be necessary to optimize several parameters to ensure maximal sensitivity while maintaining initial rate conditions. As a general guideline, less than 10% of the initial mass of substrate should be consumed in any incubation. Metabolite formation should be verified to be linear with respect to incubation time and protein concentration at the lowest substrate concentration that will be used. For some slower activities, linearity can be observed for up to 6 h incubation. Compared with CYPs, UGTs generally are much more stable under in vitro incubation conditions. Relatively high protein concentrations (over 1 mg/mL) should be avoided because of nonspecific binding of substrate to microsomes. The amount of alamethicin added to the incubation (usually 20–100 µg/mg of microsomal protein) should also be confirmed to result in maximal activation (usually a two- to threefold increase for HLMs). Alamethicin is a pore-forming antibiotic that activates UGTs by enhancing substrate access to the enzyme active site at the microsomal interior ***(6)***. Saccharolactone (2–10 m*M*) may also be required for some activities to inhibit endogenous β-glucuronidase activity. However, inhibition by saccharolactone has also been observed for some activities ***(7,8)***. Incubate pH can also affect enzymatic activity, but most investigators tend to use a pH within the physiological range (7.0–7.5). Magnesium and UDPGA are essential cofactors that are usually used at saturating concentrations (2–20 m*M*). An internal standard should also be used to enhance HPLC assay precision and accuracy (*see* **Note 11**).

3.2. Glucuronidation by Recombinant UGTs (rUGTs)

Currently, out of the 18 known UGT isoforms, 12 rUGTs are available through commercial sources, including the majority of isoforms expressed in hepatic tissue (*see* **Table 1**). Hepatic isoforms that are not available include UGT2B10 and UGT2B11, which are somewhat restricted in substrate specificity to endogenous arachidonic acid metabolites ***(9)***, and UGT2B28, which may be limited in importance because of aberrant mRNA splicing ***(10)***.

3.2.1. Activity Screen With rUGTs

Initially, all rUGTs should be screened for glucuronidation of the candidate drug using the method developed in the previous section. At least two substrate concentrations should be used, with one concentration approximating the K_m value for HLMs and one concentration 10 times the K_m value. The use of two concentrations will provide preliminary information with regard to the relative affinities of each UGT. Ideally, only one UGT is identified that is capable of glucuronidating the candidate drug, with a K_m value that is identical for both rUGT and HLM preparations (*see* next section), thereby simplifying the identification process. We have recently shown this to be the case for serotonin glucuronidation by HLMs ***(11)***. In most instances, multiple UGTs will show activity, and it will be necessary to try and identify the major isoform responsible for the activity. Unfortunately, direct comparisons of rUGT activities can be misleading because the relative abundance of the hepatic UGTs in liver tissue is currently unknown, and so the contribution of a highly abundant isoform may be underpredicted by the recombinant system. A recent study of UGT mRNA expression in liver by quantitative polymerase chain reaction (PCR) indicates that the relative content of UGT messenger ribonucleic acid (mRNA) is 2B4 > 1A3 > 1A4 > 2B15 > 1A6 > 2B7 > 2B17 > 1A9 > 1A1 ***(12)***. However, there may be differences between isoforms in the extent to which mRNA content reflects UGT protein content and activity.

3.2.2. Comparative Enzyme Kinetic Analysis

Comparison of enzyme kinetic parameters for rUGTs (the most active and those with at least 10% of the most active) with parameters measured for HLMs under identical experimental conditions also assists in isoform identification. Intrinsic clearance values (V_{max}/K_m) can be calculated and compared, but the same stipulations with regard to relative isoform abundance differences between recombinant enzymes and liver apply. Direct comparison of K_m values will help to exclude low-affinity isoforms (K_m for rUGT > HLMs) that are unlikely to contribute to HLM activity substantially and to identify high-affinity isoforms (K_m for rUGT < HLMs) that may contribute significantly at low (clinically relevant) substrate concentrations. The shape of kinetic plots may also assist in identification in that atypical kinetics (such as homotropic activation or substrate inhibition) may be observed for HLMs and also for one of the rUGTs evaluated. High nonspecific binding of substrate to microsomes can be a cause of atypical kinetics and differences in K_m values between HLMs and rUGTs *(3)*. This is most likely to occur with basic and highly lipophilic compounds and at relatively high protein concentrations (>1 mg/mL).

1. At least 10 different substrate concentrations should be used spanning the K_m value determined in preliminary experiments. UDPGA concentration should be saturating (20 m*M*).
2. Determine glucuronidation activities using pooled HLMs and rUGTs with the assay method developed in the previous section (*see* **Note 12**).
3. Evaluate plots of reaction velocity vs substrate concentration (Michaelis-Menten plot) and of reaction velocity divided by substrate concentration versus reaction velocity (Eadie-Hofstee plot) to determine which kinetic models should be used to fit the data. Typical kinetic models include the Michaelis-Menten (**Eq. 1**), Hill (**Eq. 2**), uncompetitive substrate inhibition (**Eq. 3**), and two-enzyme (**Eq. 4**) models.

$$V = V_{max} \times S/(K_m + S) \tag{1}$$

$$V = V_{max} \times S^n/(S_{50}{}^n + S^n) \tag{2}$$

$$V = V_{max} \times S/[K_m + S \times (1 + S/Ks)] \tag{3}$$

$$V = V_{max1} \times S/(K_m1 + S) + V_{max2} \times S/(K_m2 + S) \tag{4}$$

where V is the reaction velocity, S is the substrate concentration, V_{max} is the maximal reaction velocity, K_m and S_{50} are the substrate concentrations at half-maximal velocity, n is an exponent indicative of the degree of curve sigmoidicity, and K_s is an inhibition constant.

4. Fit the kinetic model parameters to the data by nonlinear least squares regression (e.g., GraphPad Prism v3.00 for Windows, GraphPad Software, San Diego, CA).

5. Evaluate the goodness of fit of the kinetic model to the data by overlaying a curve connecting predicted data points with the observed data points. If a model other than **Eq. 1** is used, then choice of that model (over **Eq. 1**) needs to be justified by an objective method such as the F test ($p < 0.05$) or the Akaike information criterion (AIC), which takes into account model complexity.

3.3. Isoform-Selective Glucuronidation Activities

A second approach is to use the intrinsic variability in expression of different UGTs in a bank of HLMs. Isoform-selective marker activities for each of the hepatic UGT isoforms are measured using the HLM bank and then correlated to the glucuronidation activities for the candidate drug measured using the same set of HLMs. The highest correlation should be with the marker activity for the relevant UGT isoform. Although correlations may be observed with HLM banks containing as few as 10 individuals, larger size HLM banks (>20 individuals) are more useful for this purpose. Validated marker activities (*see* **Table 2**) include estradiol-3-glucuronidation (UGT1A1), trifluoperazine glucuronidation (UGT1A4), serotonin glucuronidation (UGT1A6), propofol glucuronidation (UGT1A9), AZT glucuronidation (UGT2B7), and *S*-oxazepam glucuronidation (UGT2B15). Additional supportive evidence may also be provided by correlation to immunoquantified UGT protein content determined by Western blotting, although as yet form-specific antibodies are only available for UGT1A1, 1A6, and 2B7. The main limitation with correlation analysis is significant coregulation of expression of different UGT isoforms. Indeed, a recent study in this laboratory suggests that many of the UGT1A isoforms may be coregulated ***(11)***.

3.3.1. Correlation Analysis

1. Measure glucuronidation activities for the candidate drug using individual HLMs from the HLM bank with the assay method developed in the previous section. The substrate concentration should approximate the K_m value of the drug for pooled HLMs.
2. Measure UGT marker activities in the HLM bank using the incubation parameters given in **Table 3** and the HPLC assay methods outlined in **Table 4**. Incubations with propofol should be performed in glass vials because this compound is highly lipophilic and tends to adsorb to plastic containers. Glucuronides of trifluoperazine, serotonin, propofol, and oxazepam are not currently available commercially and so should be quantitated using standard curves of the parent compound. Oxazepam glucuronidation yields two glucuronide stereoisomers that can be readily separated by HPLC. The *S*-oxazepam glucuronide is the major metabolite that elutes immediately after the *R*-oxazepam glucuronide.
3. Correlate the candidate drug activities with data generated for each of the marker activities using an appropriate computer program (e.g., GraphPad Prism v3.00 for Windows, GraphPad Software, San Diego, CA). Nonparametric Spearman

Table 2
Specificity of Six Glucuronidation Activities Evaluated Using Recombinant UGTs

	Glucuronidation activity (pmol/min/mg protein)					
UGT	Estradiol-3-glucuronidation	Trifluoperazine glucuronidation	Serotonin glucuronidation	Propofol glucuronidation	AZT glucuronidation	*S*-Oxazepam glucuronidation
Vector	0	0	0	0	0	0
1A1[a]	**1069**	0	0	0	0	<1
1A3	210	0	0	0	0	0
1A4[a]	0	**950**	0	0	0	0
1A6[a]	0	0	**2200**	0	0	<1
1A7	0	0	0	301	0	0
1A8	306	0	0	61	0	0
1A9[a]	0	0	0	**1110**	0	0
1A10	114	0	0	84	0	0
2B4	—	—	—	—	19	0
2B7[a]	0	0	0	0	**107**	0
2B15[a]	0	0	0	0	0	**10**
2B17	—	—	—	—	17	0
Reference	***13***	***14***	***11***	Unpublished	Unpublished	***15***

[a]These are considered important hepatic UGT isoforms with regard to drug metabolism.

—, not determined because these isoforms were not available at the time the assays were conducted. Bold numbers indicate the highest value in each column.

Table 3
Details of In Vitro Incubation Methods Used for UGT Marker Activities

Marker activity	Substrate concentration	Protein concentration	Incubation time	Internal sandard
Estradiol-3-glucuronidation	100 μ*M*	0.25 mg/mL	30 min	Phenacetin
Trifluoperazine glucuronidation	200 μ*M*	0.25 mg/mL	30 min	Acetaminophen
Serotonin glucuronidation	4 m*M*	0.05 mg/mL	30 min	Acetaminophen
Propofol glucuronidation	100 μ*M*	0.25 mg/mL	30 min	Thymol
AZT glucuronidation	500 μ*M*	0.5 mg/mL	120 min	3-Acetamidophenol
S-Oxazepam glucuronidation	100 μ*M*	0.5 mg/mL	120 min	Phenacetin

Table 4
Details of HPLC Methods Used to Assay for Glucuronides Generated by UGT Marker Activities

Marker activity	Separation conditions[a]	UV detection wavelength	Glucuronide RT	Substrate RT	IS RT
Estradiol-3-glucuronidation	20–30% Solvent A over 15 min; balance with solvent D	280 nm	9 min: E-3-glu; 10 min: E-17-glu	19 min	13 min
Trifluoperazine glucuronidation	10–70% Solvent A over 20 min; balance with solvent C	254 nm	14 min	15 min	7 min
Serotonin glucuronidation	5% Solvent A for 8 min, 50% Solvent A over 9 min; balance with solvent D	270 nm (225 nm ex/330 nm em[b])	5 min	8 min	14 min
Propofol glucuronidation	20–100% Solvent A over 20 min; balance with solvent D	214 nm	7 min	16 min	14 min
AZT glucuronidation	15% Solvent A for 15 min, 15–50% Solvent A over 10 min; balance with solvent B	266 nm	7 min	11 min	8 min
S-Oxazepam glucuronidation	25% Solvent A for 15 min, 25–60% Solvent A over 10 min; balance with solvent D	214 nm	8 min: *R*-oxaz-glu; 9 min: *S*-oxaz-glu	25 min	17 min

[a]Flow rate is 1 mL/min.

[b]The use of an additional fluorescence detector is optional but provides higher sensitivity and ready identification of serotonin glucuronide. Serially connected UV detector is still needed for quantitation of the internal standard.

RT, retention time; IS, internal standard; ex, excitation; em, emission; solvent A, acetonitrile; solvent B, 20-m*M* potassium phosphate buffer in water, pH 2.2; solvent C, 0.1% trifluoroacetic acid in water; solvent D, 20-m*M* potassium phosphate buffer in water, pH 4.5.

correlation analysis is preferred over the parametric Pearson correlation method because data frequently are not normally distributed. Significant correlations are indicated by Spearman correlation coefficients (*rs*) greater than 0.5 and *p* values less than 0.001.

3.4. Isoform-Selective Inhibition

The final approach is to use UGT isoform-selective inhibitors of HLM activity. None of the chemical inhibitors currently used for the UGTs has been rigorously evaluated for isoform selectivity. Inhibitors that have shown potential for selectivity include tangeritin (IC_{50}, 1 µ*M*), nobiletin, and bilirubin for UGT1A1 ***(16)***; hecogenin (K_i, 11 µ*M*) for UGT1A4 ***(14)***; and suprofen, *S*-flurbiprofen, and naproxen for UGT2B7 (unpublished data). Propofol may also be useful as a UGT1A9 inhibitor, whereas all of the UGT1A6 inhibitors evaluated to date (4-nitrophenol, 1-naphthol, etc.) appear to be nonselective. Inhibitors of UGT2B15 have not been reported.

Inhibition of glucuronidation of the candidate drug should be attempted using both HLMs and rUGTs. Specific inhibition of the relevant UGT would be reflected by equipotent inhibition of both the HLMs and a single rUGT. Nonspecific inhibition would be indicated by equal or greater inhibition of glucuronidation by rUGTs other than those that the inhibitor is intended to affect. Immunoinhibition, although theoretically possible, is not feasible at present because of a lack of commercially available antibodies.

3.4.1. Chemical Inhibition

1. Prepare incubation tubes containing substrate (control activity) and substrate combined with each of the inhibitors. The substrate concentration should approximate the K_m value of the drug for pooled HLMs. Inhibitor concentrations should span a range of at least 3 log orders encompassing the predicted IC_{50} concentration.
2. Measure activities as in the previous section (*see* **Note 13**).
3. Calculate reaction velocities as a percentage of control (i.e., no inhibitor) activity ($V\%$) and derive IC_{50} values by a nonlinear curve-fitting program (e.g., GraphPad Prism v3.00 for Windows, GraphPad Software, San Diego, CA) with **Eq. 5**:

$$V\% = IC_{50}/(I + IC_{50}) \times 100, \tag{5}$$

where I is the inhibitor concentration.

4. Notes

1. Optional enhancements to the basic HPLC system would include a diode array detector, which is useful for glucuronide peak identification, and a fluorescence detector, which provides superior sensitivity for fluorescent compounds such as serotonin. Standard 25-cm × 4.6-mm 5 µ C18 columns work well for most of the described assays.

2. Phosphate buffers need to be refrigerated and checked prior to use for cloudiness, indicative of microbial growth. Tris buffer can be substituted for the phosphate incubation buffer. Slightly higher glucuronidation activities have been reported for Tris vs phosphate ***(17)***. Higher ionic strengths (>50 m*M*) should be avoided because of significant inhibition.
3. Heating to 45°C speeds solvent evaporation. Some compounds, though, may be heat labile. A refrigerated vacuum centrifuge can also be used for this purpose.
4. Agitation of the incubation tubes is not usually necessary unless relatively high incubation volumes (>250 µL) or high protein concentrations (>1 mg/mL) are used.
5. Appropriate working concentrations are about 10 times the K_m value (if known) for the substrate and about the K_m value for the glucuronide. Some glucuronides will not dissolve completely in pure methanol and may require addition of up to 10% water.
6. This is a general HPLC method that we have found useful for initial analysis of glucuronide metabolites. Modifications that may be needed for some analytes include use of a higher pH (4.5 or 7.0) or use of a different buffer (0.1% trifluoroacetic acid).
7. The λ max for the glucuronide can be determined either (1) from published values for the glucuronide (or substrate), (2) by running a UV absorbance scan of the glucuronide (or substrate) with a spectrophotometer, or (3) by using the peak spectral capability of a diode array UV absorbance detector.
8. Once the analyte peaks are positively identified, the HPLC method can be optimized to provide adequate peak separation while minimizing total runtimes. The stability of analytes can be verified by repeated injection of the same sample over the course of the study.
9. The chromatogram "overlay" capability of modern HPLC systems is particularly useful for this purpose. Comparison of peak spectra is also helpful if a diode array UV detector is available. The success of this approach is highly dependent on the consistency of HPLC peak retention times, which should be ensured by proper HPLC pump maintenance.
10. Some glucuronides (such as propofol glucuronide) are resistant to β-glucuronidase treatment. In addition, spontaneous isomerization of some acyl-glucuronides yields a compound that is insensitive to enzymatic hydrolysis.
11. Although it is desirable to use an internal standard that is similar structurally to the analyte, this is usually not necessary if the described direct injection HPLC assay method is used (i.e., no extraction step). The easiest approach to identify an appropriate internal standard is to optimize the HPLC method for the glucuronide and then screen all available compounds for retention times that are similar to but distinct from the analytes. For the assay, the internal standard can be dissolved in the acetonitrile stop solution.
12. Ensure linearity of glucuronidation with respect to time and protein concentration at the lowest substrate concentration used. The amount of glucuronide formed is determined using a standard curve generated by measuring a series of known amounts of glucuronide (or substrate, if glucuronide is unavailable) dissolved in incubation buffer. Recovery of glucuronides from microsomes is usually 100%

but can be checked by comparison of standard curves with and without microsomes.

13. Adjustment of the HPLC method may be necessary because of interfering peaks from the inhibitor and inhibitor metabolites.

References

1. Fisher, M. B., Paine, M. F., Strelevitz, T. J., and Wrighton, S. A. (2001) The role of hepatic and extrahepatic UDP-glucuronosyltransferases in human drug metabolism. *Drug Metab. Rev.* **33,** 273–97.
2. Rodrigues, A. D. (1999) Integrated cytochrome P450 reaction phenotyping: attempting to bridge the gap between cDNA-expressed cytochromes P450 and native human liver microsomes. *Biochem. Pharmacol.* **57,** 465–480.
3. Venkatakrishnan, K., von Moltke, L. L., and Greenblatt, D. J. (2001) Human drug metabolism and the cytochromes P450: application and relevance of in vitro models. *J. Clin. Pharmacol.* **41,** 1149–1179.
4. Iyer, L., Hall, D., Das, S., Mortell, M. A., Ramirez, J., Kim, S., et al. (1999) Phenotype-genotype correlation of in vitro SN-38 (active metabolite of irinotecan) and bilirubin glucuronidation in human liver tissue with UGT1A1 promoter polymorphism. *Clin. Pharmacol. Ther.* **65,** 576–582.
5. Soars, M. G., Mattiuz, E. L., Jackson, D. A., Kulanthaivel, P., Ehlhardt, W. J., and Wrighton, S. A. (2002) Biosynthesis of drug glucuronides for use as authentic standards. *J. Pharmacol. Toxicol. Methods* **47,** 161–168.
6. Fisher, M. B., Campanale, K., Ackermann, B. L., VandenBranden, M., and Wrighton, S. A. (2000) In vitro glucuronidation using human liver microsomes and the pore-forming peptide alamethicin. *Drug Metab. Dispos.* **28,** 560–566.
7. Kemp, D. C., Fan, P. W., and Stevens, J. C. (2002) Characterization of raloxifene glucuronidation in vitro: contribution of intestinal metabolism to presystemic clearance. *Drug Metab. Dispos.* **30,** 694–700.
8. Alkharfy, K. M., and Frye, R. F. (2001) High-performance liquid chromatographic assay for acetaminophen glucuronide in human liver microsomes. *J. Chromatogr. B Biomed. Sci. Appl.* **753,** 303–308.
9. Turgeon, D., Chouinard, S., Belanger, P., Picard, S., Labbe, J. F., Borgeat, P., et al. (2003) Glucuronidation of arachidonic and linoleic acid metabolites by human UDP-glucuronosyltransferases. *J. Lipid Res.* **44,** 1182–1191.
10. Levesque, E., Turgeon, D., Carrier, J. S., Montminy, V., Beaulieu, M., and Belanger, A. (2001) Isolation and characterization of the UGT2B28 cDNA encoding a novel human steroid conjugating UDP-glucuronosyltransferase. *Biochemistry* **40,** 3869–3881.
11. Krishnaswamy, S., Duan, S. X., von Moltke, L. L., Greenblatt, D. J., and Court, M. H. (2003) Validation of serotonin (5-hydroxtryptamine) as an in vitro substrate probe for human UDP-glucuronosyltransferase (UGT) 1A6. *Drug Metab. Dispos.* **31,** 133–139.
12. Congiu, M., Mashford, M. L., Slavin, J. L., and Desmond, P. V. (2002) UDP glucuronosyltransferase mRNA levels in human liver disease. *Drug Metab. Dispos.* **30,** 129–134.

13. Patten, C. J., Code, E. L., Dehal, S. S., Gange, P. V., and Crespi, C. L. (2001) Analysis of UGT enzyme levels in human liver microsomes using form specific anti-peptide antibodies, probe substrate activities and recombinant UGT enzymes [abstract]. *Drug Metab. Rev.* **33,** 165.
14. Dehal, S. S., Gange, P. V., Crespi, C. L., and Patten, C. J. (2001) Characterization of a probe substrate and an inhibitor of UDP-glucuronosyltransferase 1A4 activity in human liver microsomes and cDNA-expressed UGT-enzymes [abstract]. *Drug Metab. Rev.* **33,** 162.
15. Court, M. H., Duan, S. X., Guillemette, C., Journault, K., Krishnaswamy, S., Von Moltke, L. L., et al. (2002) Stereoselective conjugation of oxazepam by human UDP-glucuronosyltransferases (UGTs): S-oxazepam is glucuronidated by UGT2B15, while R-oxazepam is glucuronidated by UGT2B7 and UGT1A9. *Drug Metab. Dispos.* **30,** 1257–1265.
16. Williams, J. A., Ring, B. J., Cantrell, V. E., Campanale, K., Jones, D. R., Hall, S. D., et al. (2002) Differential modulation of UDP-glucuronosyltransferase 1A1 (UGT1A1)-catalyzed estradiol-3-glucuronidation by the addition of UGT1A1 substrates and other compounds to human liver microsomes. *Drug Metab. Dispos.* **30,** 1266–1273.
17. Boase, S. and Miners, J. O. (2002) In vitro–in vivo correlations for drugs eliminated by glucuronidation: investigations with the model substrate zidovudine. *Br. J. Clin. Pharmacol.* **54,** 493–503.

13

In Vitro CYP Induction in Human Hepatocytes

Daniel R. Mudra and Andrew Parkinson

Summary

The processes of modern drug discovery and development rely on the ability to obtain information regarding new chemical entities as quickly and inexpensively as possible. For this reason, laboratories have developed various in vitro techniques that can help to minimize undue investment in developmental compounds that may have undesirable pharmacokinetic properties and/or the potential to cause adverse effects, such as toxicity and drug–drug interactions. The primary culture of human hepatocytes offers a reliable in vitro system to test a compound's ability to induce the expression of cytochrome P450 enzymes, a primary route of metabolism for many pharmaceuticals. The methods in this chapter describe the isolation of primary hepatocytes from nontransplantable human liver followed by their culture and treatment with new chemical entities and/or known inducers of cytochrome P450. Enzyme induction in cultured human hepatocytes can be assessed by measuring the levels of messenger ribonucleic acid, immunoreactive protein, and/or cytochrome P450 enzyme activity as outlined in this chapter.

Key Words: Cell culture; cytochrome P450; drug development; enzyme induction; human hepatocytes; in vitro; liver; microsomes.

1. Introduction

In an effort to minimize unexpected drug–drug interactions caused by a new drug candidate, it has become increasingly important to screen new chemical entities for their ability to induce cytochrome P450 (CYP) and other drug-metabolizing enzymes (as well as drug transporters). Primary hepatocytes isolated from the livers of laboratory animals or from nontransplantable human livers and cultured in a sandwich configuration (i.e., between two layers of extracellular matrix) can be used to assess the P450 induction potential of new

From: *Methods in Pharmacology and Toxicology*
Optimization in Drug Discovery: In Vitro Methods
Edited by: Z. Yan and G. W. Caldwell © Humana Press Inc., Totowa, NJ

drug candidates. When primary hepatocytes are cultured in vitro, in an environment that allows for adequate confluency, cuboidal morphology, and the expression of liver specific functions, the degree of P450 induction caused by known inducers, at clinically relevant concentrations, is comparable (both qualitatively and quantitatively) to that observed following in vivo treatment with the same prototypical inducers ***(1–4)***. Consequently, primary cultures of hepatocytes have become widely accepted in the pharmaceutical industry and by regulatory agencies as the preferred test system to ascertain a chemical's ability to induce cytochrome P450 enzymes ***(5–10)***.

Primary cultures of hepatocytes are also well suited for examining species differences in P450 induction. For example, the antibiotic rifampin induces CYP3A in humans but not in rat or mouse; similarly, the H^+/K^+ adenosine triphosphatase (ATPase) (proton pump) inhibitor omeprazole induces CYP1A in human but not in rat or mouse ***(2,11,12)***. Species differences such as this are often attributable to the specificity with which a compound activates the nuclear receptor (e.g., pregnane X-receptor [PXR]) and genetic response element(s) belonging to a particular species ***(13,14)***. This makes human hepatocytes particularly useful in predicting the potential clinical inductive effects of developmental compounds ***(12,15–19)***. When primary human hepatocytes are seeded on collagen, overlaid with Matrigel®, and cultured for up to 10 d treatment over 2 to 3 d with prototypical inducers, this results in the marked induction of CYP1A (induced by β-naphthoflavone [β-NF], typically 13-fold), CYP2B (induced by phenobarbital and rifampin, typically 6.5- and 13-fold, respectively), and CYP3A (induced by phenobarbital and rifampin, typically 3.3- and 10-fold, respectively) ***(4)***. It should be understood that with any enzyme induction study in human hepatocytes, there is considerable variability in the magnitude of enzyme induction between individual donors. For example, although treatment with β-naphthofalvone causes on average a 13-fold induction of CYP1A2 activity, individual values range from as low as 2.3-fold to as high as 56-fold ***(4)***. Other inducible human cytochrome P450 enzymes include CYP2A6, CYP2C8, CYP2C9, CYP2C19, and CYP2E1. However, the variability of response between individuals tends to be greater with these particular enzymes to the point where no induction of these enzymes may be apparent in preparations of hepatocytes in which other P450 enzymes are inducible ***(4)***. Based on this variability, it is recommended that P450 induction be investigated in hepatocytes from multiple (typically three to five) human donors ***(5–10)***.

The choice of cell culture medium and extracellular matrix can have profound effects on the performance of hepatocyte monolayers, and such is the case with P450 enzyme induction. For example, the induction of CYP2B is highly dependent on matrix composition and medium formulation ***(20,21)***, and the presence of the glucocorticoid dexamethasone appears to be critical in establishing the proper response of several CYP enzymes, including CYP3A ***(22)***. In general, culture media should be properly modified to support hepatocyte-specific functions (e.g., albumin synthesis and CYP induction) and include components such as insulin (6.25 μg/mL), transferrin (6.25 μg/mL), selenous acid (6.35 ng/mL), and dexamethasone (25–100 n*M*).

In most cases, induction of a particular P450 enzyme involves a receptor-mediated increase in gene expression, which can be monitored by measuring the level of messenger ribonucleic acid (mRNA) transcripts, immunoreactive proteins, and/or the metabolism of P450-specific substrates. When analyzing enzymatic activities, it is important to consider species-specific metabolic profiles. For example, the *O*-dealkylation of 7-pentoxyresorufin can be used to monitor CYP2B enzymes in rat but not humans ***(23,24)***; the human CYP2B enzyme is monitored by measuring the hydroxylation of bupropion ***(25)*** or the *N*-demethylation of *S*-mephenytoin ***(26)***. In addition, human P450 enzymes primarily oxidize testosterone in the 6β-position, whereas rat P450 enzymes oxidize testosterone (in a gender-specific manner) to several different metabolites, including 2α-, 6β- 7α-, 16α-, and 16β-hydroxytestosterone ***(27,28)***. The methods described in this chapter highlight several principles, recommended by academic and industrial experts alike ***(3–10,19)***, with respect to in vitro induction studies in human hepatocytes, including the following:

- Removal of nonviable cells from the culture.
- Application of a suitable extracellular matrix (e.g., Matrigel®).
- Use of a 2- to 3-d recovery/adaptation period following hepatocyte isolation to ensure the use of cells that exhibit suitable morphology and confluency.
- Optimization of medium composition to establish liver-specific functions.
- Exposure to vehicle, test compounds, or inducers for up to 3 d.
- Inclusion of prototypical enzyme inducers (e.g., phenobarbital or rifampin) as positive controls in each experiment.
- The use of enzyme activities as the primary measure of cytochrome P450 induction.

Our methods use these principles in describing the steps necessary to (1) perfuse a portion of a previously excised liver, (2) isolate hepatocytes, (3) culture and treat hepatocytes, and (4) harvest cells for subsequent analysis of CYP expression.

2. Materials

2.1. Liver Perfusion

Liver perfusion buffers 1 and 2 (PB-1 and PB-2, respectively) should be prepared according to **Table 1**. Both solutions should be warmed (typically via a shaking water bath) to 37 ± 5°C before use (warming the buffers to a slightly

Table 1
Preparation of Liver Perfusion Buffers

Reagent	Amount	Final concentration (in 2 L)
Perfusion buffer 1		
NaCl	13.8 g	118 m*M*
KCl	0.7 g	4.7 m*M*
KH_2PO_4	0.33 g	1.2 m*M*
$NaHCO_3$	4.2 g	25 m*M*
Glucose	2.0 g	5.5 m*M*
Ethylene glycol-bis (β-aminoethyl ester)-*N*,*N*,*N*',*N*'-tetraacetic acid (EGTA)	0.4 g	0.5 m*M*
Perfusion buffer 2		
NaCl	13.8 g	118 m*M*
KCl	0.7 g	4.7 m*M*
KH_2PO_4	0.33 g	1.2 m*M*
$NaHCO_3$	4.2 g	25 m*M*
Glucose	2.0 g	5.5 m*M*
$CaCl_2$	4.0 mL of 1.0 *M* solution	2.0 m*M*
$MgSO_4$	2.4 mL of 1.0 *M* solution	1.2 m*M*

higher temperature, e.g., 43 ± 5°C, will allow for any loss in temperature when the buffers reach the core of the organ that is often well below room temperature). Any remaining volumes should be stored at 4°C.

2.2. Hepatocyte Isolation

2.2.1. Dulbecco's Modified Eagle's Medium

Dissolve two packages (13.4 g/package) of Dulbecco's modified Eagle's medium (DMEM) without phenol red (Gibco BRL, Grand Island, NY) in approx 1.8 L of water. Add 7.4 g $NaHCO_3$, 20 mL of 200 m*M* GlutaMAX-1 (Gibco BRL, Grand Island, NY), and 20 mL of 10 m*M* minimal essential media–nonessential amino acids (MEM-NEAA; Gibco BRL, Grand Island, NY) to approx 1.8 L of water. Adjust the pH to 7.4 with sodium hydroxide or hydrochloric acid as needed and adjust the final volume to 2 L with water. (Final concentrations: 44 m*M* $NaHCO_3$, 2 m*M* GlutaMAX-1, 0.1 m*M* MEM-NEAA.) Filter-sterilize and store up to 6 mo at 4°C. Medium must be supplemented before use.

Supplementation of DMEM (DMEM+). Add the following to 500 mL DMEM: 25 mL fetal bovine serum (FBS, heat inactivated), 781 µL of 4 mg/mL insulin, 5 mL of penicillin-streptomycin (5000 U/mL penicillin, 5000 µg/mL streptomycin), 50 µL of 10 m*M* dexamethasone in dimethylsulfoxide (DMSO). (Final concentrations: 5% (v/v) FBS, 6.25 µg/mL insulin, 50 U/mL penicillin, 50 µg/mL streptomycin, 1 µ*M* dexamethasone.) Store for up to 1 mo at 4°C. *Note: DMEM and DMEM⁺ are light sensitive and should be stored in a dark environment.*

2.3. Hepatocyte Culture and Treatment

2.3.1. Collagen-Coated Culture Dishes

Prepare a 3.33% (v/v) solution of Vitrogen 100™ (Cohesion Technologies, Palo Alto, CA) dissolved in 1-cyclohexyl-3-(2-morpholino-ethyl) carbodiimide metho-p-toluenesulfonate (MCDI, 130 µg/mL). Deliver 2 mL of this solution to each 60-mm Permanox Petri dish. Swirl to cover the entire bottom of the dish. Incubate for at least 6 h but no more than 12 h at 37 ± 1°C in a humidified chamber with 95%/5% (air/CO_2), then aspirate the MCDI/Vitrogen solution and replace with sterile 1X PBS (to maintain sterility, 1X PBS containing penicillin-streptomycin can be used). Repeat the rinse step. Leave the second 1X PBS wash on the dishes and store them for up to 3 mo at 37 ± 1°C in a humidified chamber with 95%/5% (air/CO_2). Check 1X PBS levels on a regular basis and replenish the 1X PBS as needed. Discard dishes if 1X PBS has dried on any area of the dish. Dishes should be prepared and handled in a biohazard safety cabinet to maintain sterility.

2.3.2. Modified Chee's Medium (MCM)

Dissolve two packages (19.1 g/package) of modified Chee's medium (MCM) without phenol red (Gibco BRL, Grand Island, NY) in approx 1.8 L of water. Add 4.4 g $NaHCO_3$, 0.336 g L-arginine, 1.17 g L-glutamine, and 0.02 g thymidine to approx 1.8 L of water. Adjust the pH to 7.4 with sodium hydroxide or hydrochloric acid as needed and adjust the final volume to 2 L with water. (Final concentrations: 26.2 m*M* $NaHCO_3$, 965 µ*M* L-arginine, 4 m*M* L-glutamine, 41 µ*M* thymidine.) Filter-sterilize and store up to 6 mo at 4°C. Medium must be supplemented before use.

Supplementation of MCM (MCM+). Add the following to 500 mL MCM: 5 mL of ITS⁺ (Fisher Scientific, Pittsburgh, PA), 5 mL of penicillin-streptomycin (5000 U/mL penicillin, 5000 µg/mL streptomycin), and 5 µL of 10 m*M* dexamethasone in DMSO. (Final concentrations: 6.13 µg/mL insulin, 6.13 µg/mL tranferrin, 6.23 ng/mL selenous acid, 50 U/mL penicillin, 50 µg/mL streptomycin, 0.1 µ*M* dexamethasone.) Store for up to 1 mo at 4°C.

2.4. Harvest

2.4.1. Homogenization Buffer (pH 7.4)

To prepare 2 L of the homogenization buffer, add the following reagents to approx 1.8 L of water to the final concentrations indicated: Tris-HCl (50 m*M*), potassium chloride (150 m*M*), and ethylenediaminetetraacetic acid, tetrasodium salt (EDTA, pH 7.4 [at room temperature], 2 m*M*). After preparation, verify that the pH is approx 7.4 at ~4°C and store for up to 2 mo at 4°C in a polypropylene, polyethylene, or glass container.

3. Methods

3.1. Liver Perfusion

1. If possible, insert a single perfusion line into the exposed blood vessels. In the case of a cut portion of a liver, it may be necessary to use the plastic cannula from a surgical catheter (or equivalent) to access the portal vein. Use up to four cannulae and attach each cannula to a branch of the perfusion tubing.
2. Seal any remaining vessels on the face of the liver with medical adhesive and allow the adhesive to set for the time indicated by the manufacturer (*see* **Note 1**).
3. Start the perfuser at a slow flow rate and gradually increase to between 100 and 500 mL/min.
4. Maintain perfusion with oxygenated PB-1 for 10 to 20 min.
5. Add collagenase type I (Worthington, Freehold, NJ) (approx 90 U/mL) to PB-2.
6. Switch the perfusion apparatus to deliver oxygenated PB-2 containing collagenase.
7. Maintain perfusion with PB-2 (with collagenase) for 10 to 20 min (if desired, the waste collected during this step may be recirculated through the perfusion apparatus).
8. Slowly decrease the flow rate on the perfusion apparatus and cease the perfusion.
9. Place the digested liver in an autoclaved or presterilized container for cell isolation.

3.2. Hepatocyte Isolation

Perform the following steps in a sterile environment:

1. Dispense DMEM$^+$ onto the digested liver such that 75% to 100% of the tissue is covered with medium.
2. Release the hepatocytes into the surrounding medium by tearing Glisson's capsule (outer membrane) using sterile surgical instruments (*see* **Note 2**).
3. Filter the suspension using a sterile 100-mesh nylon net or, for suspensions of 300 mL or larger, a dual layer of sterile cheesecloth.
4. Divide the filtered suspension between several presterilized centrifuge tubes (approximate 50-mL capacity recommended) (*see* **Note 3**).
5. Centrifuge at 40 to 60*g* for 3 ± 1 min at room temperature.
6. Discard the supernatant fraction by aspiration and add a small volume of DMEM$^+$ (5–10 mL) to each cell pellet and gently resuspend the cells.

7. Prepare a dilution (8:1:1 (v/v/v)) of PBS, Trypan blue (0.04% (v/v), Sigma Chemical Co., St. Louis, MO), and the cell suspension (*see* **Note 4**).
8. Count hepatocytes using a bright field light microscope and a hemocytometer.
9. Add isotonic percoll (Sigma Chemical Co., St. Louis, MO) to obtain a final percoll concentration of 15% to 25% (v/v) and gently mix by inversion (*see* **Note 5**).
10. Centrifuge at 40 to 60*g* for 5 ± 1 min at room temperature.
11. Discard the supernatant fraction by aspiration and add a small volume of DMEM$^+$ (5–10 mL) to each cell pellet and gently resuspend.
12. Combine all remaining cells into one tube, if possible (*see* **Note 6**).
13. Centrifuge at 40 to 60*g* for 3 ± 1 min at room temperature.
14. Discard the supernatant fraction by aspiration.
15. Add a small volume of DMEM$^+$ and resuspend gently.
16. Combine cell suspension into one vessel.
17. Prepare a dilution (8:1:1 [v/v/v]) of PBS, Trypan blue solution, and the resuspended cell suspension.
18. Count hepatocytes with a hemocytometer and a bright field microscope.

3.3. Hepatocyte Culture and Treatment

Perform the following steps in a sterile environment:

1. Dilute cells with DMEM$^+$ to 1.0–2.0 × 10^6 hepatocytes/mL (*see* **Note 7**).
2. Add 3 ± 0.5 mL of cell suspension in each culture dish (*see* **Note 8**).
3. Place hepatocytes in a humidified chamber at 37 ± 1°C with 95%/5% air/CO_2 and allow the cells to attach for 2 to 3 h (*see* **Note 9**).
4. Following the 2- to 3-h attachment period, swirl culture dishes and aspirate the medium containing unattached cells. Be gentle with the cells, however; be sure to swirl the dish sufficiently to suspend any unattached cells.
5. Add 3 mL of ice-cold, supplemented Chee's medium (MCM$^+$) containing 0.2 to 0.3 mg/mL Matrigel® (Fisher Scientific, Pittsburgh, PA) to each dish and return cultures to the humidified chamber (37 ± 1°C).
6. Replace media with 3 mL fresh MCM$^+$ (without Matrigel®) within 12 to 24 h.
7. Change MCM$^+$ on a daily basis (i.e., within 20–28 h).
8. After 2 to 3 d, if the hepatocytes exhibit near-normal morphology and adequate confluency (*see* **Note 10**), they may be exposed to chemicals (i.e., test compounds) for the purposes of investigating P450 induction.
9. Following evaluation of the cells for use in the in vitro enzyme induction study, cells should be treated with test compounds on a daily basis for 2 to 3 d.
10. To treat hepatocytes, spike media (MCM$^+$) with test compounds solubilized in a solvent (*see* **Notes 11** and **12**).
11. The media containing test compound should be removed and replaced with fresh media (also containing test compound) on a daily basis (e.g., 20–28 h) for the duration of the treatment period (typically 2–3 d).

3.4. Cell Harvest

The following steps *need not* be performed in a sterile environment:

1. Harvest hepatocytes at the end of the culture/treatment period by discarding media from dishes and rinsing the cells two to three times with 0.25 to 1.0 mL/dish ice-cold 1X PBS, being careful not to dislodge the cells. This step ensures that any unbound test article and media components will be washed away.
2. Invert the culture dish to allow excess 1X PBS to drain.
3. For preparation of microsomal samples, add 0.25 to 1.0 mL/dish of ice-cold homogenization buffer to dishes from each group. Preparation of other subcellular fractions (e.g., mRNA) may require the use of alternate buffers and reagents.
4. Scrape each dish with a rubber policeman and collect cells; cells from the same group may be pooled.
5. The collected cells may be analyzed for mRNA analysis or levels and activities of cytosolic and/or microsomal enzyme activities (*see* **Note 13**).

4. Notes

1. For best results, apply a sufficient amount of medical adhesive to seal all cut portions of the liver. This will increase the internal vascular pressure, leading to increased perfusion efficiency.
2. Depending on the efficiency of tissue digestion, scissors or knives may be employed to cut the tissue into fine pieces.
3. Optimal cell pellets will be obtained, provided the cell concentration does not exceed 7×10^6 cells/mL.
4. To obtain an accurate cell count, it is critical that the cell suspension from which the aliquot is taken be homogeneous. To obtain the most homogeneous suspension possible, gently manipulate the solution within the centrifuge tube and verify the homogeneity by visual inspection immediately prior to removing the counting aliquot.
5. Do not exceed 5 mL of the cell pellet in one 50-mL centrifuge tube. Divide the cell suspension into additional tubes if necessary.
6. Do not exceed 10 mL of pellet in one 50-mL centrifuge tube.
7. The concentration of cells is dependent on the viability and total number of dishes needed. In general, a cell preparation with a lower viability can benefit from culturing at a higher cell density.
8. For optimal attachment and survival in culture, hepatocytes should be seeded on culture dishes containing a collagen substratum. Coated culture dishes may be purchased commercially, but for best results, we recommend that Permanox-style culture dishes (60-mm dishes) (Fisher Scientific, Pittsburgh, PA) be custom coated according to the procedure in **Subheading 2.3.**
9. For optimal dispersion of cells, it is recommended to gently swirl each culture dish in a "figure 8" pattern approx 3 to 4 times before placing in the incubator.
10. In most cases, primary cultures of hepatocytes are maintained for 2 to 3 d before initiating experiments with inducers. In vitro induction studies should have only

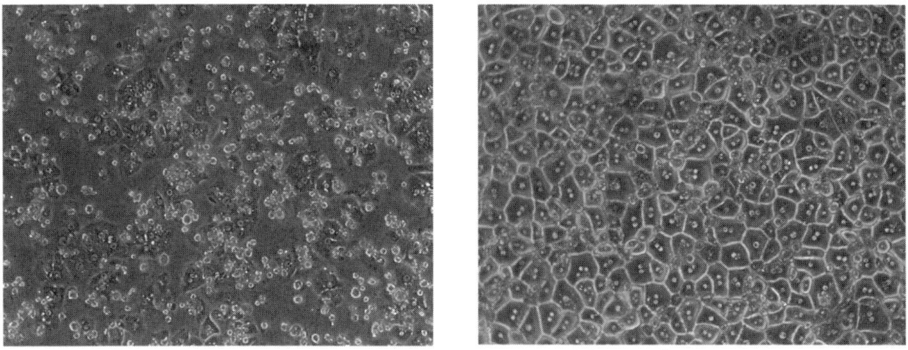

Poor confluency   Acceptable confluency

Fig. 1. Cultured primary human hepatocytes.

hepatocyte cultures that exhibit "acceptable confluency" (*see* **Fig. 1**). Cells with "poor confluency" will likely not exhibit the hepatocyte-specific functions required for reliable analysis of P450 induction profiles and should not be used in P450 induction studies.

11. It is expected to have a high degree of variability of response between human donors. Depending on the enzyme in question, this may result in differing magnitudes of response (i.e., fold-induction) and/or absolute rates of enzymatic activity (measured as pmol/mg/min or similar units). For this reason, it is imperative that the proper positive control inducers be included with each experiment. **Table 2** provides a guideline of known inducers for each human P450 enzyme and the appropriate concentration with which to treat cultured hepatocytes.
12. DMSO is the recommended solvent for delivery of the inducer (i.e., test compound). Treatment of human hepatocytes with DMSO has been shown to cause induction of CYP3A4 *(3)*. Therefore, to avoid elevated P450 activities (e.g., CYP3A) in treated cultures, the final vehicle (DMSO) concentration should not exceed 0.1% (v/v).
13. The following are recommended methods for preparation and measurement of microsomal cytochrome P450 from cultured hepatocytes.

Method	Literature reference
Preparation of microsomes from cultured hepatocytes	***3,4,18***
7-Ethoxyresorufin *O*-dealkylation (a marker for CYP1A2)	***4,23,24,29***
Burpoprion hydroxylation (a marker for CYP2B6)	***25***
Diclofenac 4-hydroxylation (a marker for CYP2C9)	***4,29***
S-Mephenytoin 4'-hydroxylation (a marker for CYP2C19)	***4,26,29***
Testosterone 6β-hydroxylation (a marker for CYP3A4/5)	***4,27,28,29***
Western immunoblot	***30,31***
Measurement of mRNA using branched DNA technology	***32***

Table 2
Prototypical Inducers of Human Cytochrome P450 Enzymes

Human cytochrome P450 ezyme	Prototypical inducer[a]	Treatment concentration to obtain maximal induction[a]
CYP1A2	β-Naphthoflavone	33 μ*M*
	Omeprazole	100 μ*M*
CYP2A6[b]	Phenobarbital[b]	750 μ*M*[b]
	Rifampin[b]	20 μ*M*[b]
CYP2B6	Phenobarbital	750 μ*M*
	Rifampin	20 μ*M*
CYP2C9	Rifampin	20 μ*M*
CYP2C19	Rifampin	20 μ*M*
CYP2E1	Isoniazid[c]	100 μ*M*
CYP3A4	Phenobarbital	750 μ*M*
	Rifampin	20 μ*M*

[a]Sources: **refs. *4*, *11*, *13***, and ***21***.

[b]Variance in enzymatic rates in individual human liver microsomes suggests that CYP2A6 is an inducible enzyme ***(11,22)***, but no optimal prototypical inducer of this enzyme has yet been identified.

[c]It is expected that, on average, hepatocyte cultures from only about one-half of human donors will respond to isoniazid with induction of CYP2E1 ***(10)***.

References

1. Abdel-Rahman, S. M. and Leeder, S. J. (2000) Drugs as inducers of metabolic enzymes: phenobarbital, phenytoin, and carbamezine, in *Metabolic Drug Interactions*, (Levy, R. H., Thummel, K. E., Trager, W. F., et al., eds.), Lippincott Williams & Wilkins, Philadelphia, pp. 673–690.
2. Jang, G. R. and Maurel, P. J. P. (2000) Drugs as inducers of metabolic enzymes: rifampin, dexamethasone, and omeprazole, in *Metabolic Drug Interactions*, (Levy, R. H., et al., eds.), Lippincott Williams & Wilkins, Philadelphia, pp. 691–705.
3. LeCluyse, E., Madan, A., Hamilton, G., Carroll, K., DeHaan, R., and Parkinson, A. (2000) Expression and regulation of cytochrome P450 enzymes in primary cultures of human hepatocytes. *J. Biochem. Mol. Toxicol.* **14,** 177–188.
4. Madan, A., Graham, R. A., Carroll, K. M., Mudra, D. M., Burton, L. A., Krueger, L. A., et al. (2003) Effects of prototypical microsomal enzyme inducers on cytochrome P450 expression in cultured human hepatocytes. *Drug Metab. Dispos.* **31,** 421–431.
5. Tucker, G. T., Houston, J. B., and Huang, S.-M. (2001) Optimizing drug development: strategies to assess drug metabolism/transporter interaction potential—toward a consensus. *Pharm. Res.* **18,** 1071–1080.
6. Tucker, G. T., Houston, J. B., and Huang, S.-M. (2001) Optimizing drug development: strategies to assess drug metabolism/transporter interaction potential—toward a consensus. *Clin. Pharmacol. Ther.* **70,** 103–114.

7. Tucker, G. T., Houston, J. B., and Huang, S.-M. (2001) Optimizing drug development: strategies to assess drug metabolism/transporter interaction potential—toward a consensus. *Br. J. Clin. Pharmacol.* **52,** 107–117.
8. Tucker, G. T., Houston, J. B., and Huang, S.-M. (2001) Optimizing drug development: strategies to assess drug metabolism/transporter interaction potential—toward a consensus. *Eur. J. Pharm. Sci.* **13,** 417–428.
9. Bjornsson, T. D., Callaghan, J. T., Einolf, H. J., Fischer, V., Gan, L., Grimm, S., et al. (2003) The conduct of in vitro and in vivo drug-drug interaction studies: a Pharmaceutical Research and Manufacturers of America (PhRMA) perspective. *Drug Metab. Dispos.* **31,** 815–832.
10. Bjornsson, T. D., Callaghan, J. T., Einolf, H. J., Fischer, V., Gan, L., Grimm, S., et al. (2003) The conduct of in vitro and in vivo drug-drug interaction studies: a PhRMA perspective. *J. Clin. Pharmacol.* **43,** 443–469.
11. Shih, H., Pcikwell, G. V., Guenette, D. K., Bilir, B., and Quattrochi, L. C. (1999) Species differences in hepatocyte induction of CYP1A1 and CYP1A2 by omeprazole. *Hum. Exp. Toxicol.* **18,** 95–105.
12. Lu, C. and Li, A. P. (2001) Species comparison in P450 induction: effects of dexamethasone, omeprazole, and rifampin on P450 isoforms 1A and 3A in primary cultured hepatocytes from man, Sprague-Dawley rat, minipig and beagle dog. *Chem. Biol. Interact.* **134,** 271–281.
13. Jones, S. A., Moore, L. B., Shenk, J. L., Wisely, G. B., Hamilton, G. A., McKee, D. D., et al. (2000) The pregnane X receptor: a promiscuous xenobiotic receptor that has diverged during evolution. *Mol. Endocrinol.* **14,** 27–39.
14. LeCluyse, E. L. (2001) Pregnane X receptor: molecular basis for species differences in CYP3A induction by xenobiotics. *Chem. Biol. Interact.* **134,** 283–289.
15. Diaz, D., Fabre, I., Daujat, M., Saint Aubert, B., Bories, P., Michel, H., et al. (1990) Omeprazole is an aryl hydrocarbon-like inducer of human hepatic cytochrome P450. *Gastroenterology* **99,** 737–747.
16. Pichard, L., Fabre, I., Fabre, G., Domergue, J., Saint Aubert, B., Mourad, G., et al. (1990) Cyclosporin A drug interactions: screening for inducers and inhibitors of cytochrome P-450 (cyclosporin A oxidase) in primary cultures of human hepatocytes and in liver microsomes. *Drug Metab. Dispos.* **18,** 595–606.
17. Curi-Pedrosa, R., Daujat, M., Pichard, L., Ourlin, J. C., Clair, P., Gervot, L., et al. (1994) Omeprazole and lansoprazole are mixed inducers of CYP1A and CYP3A in human hepatocytes in primary culture. *J. Pharmacol. Exp. Ther.* **269,** 384–392.
18. Robertson, P., DeCory, H. H., Madan, A., and Parkinson, A. (2000) In vitro inhibition and induction of human hepatic cytochrome P450 enzymes by modafinil. *Drug Metab. Dispos.* **28,** 664–671.
19. LeCluyse, E. (2001) Human hepatocyte culture systems for the in vitro evaluation of cytochrome P450 expression and regulation. *Eur. J. Pharm. Sci.* **13,** 343–368.
20. Sidhu, J. S., Farin, F. M., and Omiecinski, C. J. (1993) Influence of extracellular matrix overlay on phenobarbital-mediated induction of CYP2B1, 2B2, and 3A1 genes in primary adult rat hepatocyte culture. *Arch. Biochem. Biophys.* **301,** 103–113.
21. LeCLuyse, E., Bullock, P., Madan, A., Carroll, K., and Parkinson, A. (1999) Influence of extra-cellular matrix overlay and medium formulation on the induc-

tion of cytochrome P450 2B in primary cultures of rat hepatocytes. *Drug Metab. Dispos.* **27,** 909–915.

22. Pascussi, J. M., Drocourt, L., Gerbal-Chaloin, S., Fabre, J. M., Maurel, P., and Vilarem, M. J. (2001) Dual effect of dexamethasone on CYP3A4 gene expression in human hepatocytes: sequential role of glucocorticoid receptor and pregnane X receptor. *Eur. J. Biochem.* **268,** 6346–6358.
23. Burke, M. D. and Mayer, R. T. (1974) Ethoxyresorufin: direct fluorimetric assay of a microsomal O-dealkylation which is preferentially inducible by 3-methylcholanthrene. *Drug Metab. Dispos.* **2,** 583–588.
24. Burke, M. D., Thompson, S., Weaver, R. J., Wolf, C. R., and Mayer, R. T. (1994) Cytochrome P450 specificities of alkoxyresorufin O-dealkylation in human and rat liver. *Biochem. Pharmacol.* **48,** 923–936.
25. Faucette, S. R., Hawke, R. L., Lecluyse, E. L., Shord, S. S., Yan, B., Laethem, R. M., et al. (2000) Validation of bupropion hydroxylation as a selective marker of human cytochrome P450 2B6 catalytic activity. *Drug Metab. Dispos.* **28,** 1222–1230.
26. Meier, U. T., Dayer, P., Male, P. J., Kronbach, T., and Meyer, U. A. (1985) Mephenytoin hydroxylation polymorphism: characterization of the enzymatic deficiency in liver microsomes of poor metabolizers phenotyped in vivo. *Clin. Pharmacol. Ther.* **38,** 488–494.
27. Sonderfan, A. J., Arlotto, M. P., Dutton, D. R., McMillen, S. K., and Parkinson, A. (1987) Regulation of testosterone hydroxylation by rat liver microsomal cytochrome P-450. *Arch. Biochem. Biophys.* **255,** 27–41.
28. Sonderfan, A. J. and Parkinson, A. (1988) Inhibition of steroid 5 alpha-reductase and its effects on testosterone hydroxylation by rat liver microsomal cytochrome P-450. *Arch. Biochem. Biophys.* **265,** 208–218.
29. Pearce, R. E., McIntyre, C. J., Madan, A., Sanzgiri, U., Draper, A. J., Bullock, P. L., et al. (1996) Effects of freezing, thawing, and storing human liver microsomes on cytochrome P450 activity. *Arch. Biochem. Biophys.* **331,** 145–169.
30. Laemmli, U. K. (1970) Cleavage of structural proteins during the assembly of the head of bacteriophage T4. *Nature* **227,** 680–685.
31. Towbin, H., Staehelin, T., and Gordon, J. (1979) Electrophoretic transfer of proteins from polyacrylamide gels to nitrocellulose sheets: procedure and some applications. *Proc. Natl. Acad. Sci. USA* **76,** 4350–4354.
32. Czerwinski, M., Opdam, P., Madan, A., Carroll, K., Mudra, D. R., Gan, L. L., et al. (2002) Analysis of CYP mRNA expression by branched DNA technology. *Methods Enzymol.* **357,** 170–179.

14

High-Throughput Screening of Human Cytochrome P450 Inhibitors Using Fluorometric Substrates

Methodology for 25 Enzyme/Substrate Pairs

David M. Stresser

Summary

This chapter provides a detailed description of methodology used to assess the cytochrome P450 inhibition potential of small molecules using fluorometric substrates in a multiwell plate format. Inhibition of cytochromes P450 can result in drug–drug interactions or, in some cases, therapeutic benefit. Because of the safety and economic concerns (clinical failure or product withdrawal), screening of drug candidates for cytochrome P450 inhibition potential is nowadays conducted much earlier in the drug development process. At this stage, much larger numbers of drug candidates are in need of evaluation. Thus, safety, economic, and throughput pressures have forced the development of assays that are rapid throughput but have high predictive value. Fluorometric assays incorporating recombinant human enzymes are ideally suited for this purpose.

Key Words: P450s; CYPs; inhibition.

1. Introduction

1.1. Biological Importance of Cytochrome P450 Inhibition

Cytochrome P450 (CYP) is a superfamily of heme-containing enzymes *(1)* that mediates the metabolism and inactivation of many drugs but can also generate toxicologically or hormonally active metabolites from exogenous or endogenous molecules *(2,3)*. Drugs that inhibit cytochromes P450 may cause the toxic accumulation of a coadministered drug (or itself), resulting in a drug-drug interaction *(4)*. Inhibition of cytochrome P450 by drugs or other

From: *Methods in Pharmacology and Toxicology*
Optimization in Drug Discovery: In Vitro Methods
Edited by: Z. Yan and G. W. Caldwell © Humana Press Inc., Totowa, NJ

xenobiotics can also affect endogenous molecule metabolism. This can result in therapeutic benefit *(5)* but might also disrupt endocrine homeostasis *(6,7)*.

1.2. Fluorometric Cytochrome P450 Inhibition Assays: Concepts

Over the past decade, economic and competitive pressures as well as technological advances in robotics, chemistry, and genetic engineering have driven the development of high-throughput drug metabolism and pharmacokinetic screening methods *(8,9)*. A fluorometric, microplate method to screen for inhibition of the major human drug-metabolizing CYPs was published in 1997 by Crespi et al. *(10)*, capitalizing on earlier advances in fluorescent CYP probe development *(11)*, genetic engineering *(12)*, and plate-based CYP fluorometric assays *(13)*. Since then, the assay has been optimized, validated, and expanded to include many other enzyme/substrate pairs *(14–29)*, including CYP enzymes involved in carcinogen and endogenous molecule metabolism. The cornerstone of these assays is the use of a "surrogate" substrate representing a coadministered drug or endogenous substrate. Surrogates are necessary because it is not practical to test all possible drug–drug or drug–endobiotic pairings that an individual may encounter. Substrates that yield a fluorescent metabolite offer a means of measuring CYP activity (and thus inhibition of activity) in vitro without the need for chromatography. Most fluorometric substrates are metabolized by more than one P450 isoform present in human liver *(30)*. Therefore, the use of complementary deoxyribonucleic acid (cDNA)-expressed enzymes allows an assessment of inhibition potential against a single enzyme without the complications of having other enzymes present that may metabolize the substrate or drug candidate.

1.3. Getting Started

The commercial availability of CYP inhibition assay kits has greatly facilitated establishing the assay for the beginner (e.g., BD Biosciences, Woburn, MA; Panvera, Madison, WI) and may be the simplest way to get started. Kits available from our laboratory contain all components necessary to perform the assay except acetonitrile (or, with fluorescein substrates, sodium hydroxide solution) and multiwell plates. Kits also include detailed instruction manuals that will not be duplicated here. However, not all enzyme/substrate pairings are available in kit form. Therefore, the methodology described below is designed for researchers interested in a wider range of enzyme/substrate pairings or those who wish to obtain assay components individually. It is strongly recommended to review the methodology in its entirety before beginning experimental work.

2. Materials

2.1. Assay Components and Consumables

1. 0.5 *M* Potassium phosphate buffer, pH 7.4, or 0.5 *M* Tris-HCl, pH 7.5, stored at room temperature.
2. cDNA-expressed cytochrome P450 (BD Supersomes™ enzymes, BD Biosciences), stored at –80°C.
3. Insect cell "control" protein (BD Biosciences), stored at –80°C.
4. Fluorometric substrates (BD Biosciences). A list of substrates and suggested stock concentrations prepared in acetonitrile is shown in **Table 1**.
5. Metabolites for each substrate (BD Biosciences). A list of metabolites and their excitation and emission properties is shown in **Table 1**.
6. 20X Cofactors solution (a "20X" solution refers to a solution that requires a 20-fold dilution to obtain the final concentration in the assay).

   Cofactor solution "20/20." This solution contains 20 mg nicotinamide adenine dinucleotide phosphate (NADP+) (*see* **Note 1**), 20 mg glucose-6-phoshate, and 13.3 mg magnesium chloride hexahydrate per 1 mL of distilled water. This solution may be purchased (BD Biosciences) or prepared by making a single reagent solution in water, using the resultant solution in place of water for the second reagent, and then using this resultant solution in place of water for the third reagent. Store at –20°C.

   Cofactor solution "1/20." For CYP2D6 and CYP2A6 assays, prepare the same solution but reduce by 20-fold the amount of NADP+ added.
7. Glucose-6-phosphate dehydrogenase (G6PDH) solution (100X).

   This solution contains 40 U G6PDH (type XV) per milliliter of 5 m*M* sodium citrate. This solution may be purchased (BD Biosciences) or prepared. Store at –20°C.
8. Incubator or heating platforms capable of heating to 37°C.
9. Assay stop solutions.

   Acetonitrile/0.5 *M* Tris base (80:20 [v/v]). Store at room temperature.

   2 *N* sodium hydroxide. Store at room temperature.
10. Troughs or Petri dishes suitable for multichannel pipetting.
11. 2.0-mL, 15-mL, and 50-mL conical tubes.
12. Timer.
13. Multiwell plates (e.g., 96-well black plates, BD cat. no. 353241).
14. Lids for plates (e.g., BD cat. no. 353958).

2.2. Instrumentation

Fluorometric plate reader. A plate reader with top-reading capability is preferable and required for opaque-bottom plates (*see* **Note 2**).

Table 1
Fluorometric Substrates, Metabolites, and Their Properties

Substrate	Acronym	Stock concentrations (m*M* in acetonitrile)	Metabolite	Ex	Em
Resorufin benzyl ether	BzRes	10	Resorufin	530	590
7-Ethoxy-3-cyanocoumarin	CEC	20	7-Hydroxy-3-cyanocoumarin	410	460
7-Ethoxyresorufin	ER	4.1	Resorufin	530	590
Coumarin	Cou	1.1	7-Hydroxycoumarin	390	460
7-Ethoxy-4-trifluoromethylcoumarin	EFC	25	7-Hydroxy-4-trifluoromethylcoumarin	410	538
Dibenzylfluorescein	DBF	2	Fluorescein	485	538
7-Methoxy-4-trifluoromethylcoumarin	MFC	25	7-Hydroxy-4-trifluoromethylcoumarin	410	538
7-Benzyloxy-4-trifluoromethylcoumarin	BFC	50	7-Hydroxy-4-trifluoromethylcoumarin	410	538
3-*O*-methylfluorescein	OMF	2	Fluorescein	485	538
3-[2-(*N*,*N*-Diethyl-*N*-methylamino) ethyl]-7-methoxy-4-methylcoumarin	AMMC	1	(3-[2-(*N*,*N*-diethyl-*N*-methylammonium)ethyl]-7-hydroxy-4-methylcoumarin)[a]	390	460
7-Methoxy-4-(aminomethyl)coumarin	MAMC	10	7-Hydroxy-4-(aminomethyl)coumarin	390	460
7-Benzyloxyquinoline	BQ	16	7-Hydroxyquinoline	410	538

[a]–3-[2-(*N*,*N*-diethyl-*N*-methylamino) ethyl]-7-hydroxy-4-methylcoumarin is used as an external standard for quantification of (3-[2-(*N*,*N*-diethyl-*N*-methylammonium)ethyl]-7-methoxy-4-methylcoumarin). Ex, excitation; Em, emission.

3. Methods

3.1. Preparation of Solutions

The methods outlined below describe the preparation of assay components in volumes suitable for testing three chemicals in duplicate and a positive control chemical in 96-well plates (200-µL assay volume). Volumes may be scaled to achieve the desired assay volume (*see* **Note 3**). Assay solution components include (1) test substance, (2) cofactor mix, (3) enzyme/substrate mix, and (4) assay stop solution. To perform the assay, the test substances and cofactor mix are first combined and dilutions prepared. Then, the reaction is initiated by addition of the enzyme/substrate mix and, after a suitable incubation period, terminated by the addition of stop solution. The last step may be omitted if one chooses to monitor metabolite formation continuously.

3.1.1. Preparation of the Test Substance Stock Solution

Test substances must be dissolved fully in a suitable solvent for addition to the assay. Dissolving compounds in aqueous buffer (neutral, weakly acidic, or basic) or water is preferable but often not practical to achieve a suitable upper concentration while allowing volume for addition of other assay components. Consequently, organic solvents are used most often to prepare concentrated solutions (e.g., 10–100 m*M*) to allow addition of high concentrations to the assay but in a small volume. Because organic solvents may activate or, more often, inhibit enzyme catalytic activity, the volume of organic solvent used is kept low. The volume tolerated varies with the enzyme/substrate pair. Guidance for solvent tolerance is available (*see* **Note 4**). Use of a solvent, such as acetonitrile, that is well tolerated by the enzyme allows a higher final percentage and facilitates accurate addition of the test substance solution to the assay for small assay volumes. The test substance stock solution in organic solvent is typically prepared in volumes between 0.1 and 1 mL.

3.1.2. Preparation of the 2X Cofactor Mix

All CYP enzymes require reducing equivalents (e.g., nicotinamide adenine dinucleotide phosphate [NADPH]) for catalytic activity. The procedure below describes the preparation of 15 mL of a 2X NADPH-regenerating system mix. Most of this solution will be used for the serial dilution step described in **Subheading 3.4.**. However, a portion must be set aside to prepare the cofactor/test substance mix in **Subheading 3.1.4.**. The volume to be set aside will depend on the accuracy of the pipet and the tolerance of the assay to organic solvent.

1. In a 50-mL conical tube, add 1.5 mL of 0.5 *M* potassium phosphate, pH 7.4 buffer. For CYP2A6, substitute 0.5 *M* Tris buffer, pH 7.5.

2. Add the cofactor solution. The cofactor solution varies in NADPH content by enzyme. For assays other than CYP2A6 and CYP2D6, add 1.5 mL of the "20/20" cofactor solution. For CYP2A6, add 1.5 mL of the "1/20" cofactor solution. For CYP2D6 assays, add 0.188 mL of the "1/20" solution.
3. Add 0.3 mL of the G6PDH solution.
4. Add 0.3 mL of insect cell control protein (*see* **Note 5**).
5. Bring to 15 mL with distilled water.
6. Remove an adequate volume of this solution for use in **Subheading 3.1.4.**.
7. To the remaining solution, add 2X volume of the same solvent used to dissolve the test substances (*see* **Note 6**). For example, add 0.04 parts acetonitrile to 0.96 parts 2X cofactor mix.
8. Warm the mix to 37°C in a water bath.

3.1.3. Preparation of the 2X Enzyme/Substrate Mix

This mix contains 10 mL of a 2X enzyme/substrate mix. Combining this solution with the 2X cofactor mix starts the reaction.

1. In a 15-mL conical tube, add buffer and water to prepare a 2X mix. The final concentration of buffer in the 2X mix is 0 to 0.35 *M*, depending on the enzyme (*see* **Note 7**).
2. Add sufficient water to bring the volume up to 10 mL – *X*, where *X* is the volume occupied by the enzyme, control protein, and substrate described in the following steps.
3. Add insect cell control protein to bring the concentration in the 2X mix to 0.4 mg/mL–*Y*, where *Y* is the protein concentration contributed by the enzyme described in **step 5**.
4. Add substrate according to **Table 2** to prepare a 2X solution (e.g., for CYP1A1, add 250 nmol BzRes).
5. Add BD Gentest Supersomes™ enzyme according to **Table 2** to prepare a 2X solution (e.g., for CYP1A1, add 250 pmol enzyme).
6. Warm the mix to 37°C in a water bath. Use within 1 h; otherwise, maintain on ice for up to 4 h prior to addition to the water bath.

3.1.4. Preparation of the Cofactor/Test Substance Mix

Using the cofactor mix set aside in **step 6** in **Subheading 3.1.2.**, prepare a 2X solution of the upper concentration of each test substance. This solution will be used as a reservoir from which to conduct the serial dilution steps described in **Subheading 3.4.**. The solution may be prepared either within the reaction vessel (e.g., the first well in a row of a multiwell plate) or in a separate vessel prior to addition to the plate. The choice may depend on the ease of adding small volumes of organic solvent to the mix. Volumes depend on the type of solvent used (*see* **Note 4** for tolerance recommendations). Scaling up the volumes may circumvent accuracy concerns (e.g., 6 µL dimethylsulfoxide [DMSO] test substance stock solution to 1494 µL cofactor mix "off plate,"

Table 2
Enzyme/Substrate Pairings and Guidelines for Use

Enzyme	Substrate	Substrate concentration (μ*M*)	Incubation time (min)	Enzyme concentration (n*M*)	Stop solution
CYP1A1	BzRes	12.5	30	12.5	ACN/Tris
CYP1A2	CEC	2.5	15	1	ACN/Tris
CYP1A2	ER	0.25	3	1.5	ACN/Tris
CYP1B1	BzRes	12.5	15	12.5	ACN/Tris
CYP2A6	Cou	3	10	5	ACN/Tris
CYP2B6	EFC	2.5	30	5	ACN/Tris
CYP2C8	DBF	1	30	20	NaOH
CYP2C9	CEC	15	45	25	ACN/Tris
CYP2C9	MFC	50	45	10	ACN/Tris
CYP2C9	DBF	1	30	10	NaOH
CYP2C19	CEC	6	30	5	ACN/Tris
CYP2C19	DBF	2	30	5	NaOH
CYP2C19	BFC	25	45	25	ACN/Tris
CYP2C19	OMF	2	30	5	NaOH
CYP2D6	AMMC	0.5	30	5	ACN/Tris
CYP2D6	MAMC	7.5	60	10	ACN/Tris
CYP2E1	MFC	100	45	10	ACN/Tris
CYP3A4	BFC	50	30	5	ACN/Tris
CYP3A4	DBF	1	10	1	NaOH
CYP3A4	BQ	40	30	25	ACN/Tris
CYP3A4	BzRes	50	45	25	ACN/Tris
CYP3A5	BFC	50	30	40	ACN/Tris
CYP3A7	BFC	50	45	25	ACN/Tris
CYP19	DBF	0.2	30	2	NaOH
CYP19	MFC	25	30	7.5	ACN/Tris

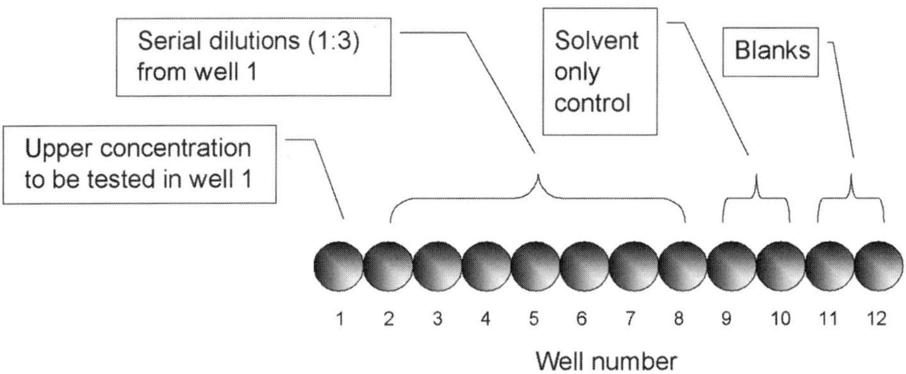

Fig. 1. Example assay map showing one row of a 96-well plate.

rather than 0.6 μL DMSO test substance stock solution to 149.4 μL cofactor mix directly within the plate well). Preparing this mix "off plate" also allows the opportunity to inspect the solution for insoluble material (*see* **Note 8**).

3.2. Plate Setup

A suggested plate map design incorporates 12 wells lengthwise across a 96-well plate for a single test. **Figure 1** shows an example design for one row of a plate. Well 1 contains the uppermost concentration of test substance, and wells 2 through 8 are reserved for serial dilutions, typically with 1:3 spacing. Wells 9 and 10 contain duplicate solvent-only controls that will represent the uninhibited control enzyme activity to which inhibited activity will be compared. Wells 11 and 12 are blank wells, in which stop solution is added prior to the addition of the enzyme/substrate mix and controls for background fluorescence imparted by the reaction components.

3.4. Performing the Serial Dilution of the Test Substance

The serial dilution step is carried out to examine inhibitory potential of a wide range of test substance concentrations. A 1:3 serial dilution allows for testing concentrations spanning over three orders of magnitude and is usually sufficient to bracket the IC_{50} without prior knowledge of inhibitory potency. The procedure below describes the serial dilution using the aqueous 2X cofactor mix in **Subheading 3.1.2.** as the receiving solution, assuming one row for each test.

1. Add 100 μL of 2X cofactor mix to all wells except well 1.
2. Add 150 μL of the cofactor/test substance mix to well 1 (cofactor mix and test substance solution may be added individually within the well or prepared "off plate"; *see* **Subheading 3.1.4.**).
3. Remove 50 μL from well 1 and dispense into well 2. Mix thoroughly by aspirating and dispensing 50 μL. One aspiration/dispense cycle is sufficient to provide adequate mixing.
4. Continue across the row as in **step 3**, discarding the last 50 μL after well 8.
5. Change the pipet tip after well 4 to minimize potential carryover of compounds with questionable solubility.
6. Warm the plates to 37°C.

3.5. Initiate the Reaction by Addition of the Enzyme/Substrate Mix

The reaction is initiated by adding the prewarmed enzyme substrate mix. Adding in the 2X volume ensures rapid and thorough mixing.

1. Add 100 μL of the enzyme substrate mix to all wells in the row except wells 11 and 12.
2. Incubate plates at 37°C for the time periods as described in **Table 2**.

3.6. Stop Reaction by Addition of Appropriate Assay Stop Solution

1. At the end of the incubation period, add 0.075 mL of stop solution, as recommended in **Table 2**, to all wells in the row. Alternatively, one may collect data continuously within the plate reader (maintained at 37°C) for all substrates except OMF and DBF (*see* **Note 9**). This approach ensures reaction velocity linearity and allows monitoring of time-dependent changes in IC_{50} values that may indicate irreversible inhibition *(28)*. However, assay sensitivity (especially at earlier time-points) and throughput will be lower as the plate reader would be more often occupied.
2. Add 100 µL of enzyme/substrate mix to wells 11 and 12 (blanks).

3.7. Acquire the Data by Reading the Plate on a Fluorometric Plate Reader

1. Scan the plate using a fluorometric plate reader set for appropriate excitation and emission wavelengths (*see* **Table 1**). *See* **Note 10**. Plates may be read up to 8 h after stopping the reaction without significant changes occurring to either signal-to-background ratios or IC_{50} values. If 2 *N* sodium hydroxide is used as the stop solution (for fluorescein derivates only), read the plates after a suitable signal development period (2 h, with plates kept at 37°C recommended).

3.8. Determine the Percent Inhibition and Calculate the IC_{50} Values

1. After subtracting background fluorescence, determine the percent inhibition of catalytic activity caused by the test substance relative to the mean of the duplicate solvent-only wells (*see* **Note 11**).
2. If percent inhibition exceeds 50%, the IC_{50} value may be calculated. There are many commercially available curve-fitting software packages for this purpose (e.g., BD Gentest™ Multiwell plate manager, BD Biosciences, Woburn, MA). Alternatively, linear interpolation may be used as described below:

$$IC_{50} = [(50 - A)/(B - A)] \times (D - C) + C,$$

where A = the first point on the curve, expressed in percent inhibition, that is less than 50% (e.g., 49%); B = the first point on the curve, expressed in percent inhibition, that is greater than or equal to 50% (e.g., 76%); C = the concentration of inhibitor that gives A% inhibition (e.g., 1.23 µ*M*); and D = the concentration of inhibitor that gives B% inhibition (e.g., 3.70 µ*M*). For example,

$$IC_{50} = [(50 - 48.9)/(75.9 - 48.9)] \times (3.70 - 1.23) + 1.23 = 1.33\ \mu M.$$

3.9. Tips on Data Interpretation

Typical of binding assays, interactions can be displayed graphically, with log concentration on the abscissa and percent maximal activity on the ordinate. With most inhibitors and CYP enzymes, the shape of the concentration response curve is sigmoidal, and this is exemplified by curve A in **Fig. 2**. How-

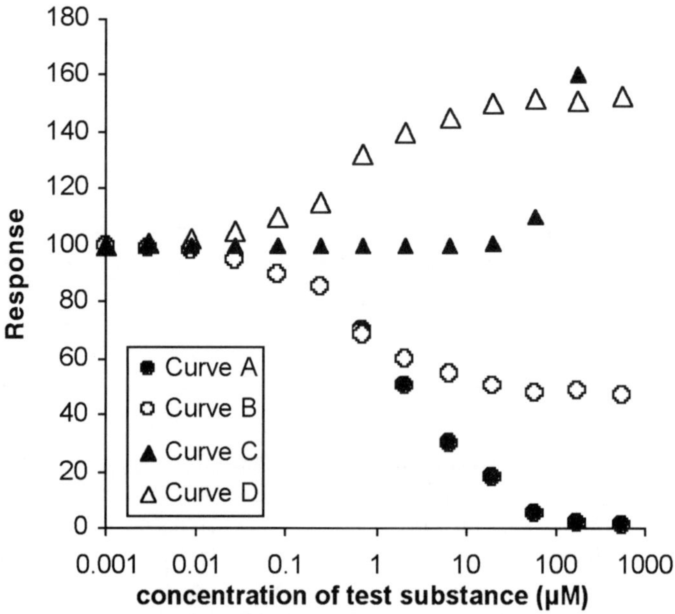

Fig. 2. Example enzyme inhibition response curves.

ever, it is important to realize that not all compounds that elicit a change in fluorescence response follow this paradigm. **Figure 2** shows a sampling of other curve shapes commonly observed. Curve B shows the response of a test substance causing partial inhibition of the enzyme. In this particular example, the curve begins to plateau near 50% inhibition. Obviously, this can profoundly influence the reproducibility of the "IC_{50}" value and illustrates the pitfalls of testing only one or two concentrations of test substance under the assumption that all activity is inhibitable. The response in curve C shows no evidence of inhibition but rather an apparent increase in enzyme activity. Another explanation is that the compound is exhibiting autofluorescence. In this case, the response is usually directly proportional to the amount of test substance present and more often occurs at relatively high concentrations, which may be beyond the concentration range of interest. Autofluorescence of the test substance or its metabolites can be examined easily by including a relevant concentration (e.g., 10 μ*M*) of test substance in an available blank well or by incubating in the absence of a fluorescent probe. Autofluorescence can often be overcome by selecting substrates yielding red-shifted metabolites (such as resorufins) if available. Curve D shows a more gradual increase in response that is not directly proportional to the amount of test substance and appears to plateau.

This response is more consistent with saturable activation of the enzyme. Often, an activation response is coupled with an inhibition response at higher concentrations of test substance. Curves B and D are frequently seen with enzymes exhibiting atypical kinetics, such as CYP3A4. In such cases, flagging the test substance for follow-up studies or checking the response with additional substrates for the same enzyme is prudent. A discussion of interpreting in vitro IC_{50} and K_i values is beyond the scope of this article. However, the reader is referred to an excellent review article as it pertains to common misconceptions and practical considerations in the prediction of inhibition responses in vivo from in vitro data ***(31)***.

3.10. Reference Data

Reference data are provided in **Table 3**. Additional reference data are widely available ***(10,14–29)***.

4. Notes

1. Reduced β-nicotimamide adenine dinucleotide phosphate (NADPH) has excitation and emission wavelengths of ~340 nm and ~450 nm, respectively, and may impart background fluorescence. Reducing the NADPH content improves the signal-to-background ratio and is required for some assays (e.g., CYP2D6, CYP2A6) that specify excitation and emission wavelengths in that range. We determined that the mean K_m ± SD of NADPH utilization was ~0.8 ± 0.9 n*M* among four different enzyme/substrate pairs. Therefore, reducing the NADPH content but maintaining the final concentration >10-fold, the K_m has a minimal impact on reaction velocity. The preparation of a 1-mg/mL NADP+ cofactor solution (i.e., "1/20" solution described in **item 6** in **Subheading 2.1.**) allows a convenient reagent to reduce final NADPH content in the assay.
2. Not all fluorometric plate readers are identical in sensitivity. Higher sensitivity instruments will allow an increased signal-to-background ratio, thus improving assay performance. We have found price to be a poor indicator of plate reader sensitivity.
3. Assay volumes may be decreased somewhat with an acceptable loss of signal-to-noise ratios for some enzyme/substrate pairs using preexisting equipment. The adaptation of the assay to a 384-well format has been described ***(22)***. Highly sensitive plate readers with laser light sources (e.g., Acquest™, Molecular Devices, Sunnyvale, CA) are required for 1536-well applications.
4. The effect of many common miscible organic solvents has been evaluated for their effect on CYP enzyme/substrate pairs (http://www.biosciences.com/discovery-labwave/gentest/products/HTS_kits/HTS/hts_appendicies.shtml). The effect of organic solvent on enzyme activity is well documented, but its effect on the inhibition potential of a given test substance has not been as extensively investigated. Unless assay tolerance has been investigated thoroughly, general

Table 3
Reference Data

Enzyme	Substrate	Test substance	IC_{50} value (μ*M*)
CYP1A1	BzRes	α-Naphthoflavone	0.19
		β-Estradiol	22
CYP1A2	CEC	α-Naphthoflavone	0.016
		Furafylline	2.11
CYP1B1	BzRes	α-Naphthoflavone	0.030
		β-Estradiol	24
CYP2A6	Cou	8-Methoxypsoralen	1.68
		Tranylcypromine	0.22
		Nicotine	307
		Diethyldithiocarbamate	105
CYP2B6	EFC	Tranylcypromine	5.0
		Methoxychlor	14
		Orphenadrine	326
		Nicotine	3498
CYP2C8	DBF	Quercetin	1.9
		Ketoconazole	4.4
		Sulfaphenazole	156
		Diclofenac	396
CYP2C9	CEC	Tienilic acid	0.15
		Sulfaphenazole	0.30
		S-Warfarin	6.41
		Tolbutamide	223
CYP2C9	DBF	Tienilic acid	0.40
		Sulfaphenazole	0.45
		S-Warfarin	13
		Tolbutamide	169
CYP2C9	MFC	Tienilic acid	0.50
		Sulfaphenazole	0.51
		S-Warfarin	>200 (activation)
		Tolbutamide	432
CYP2C19	BFC	Lansoprazole	1.42
		Ticlodipine	1.97
		Tranylcypromine	5.33
		Omeprazole	5.96
CYP2C19	CEC	Lansoprazole	1.35
		Ticlodipine	0.23
		Omeprazole	8.83
		Tranylcypromine	3.99

(*continued*)

Table 3 (Continued)
Reference Data

Enzyme	Substrate	Test substance	IC_{50} value (μM)
CYP2C19	DBF	Lansoprazole	0.36
		Ticlodipine	0.28
		Omeprazole	4.0
		Tranylcypromine	1.9
CYP2D6	AMMC	Quinidine	0.005
		Fluoxetine	0.16
		Imipramine	1.3
		Bufuralol	2.9
CYP2D6	MAMC	Quinidine	0.008
		Fluoxetine	0.36
		Imipramine	2.2
		Bufuralol	5.5
CYP2E1	MFC	Diethyldithiocarbamate	4.1
		4-Methylpyrazole	6.2
		Disulfiram	13
		Chlorzoxazone	210
CYP3A4	BFC	Mibefradil	0.005
	DBF	Mibefradil	0.055
	BQ	Mibefradil	0.066
	BzRes	Mibefradil	0.021
CYP3A5	BFC	Mibefradil	0.23
CYP3A7	BFC	Mibefradil	0.44
CYP19	DBF	4-Hydroxyandrostenedione	0.031
		Testosterone	0.18
		Aminoglutethimide	0.77
		Tranylcypromine	1.34

recommendations for final assay concentrations are 2% acetonitrile, 1% methanol, and 0.2% dimethylsulfoxide. The DMSO concentration can be increased to 0.4% for CYP1A2/CEC, CYP2D6/AMMC, and CYP3A4/BQ and 0.5% DMSO for CYP19/DBF.

5. The addition of insect control protein at this step is optional but recommended. The presence of protein aids in solubilizing some compounds and in preventing nonspecific binding to the vessel walls. This also provides a method of standardizing total protein content, a parameter known to influence the magnitude of inhibition by a compound.
6. Use the same lot of solvent if possible to avoid lot-dependent effects.
7. Buffer type and strength influence enzyme catalytic activity ***(32)***. For example,

CYP2A6 is strongly inhibited by phosphate; consequently, Tris-HCl buffer is preferred for this assay. CYP3A4 exhibits higher catalytic activity in the presence of relatively high ionic strength (e.g., 200 m*M*), whereas CYP2C9 is more active at a lower ionic strength (e.g., 25 m*M*). In general, conditions are chosen to achieve higher catalytic activity, which reduces enzyme consumption and improves signal-to-background ratios. Unfortunately, not all enzyme/substrate pairs presented here have been optimized for this parameter. We recommend the following ionic strengths of potassium phosphate buffer, pH 7.4, with the five major drug-metabolizing enzymes: 25 m*M* of CYP2C9, 50 m*M* of CYP2C19, 100 m*M* of CYP1A2 and CYP2D6, 200 m*M* of CYP3A4/5/7, and 50 m*M* or 100 m*M* for all other enzymes.

8. Because the mix represents twice the highest concentration to be tested, it is prudent to inspect the mix for insoluble material. If possible, determine the solubility of the test substance in the matrix prior to conducting the assay. The inclusion of insect cell control protein aids in solubilizing some compounds. If the compound yields an insoluble suspension that is homogeneous, a satisfactory serial transfer may be possible and allow dilution to a concentration into the soluble range.
9. The stop solution inactivates the enzyme by adding organic solvent or, in the case of the fluorescein derivatives OMF and DBF, a strong base. For OMF and DBF, the initial metabolite from the cleavage of the ether linkage requires further ester hydrolysis to maximize fluorescence. Increasing the pH also ionizes the aromatic hydroxl group, maximizing the quantum yield of the metabolite.
10. Some plate readers do not provide all necessary filters for these metabolites and may require custom preparations. In general, keeping the cutoff within 10 nm of the suggested excitation and emission wavelengths will provide adequate assay responses.
11. Quantification of the metabolite is not necessary to determine percent inhibition and calculate IC_{50} values because activity can be measured relative to the solvent-only controls. If desired, prepare a metabolite standard curve in matrix.

Acknowledgments

The author thanks Dr. Christopher J. Patten for his helpful comments and discussion. Thanks also to Stephanie Turner, Thuy Ho, Sweta Parikh, and Catherine Cargill for generating the reference data and assistance in developing the assay conditions.

References

1. http://drnelson.utmem.edu/CytochromeP450.html
2. Rendic, S. (2002) Summary of information on human CYP enzymes: human P450 metabolism data. *Drug Metab. Rev.* **34,** 83–448.
3. Geungerich, F. P. (2001) Common and uncommon cytochromes P450 reactions related to metabolism and chemical toxicity. *Chem. Res. Toxicol.* **14,** 611–650.

4. Levy, R., Thummel, K., Trager, W., Hansten, P., and Eichelbaum, M., eds. (2000) *Metabolic Drug Interactions*. Lippincott Williams & Wilkins, Philadelphia.
5. Brodie, A., Lu, Q., and Long, B. (1999) Aromatase and its inhibitors. *J. Steroid. Biochem. Mol. Biol.* **69,** 205–219.
6. Kragie, L., Turner, S. D., Patten, C. J., Crespi, C. L., and Stresser, D. M. (2002) Assessing pregnancy risks of azole antifungals using a high throughput aromatase inhibition assay. *Endocr. Res.* **28,** 129–140.
7. Zarn, J. A., Bruschweiler, B. J., and Schlatter, J. R. (2003) Azole fungicides affect mammalian steroidogenesis by inhibiting sterol 14 alpha-demethylase and aromatase. *Environ. Health Perspec.* **111,** 255–261.
8. White, R. E. (2000) High-throughput screening in drug metabolism and pharmacokinetic support of drug discovery. *Annu. Rev. Pharmacol. Toxicol.* **40,** 133–157.
9. Smith, D. A. and van de Waterbeemd, H. (1999) Pharmacokinetics and metabolism in early drug discovery. *Curr. Opin. Chem. Biol.* **3,** 373–378.
10. Crespi, C. L., Miller, V. P., and Penman, B. W. (1997) Microtiter plate assays for inhibition of human, drug-metabolizing cytochromes P450. *Anal. Biochem.* **248,** 188–190.
11. Ullrich, V. and Weber, P. (1972) The O-dealkylation of 7-ethoxycoumarin by liver microsomes: a direct fluorometric test. *Hoppe Seylers Z Physiol. Chem.* **353,** 1171–1177.
12. Crespi, C. L. (1995) Xenobiotic-metabolizing human cells as tools for pharmacological and toxicological research. *Adv. Drug Res.* **26,** 179–235.
13. Kennedy, S. W. and Jones, S. P. (1994) Simultaneous measurement of cytochrome P4501A catalytic activity and total protein concentration with a fluorescence plate reader. *Anal. Biochem.* **222,** 217–223.
14. Favreau, L. V., Palamanda, J. R., Lin, C. C., and Nomeir, A. A. (1999) Improved reliability of the rapid microtiter plate assay using recombinant enzyme in predicting CYP2D6 inhibition in human liver microsomes. *Drug Metab. Dispos.* **27,** 436–439.
15. Onderwater, R. C., Venhorst, J., Commandeur, J. N., and Vermeulen, N. P. (1999) Design, synthesis, and characterization of 7-methoxy-4-(aminomethyl)coumarin as a novel and selective cytochrome P450 2D6 substrate suitable for high-throughput screening. *Chem. Res. Toxicol.* **12,** 555–559.
16. Crespi, C. L. and Stresser, D. M. (2000) Fluorometric screening for metabolism-based drug-drug interactions *J. Pharmacol. Toxicol. Method* **44,** 325–331.
17. Stresser, D. M., Turner, S. D., Blanchard, A. B., Miller, V. P., Erve, J. C. L., Dandeneau, A. C., et al. (2000) Substrate-dependent modulation of CYP3A4 catalytic activity: analysis of 27 test compounds with four fluorometric substrates. *Drug Metab. Dispos.* **28,** 1440–1448.
18. Stresser, D. M., Turner, S. D., McNamara, J., Stocker, P., Miller, V. P., Crespi, C. L., et al. (2000) A high-throughput screen to identify inhibitors of aromatase (CYP19). *Anal. Biochem.* **284,** 427–430.
19. Bapiro, T. E., Egnell, A. C., Hasler, J. A., and Masimirembwa, C. M. (2001) Application of higher throughput screening (HTS) inhibition assays to evaluate

the interaction of antiparasitic drugs with cytochrome P450s. *Drug Metab. Dispos.* **29,** 30–35.

20. Katsunori, N., Hanna, I. H., Cai, H., Nishimura, Y., Williams, K. M., and Guengerich, F. P. (2001) Coumarin substrates for cytochrome P450 2D6 fluorescence assays. *Anal. Biochem.* **292,** 280–286.
21. Chauret, N., Dobbs, B., Lackman, R., Bateman, K., Nicoll-Griffith, D., Stresser, D. M., et al. (2001) The use of 3-[2-(n,n-diethyl-n-methylammonium)ethyl]-7-methoxy-4-methylcoumarin (AMMC) as a specific CYP2D6 probe in human liver microsomes. *Drug Metab. Dispos.* **29,** 1196–1200.
22. Kariv, I., Fereshteh, M. P., and Oldenburg, K. R. (2001) Development of a miniaturized 384-well high throughput screen for the detection of substrates of cytochrome P450 2D6 and 3A4 metabolism. *J. Biomol. Screen.* **6,** 91–99.
23. Nomeir, A. A., Ruegg, C., Shoemaker, M., Favreau, L. V., Palamanda, J. R., Silber, P., et al. (2001) Inhibition of CYP3A4 in a rapid microtiter plate assay using recombinant enzyme and in human liver microsomes using conventional substrates. *Drug Metab. Dispos.* **29,** 748–753.
24. Crespi, C. L., Miller, V. P., and Stresser, D. M. (2002) Design and application of fluorometric assays for human cytochrome P450 inhibition. *Methods Enzymol.* **357,** 276–284.
25. Marks, B. D., Smith, R. W., Braun, H. A., Goossens, T. A., Christenson, M., Ozers, M. S., et al. (2002) A high throughput screening assay to screen for CYP2E1 metabolism and inhibition using a fluorogenic vivid P450 substrate. *Assay Drug Dev. Technol.* **1,** 73–81.
26. Venhorst, J., Rooseboom, M., Vermeulen, N. P. E., and Commandeur, J. N. M. (2003) Studies on the inhibition of human cytochromes P450 by selenocysteine *Se*-conjugates. *Xenobiotica* **33,** 57–72.
27. Yakahito, Y., Suzuki, A., and Kohno, Y. (2002) Application of microtiter plate assay to evaluate inhibitory effects of various compounds on nine cytochrome P450 isoforms and to estimate their inhibition patterns. *Drug Metab. Pharmacokin.* **17,** 437–448.
28. Yan, Z., Rafferty, B., Caldwell, G. W., and Masucci, J. A. (2002) Rapidly distinguishing reversible and irreversible CYP450 inhibitors by using fluorometric kinetic analysis. *Eur. J. Drug Metab. Pharmacokinet.* **27,** 281–287.
29. Ekins, S., Stresser, D. M., and Williams, J. A. (2003) In vitro and pharmacophore insights into CYP3A enzymes. *Trends Pharmacol. Sci.* **24,** 161–166.
30. Stresser, D. M., Turner, S. D., Blanchard, A. P., Miller, V. P., and Crespi, C. L. (2002) Cytochrome P450 fluorometric substrates: identification of isoform-selective probes for rat CYP2D2 and human CYP3A4. *Drug Metab. Dispos.* **30,** 845–852.
31. Lin, J. (2000) Sense and nonsense in the prediction of drug-drug interactions. *Curr. Drug Metab.* **1,** 305–331.
32. Crespi, C. L. (1998) Effect of salt concentration on the activity of liver microsomal and cDNA-expressed human cytochromes P450. *ISSX Proc.* **13,** 74. Also available at http://www.bdbiosciences.com/discovery-labwave/gentest/products/pdf/post-002.pdf

15

Evaluation of Cytochrome P450 Inhibition in Human Liver Microsomes

Zhengyin Yan and Gary W. Caldwell

Summary

Evaluation of lead compounds for P450 inhibition in human liver microsomes has been widely accepted as an in vitro approach to assess drug interaction potential. This chapter describes a detailed traditional CYP inhibition protocol for six major isoforms: 1A2, 2C9, 2C19, 2D6, 2E1, and 3A4. Microsomal incubation conditions were optimized and kinetic parameters determined to initially establish the inhibition assay. In CYP inhibition assay, separated incubations were performed for individual CYPs, and resulting samples were pooled and analyzed by liquid chromatography/tandem mass spectrometry (LC-MS/MS). It is without doubt that results from this in vitro experiment are of great value in lead optimization in drug discovery and development. It is obvious that more efforts are still needed to establish the relevance between in vitro CYP inhibition and drug interactions in the clinic.

Key Words: CYPs; drug interactions; P450 inhibition.

1. Introduction

During the past decade, the success of pharmaceutical research has brought many agents on the market and also has expanded therapeutic indications to those existing drugs. With a wide variety of drugs available, multiple drug therapy has become a common practice in today's medicine. As a result, drug-drug interactions have been an increasing concern both in the clinic and among regulatory authorities in recent years. Such a concern has arisen with respect to refusal of approval and withdrawal from the market. As part of the effort to reduce attrition rates of new chemical entities (NCEs), it is becoming routine in drug discovery to evaluate lead compounds for drug–drug interactions prior to clinical trials in humans *(1)*.

From: *Methods in Pharmacology and Toxicology*
Optimization in Drug Discovery: In Vitro Methods
Edited by: Z. Yan and G. W. Caldwell © Humana Press Inc., Totowa, NJ

Table 1
Summary of Commonly Used In Vitro CYP Probe Substrates

CYP	Preferred substrate	Specific reaction	K_m (mM)
1A2	Phenacetin	Phenacetin *O*-deethylation	10–50
2C9	*S*-warfarin	*S*-warfarin 7'-hydroxylation	1–5
	Tolbutamide	Tolbutamide 4'-hydroxylation	100–200
2C19	*S*-mephenytoin	*S*-mephenytoin 4'-hydroxylation	30–340
2D6	Dextromethorphan	Dextromethorphan *O*-demethylation	2–10
	Bufuralol	Bufuralol 1'-hydroxylation	4–10
2E1	Chlorzoxazone	Chlorzoxazone 6'-hydroxylation	40
3A4	Midazolam	Midazolam 1'-hydroxylation	3–5
	Testosterone	Testosterone 6'-hydroxylation	50–100

Although modulation of other proteins such as P-glycoprotein and UDP-glucuronosyltransferases by coadministered drugs causes adverse side effects, inhibition of cytochrome P450s (CYPs) is currently recognized as the major mechanism for drug–drug interactions observed in the clinic. As the most important drug metabolism enzymes in humans, CYPs are responsible for metabolizing more than 95% of marketed drugs. Therefore, in vitro assessment of potential drug interactions has largely been focused on inhibition of CYPs, particularly those major isoforms such as CYP1A2, 2C9, 2C19, 2D6, 2E1, and 3A4. CYP inhibition can be evaluated in different in vitro systems, including complementary deoxyribonucleic acid (cDNA)-expressed enzymes ***(2)***, liver microsomes ***(3)***, and hepatocytes ***(4)***. Each system has its own advantages and limitations. The decision to use a particular approach depends on the goal of the evaluation. Microsomes are prepared from liver homogenates that contain a mixture of individual CYP enzymes. Therefore, inhibition of CYPs by NCEs is most frequently investigated in human liver microsomes.

In a CYP inhibition assay, test compounds are evaluated for the potency of altering the rate of a specific CYP-catalyzed reaction. As summarized in **Table 1**, many compounds are selectively metabolized by a particular P450 enzyme and are routinely used as CYP-specific probes in inhibition studies ***(5)***. The rate of a specific CYP marker reaction, as measured by the production of a specific metabolite, is often determined by liquid chromatography interfaced with UV spectrometry, fluorimetry, or tandem mass spectrometry (LC-MS/MS). Among them, LC-MS/MS is an optimal choice, largely because of its high sensitivity and selectivity and simultaneous detection capability. During the past few years, several different strategies that have been proposed to increase the throughput of P450 inhibition assays include using cocktail substrates in microsomal incubations ***(6)*** and applying ultra-fast LC runs in LC-MS/MS analysis ***(7,8)***. The current method is a traditional approach in which a single substrate is included in a separated microsomal incubation, and resulting samples are pooled and analyzed by LC-MS/MS ***(9)***. In addition, this method reflects recent consensus on CYP probe substrates and experimental design ***(10,11)***.

2. Materials

2.1. Buffers

1. Potassium phosphate, monobasic KH_2PO_4 (EM SCIENCE, Gibbstown, NJ).
2. Potassium phosphate, dibasic, trihydrate $K_2HPO_4 \cdot 3H_2O$ (Sigma, St. Louis, MO).

2.2. Reagents for the NADPH-Regenerating System

1. Glucose-6-phoshate (Sigma, St. Louis, MO).
2. β-Nicotinamide adenine dinucleotide phosphate, NADPH, reduced form (Sigma, St. Louis, MO).
3. Sodium citrate, tribasic (Sigma, St. Louis, MO).
4. Glucose-6-phosphate dehydrogenase (G6PDH) (Sigma, St. Louis, MO).
5. $MgCl_2 \cdot 6H_2O$ (Sigma, St. Louis, MO).

2.3. CYP-Specific Substrates and Metabolites (Note 1)

1. Tolbutamide, a probe substrate for CYP2C9 (Sigma, St. Louis, MO).
2. *S*-mephenytoin, a probe substrate for CYP2C19 (*Ultrafine* Chemicals, Manchester, UK).
3. Dextromethorphan, a probe substrate for CYP2D6 (Sigma, St. Louis, MO).
4. Phenacetin, a probe substrate for CYP1A2 (Sigma, St. Louis, MO).
5. Testosterone, a probe substrate for CYP3A4 (Sigma, St. Louis, MO).
6. Midazolam, a probe substrate for CYP3A4 (Sigma, St. Louis, MO).
7. Chlorzoxazone, a probe substrate for CYP2E1 (Sigma, St. Louis, MO).
8. Acetaminophen, a specific metabolite from phenacetin (Sigma, St. Louis, MO).
9. 4-Hydroxy-tolbutamide, a specific metabolite from tolbutamide (Sigma, St. Louis, MO).
10. 4-Hydroxy-*S*-mephenytoin a specific metabolite from *S*-mephenytoin (*Ultrafine* Chemicals, Manchester, UK).
11. Dextrorphan a specific metabolite from dextromethorphan (Sigma, St. Louis, MO).
12. 6β-Hydroxy-testosterone, a specific metabolite from testosterone (Sigma, St. Louis, MO).
13. 4-Hydroxy-midazolam, a specific metabolite from midazolam (*Ultrafine* Chemicals, Manchester, UK).
14. 6-Hydroxychlorzoxazone, a specific metabolite from chlorzoxazone (*Ultrafine* Chemicals, Manchester, UK).

2.4. CYP Selective Inhibitors

1. α-Naphthoflavone, a CYP1A2 selective inhibitor (Sigma, St. Louis, MO).
2. Sulfaphenazole, a CYP2C9 selective inhibitor (Sigma, St. Louis, MO).
3. Tranylcypromine, a CYP2C19 selective inhibitor (Sigma, St. Louis, MO).
4. Quinidine, a CYP2D6 selective inhibitor (Sigma, St. Louis, MO).
5. Ketoconazole, a CYP3A4 selective inhibitor (Sigma, St. Louis, MO).
6. 4-Methyl-pyrazole, a CYP2E1 selective inhibitor (Sigma, St. Louis, MO).

2.5. Materials for Microsomal Incubation

1. Pooled human liver microsomes (Gentest Corp., Woburn, MA).
2. Water bath, 37°C.
3. Assay plates: 96-well plate, polypropylene, 500 mL/well.

2.6. Solvent and Test Compounds

1. Deionized water.
2. Methanol.
3. Acetonitrile.
4. Methanol acidified with 10 m*M* acetic acid.
5. Methanol basified with 10 m*M* sodium hydroxide.
6. Acetonitrile acidified with 10 m*M* acetic acid.
7. Acetonitrile basified with 10 m*M* sodium hydroxide.
8. Test compounds.

2.7. Other Materials and Instruments for the Analysis

1. Refrigerated centrifuge.
2. Micromass Quattro Micro triple quadrupole mass spectrometer (Manchester, UK) or other triple quadrupole mass spectrometers.
3. Agilent 1100 high-performance liquid chromatography (HPLC) system or a similar instrument with an autosampler interfaced to the electrospray apparatus of the Quattro Micro triple quadrupole mass spectrometer.

3. Methods

The P450 inhibition assay can be conducted manually or robotically, depending on the throughput requirement. The current method is a manual version, but it can be easily modified to run the assay robotically. In an inhibition assay, the concentration of a probe substrate should be at or close to its Michaelis-Menten constant K_m; therefore, kinetic parameters (K_m, V_{max}) of a particular substrate should be first determined prior to performing the CYP inhibition assay. It has been noted that kinetic parameters of CYP substrates vary significantly in literature (**Table 1**), probably because of the differences in microsomal preparations and experimental conditions and procedures. To initially establish the inhibition assay, one has to first determine kinetic parameters of individual CYP-specific substrates in a microsomal preparation under certain incubation conditions. Therefore, concentrations of CYP-specific substrates in a CYP inhibition assay can be chosen based on K_m values, and K_i of a test compound can be estimated. Once kinetic parameters of CYP substrates are determined, the same experiment does not need to be repeated as long as incubation conditions are not changed.

3.1. Buffers, Cofactors, and Stop Solution

1. 0.5 *M* Potassium phosphate, KH_2PO_4, monobasic. Dissolve 34 g KH_2PO_4 in 450 mL deionized water, and bring the final volume to 500 mL with deionized water.
2. 0.5 *M* Potassium phosphate, K_2HPO_4, dibasic. Dissolve 57 g $K_2HPO_4 \cdot 3H_2O$ in 450 mL deionized water, and bring the final volume to 500 mL with deionized water.
3. 0.5 *M* Potassium phosphate, pH 7.4. Mix 60 mL 0.5 *M* KH_2PO_4 with 280 mL 0.5 *M* K_2HPO_4, and check with a pH meter for a pH of 7.4. If necessary, adjust pH with either 0.5 *M* KH_2PO_4 or 0.5 *M* K_2HPO_4 accordingly (*see* **Note 2**).
4. Sodium citrate, tribasic, 5 m*M*. Dissolve 14.7 mg sodium citrate in 100 mL deionized water. Store at –20°C.
5. Cofactors: dissolve 400 mg $NADP^+$, 400 mg glucose-6-phoshate, and 266 mg $MgCl_2 \cdot 6H_2O$ in 18 mL deionized water. Adjust the final volume to 20 mL. Aliquot and store at –20°C.
6. Glucose-6-phosphate dehydrogenase (G6PDH): 40 U/mL, prepared in 5 m*M* sodium citrate (tribasic). Aliquot and store at –20°C.
7. Stop solution: acetonitrile containing 2.0 m*M* propranolol as an internal standard for LC-MS/MS analysis (*see* **Note 3**).

3.2. Determination of Kinetic Parameters in Microsomal Incubation

To determine the kinetic parameters for CYP-specific substrates, incubation conditions were first optimized (*see* **Note 4**). In the current method, the final concentration of microsomal proteins is 0.25 mg/mL, and incubation time is set for 10 min. The concentration range of a particular substrate can be estimated according to K_m values in the literature (**Table 1**; *see* **Note 5**). Briefly, a CYP-specific substrate compound at different concentrations is mixed with microsomes in duplicate. After a short preincubation, an NADPH-regenerating solution is added to initiate the reaction. The reaction is stopped by the addition of acetonitrile. Metabolites generated from a specific CYP-catalyzed oxidation are analyzed using LC-MS/MS.

3.2.1. Substrate Stock Solutions

1. Tolbutamide, 300 m*M* dissolved in methanol.
2. *S*-mephenytoin, 40 m*M* dissolved in acetonitrile.
3. Dextromethorphan, 20 m*M* dissolved in distilled water.
4. Phenacetin, 50 m*M* dissolved in methanol.

5. Testosterone, 20 m*M* dissolved in acetonitrile.
6. Midazolam, 20 m*M* dissolved in methanol.
7. Chlorzoxazone, 20 m*M* dissolved in acetonitrile.

3.2.2. Substrate Working Solutions

1. Label eight microfuge tubes as A–H.
2. Dilute the substrate stock solution with deionized water to the highest desired concentration in tube A.
3. Add 400 mL deionized water to each of tubes B–H.
4. Transfer 200 mL of substrate solution from tube A to B and mix by vortexing.
5. Similarly, perform a serial dilution (threefold dilution) of substrate in tubes C–G.
6. Tube H contains only deionized water.

3.2.3. Microsomal Dilutions

1. Calculate the total volume of the microsomal solution (V mL, 0.5 mg/mL) based on the number of CYP substrates tested (*see* **Note 6**).
2. To make a 13-mL microsomal solution, add 2.6 mL 0.5 *M* potassium phosphate (pH 7.4) to a 15-mL tube.
3. Add 325 mL human liver microsomes (20 mg/mL proteins).
4. Supply deionized water to bring to the desired volume (13 mL).
5. Invert the tube repeatedly to mix all components and keep on ice.

3.2.4. NADPH-Regenerating Solution

NADPH is an electron donor in CYP-catalyzed oxidation reactions. Reduced NADPH at 1 m*M* can be added directly to the microsomal mixture to initiate the reaction. More commonly, NADPH is generated from $NADP^+$ by glucose-6-phosphate dehydrogenase. In the current method, a NADPH-regenerating solution is prepared as described below, which contains 2.6 m*M* $NADP^+$, 0.8 U/mL G6PDH, 6.7 m*M* glucose-6-phosphate, and 6.6 m*M* magnesium chloride.

1. Transfer 2.6 mL 0.5 *M* potassium phosphate, pH 7.4, to a 15-mL tube.
2. Add 8.84 mL deionized water to the tube.
3. Add 1.3 mL stock solution of cofactors.
4. Mix 0.26 mL of G6PDH solution (40 U/mL) to complete the NADPH-regenerating system right before use (*see* **Subheading 3.2.5.**).

3.2.5. Microsomal Incubation

1. In a 96-well plate, add 5 mL of substrate at different concentrations to corresponding wells in duplicate (well A receives the substrate at the highest concentration from tube A, and well H receives deionized water from tube H).
2. Dispense 125 mL diluted HLM to each well using a multichannel pipet.
3. Prewarm plate in a 37°C water bath for 5 min.

4. Complete preparation of NADPH-generating solution by adding the G6PDH (in **Subheading 3.2.4.**).
5. With a multichannel pipet, dispense 120 mL of NADPH-generating solution to each well to initiate the reaction.
6. Incubate the plate in a 37°C water bath for 10 min.
7. Add 80 mL of ice-cold stop solution to all wells to stop the reaction.
8. Cover the plate with an adhesive cover.
9. Centrifuge the plate at 4°C for 30 min at 5000*g* to pellet down proteins.
10. Transfer 200 mL of supernatants into HPLC vials for LC-MS/MS analysis as described in **Subheading 3.5.**.

3.3. Determination of IC_{50} Values in Human Liver Microsomes

In human liver microsomes, inhibition potency of a test compound can be assessed by determining the K_i or IC_{50} value of a CYP-specific probe substrate. After kinetic parameters of a CYP-specific substrate are determined, experiments can be performed to measure the IC_{50} value of a test compound for this particular CYP enzyme. Basically, a test compound is serially diluted to desired concentrations and then mixed with microsomes containing a CYP-specific substrate at a concentration equal or close to the K_m value of the substrate determined under optimal conditions. After incubation with NADPH, the effect of the test compound on the CYP marker activity can be evaluated by measuring a specific metabolite of the CYP substrate. For the quality control, a CYP-selective inhibitor is also included in the assay.

3.3.1. Preparation of Known CYP Inhibitors

Individual CYP-selective inhibitors can be used to initially validate the inhibition assay when the assay is first established and to verify the assay as positive controls.

1. α-Naphthoflavone, 0.1 m*M* dissolved in acetonitrile.
2. Sulfaphenazole, 1 m*M* dissolved in acetonitrile.
3. Tranylcypromine, 5 m*M* dissolved in acetonitrile.
4. Quinidine, 0.2 m*M* dissolved in acetonitrile.
5. Ketoconazole, 0.1 m*M* dissolved in acetonitrile.
6. Dilute CYP-specific inhibitors in tube H to the desired concentration (*see* **Note 7**).

3.3.2. Test Compound Solutions

1. Dissolve test compounds in an appropriate solvent (*see* **Note 8**) to prepare a 10-m*M* solution.
2. Label seven microfuge tubes as A-G.
3. Transfer 250-mL of compound stock solution to tube A.
4. Add 750 mL solvent (used to dissolve the compound) to each of tubes B–G.
5. Transfer 250 mL of compound stock solution to tube B and mix by vortexing.

6. Perform a serial dilution (fourfold dilutions) of compound in tubes C–F.
7. Tube G has only solvent but no compound.
8. Tube H will receive a CYP-specific inhibitor for quality control (*see* **Subheading 3.4.1.**).

3.3.3. Preparation of Microsome-Substrate Mixtures

1. Calculate the total volume of the microsomal solution (V mL, 0.5 mg/mL), based on the number of test compounds (*see* **Note 6**).
2. To make a 13-mL microsomal solution, add 2.6 mL 0.5 *M* potassium phosphate, pH 7.4, to a 15-mL tube.
3. Add 325 mL human liver microsomes (20 mg/mL proteins).
4. Add an appropriate amount of CYP substrate.
5. Supply deionized water to bring to the desired volume (13 mL).
6. Invert the tube repeatedly to mix all components and keep on ice.
7. Repeat the procedure for all CYP probe substrates.

3.3.4. Microsomal Incubation Procedures

1. Prepare the NADPH-regenerating solution as previously described in **Subheading 3.3.3.**
2. Dispense the 125-mL HLM-substrate mixture with a multichannel pipet to all wells.
3. Add 2.5 mL of test compound in duplicate at different concentrations to corresponding wells (well A receives test compound from tube A, and well H receives only solvent from tube H).
4. Prewarm the plate at 37°C for 5 min.
5. Complete preparation of the NADPH-generating solution by adding the G6PDH.
6. Add 122.5 mL of the NADPH generating solution to all wells.
7. Incubate in a 37°C water bath for 10 min.
8. Prepare the stop solution: acetonitrile containing 2.0 m*M* propranolol as an internal standard for LC-MS/MS analysis.
9. Add 80 mL of ice-cold stop solution to all wells to stop the reaction.
10. Repeat the procedure for all CYP substrates.
11. Centrifuge the plate at 4°C for 30 min at 5000*g* to pellet down proteins.
12. Pool supernatants in duplicate (*see* **Note 9**) and transfer 200 mL to HPLC vials for LC-MS/MS analysis, as described in **Subheading 3.5.**

3.4. Inhibition Assay With Preincubation

Inhibition of CYPs can be classified mechanistically into two categories: reversible inhibition and irreversible inhibition. In reversible inhibition, compounds directly compete at CYP active sites, and enzymatic activity of CYPs can be fully restored both in vitro and in vivo after inhibitors are depleted. As irreversible inhibitors, compounds inhibit CYP activity by irreversible binding, or they are first converted by the CYP to reactive metabolites that irreversibly bind to the sites within the active center of the enzyme. Experimentally, reversible and irreversible inhibitions are readily distinguished. Irreversible binding causes the enzyme to become inactivated with time, whereas reversible binding has no effect on enzyme activity. To distinguish reversible inhibitors from irreversible inhibitors, a preincubation of test compounds with HLM in the presence of NADPH is usually performed prior to adding CYP probe substrates. During the preincubation, irreversible inhibitors inactivate CYP enzymes; as a result, the IC_{50} value decreases significantly compared to the values obtained from the normal inhibition assay (*see* **Subheading 3.3.**).

1. Prepare the NADPH-regenerating solution and the test compound, as described previously in **Subheading 3.3.3.** and **Subheading 3.4.2.**, respectively.
2. Dispense 5 mL of test compound in duplicate at different concentrations to corresponding wells. (tube A corresponds to well A, the highest concentration, and tube G corresponds to well G, the lowest concentration. Well H receives only solvent.)
3. Add 125 mL diluted HLM solution to each well.
4. Prewarm the plate at 37°C for 5 min.
5. Complete preparation of the NADPH-generating solution by adding the G6PDH.
6. Add 120 mL of the NADPH-generating solution per well.
7. Incubate in a 37°C water bath for 10 min.
8. Add 25 mL of CYP-specific substrate to each well, and continue incubation for an additional 10 min.
9. Add 80 mL of ice-cold ACN to all wells to stop the reaction.
10. Centrifuge the plate at 4°C for 30 min at 5000*g* to pellet down the proteins.
11. Pool samples in duplicate (*see* **Note 9**), and transfer 200 mL of supernatants into HPLC vials for LC-MS/MS analysis, as described in **Subheading 3.5.**

3.5. LC-MS/MS Analyses

Analyses of CYP-specific metabolites are performed with an Agilent 1100 HPLC system interfaced with a Quattro Micro triple quadrupole mass spectrometer. LC-MS/MS analyses were conducted using electrospray ionization with positive ion detection. The mass spectrometer was first tuned using metabolite standards to achieve maximal sensitivity. A Hypersil BDS C18 column (2.1 × 150 mm) was used for chromatographic separation. The starting solvent condition was 95% water (0.5% acetic acid), and metabolites were eluted using a single gradient from 95% water to 95% acetonitrile over 12 min at a flow rate of 0.25 mL/min. At 12 min, the column was flushed with 95% acetonitrile for 2 min before reequilibration at initial conditions. The divert valve was activated to divert the HPLC eluant to waste during the first minute of elution, and then it switched the eluant to the mass spectrometer for analysis. The mass spectrometer was operated in the MRM mode to simultaneously

Table 2
MRM Transitions for the Major Metabolites of Seven CYP-Specific Substrates

CYP	Metabolite	Transition (*m/z*)	Cone (V)	Collision (eV)
1A2	Acetaminophen	152 → 110	32	20
2C9	4-Hydroxytobutamide	287 → 171	37	18
2C19	4-Hydroxymephenytoin	235 → 150	38	20
2D6	Dextrorphan	152 → 110	30	28
2E1	6-Hydroxychlorzoxazone	186 → 130	30	27
3A4	6β-Hydroxytestosterone	305 → 269	35	20
3A4	1-Hydroxymidazolam	342 → 324	35	27

detect multiple specific metabolites generated by individual CYP enzymes. The transitions monitored in MRM are given in **Table 2**.

3.6. Calculations

3.6.1. Calculation of K_m and V_{max}

The K_m and V_{max} values are obtained by nonlinear regression of a plot enzyme activity vs substrate concentration using GraphPad Prism software or other similar software. A typical Michaelis-Menten plot is shown in **Fig. 1**. However, non-Michaelis-Menten kinetics is occasionally observed for some compounds (*see* **Note 10**).

3.6.2. Determination of IC_{50} Values

The IC_{50} value of a test compound is determined by nonlinear regression of a plot enzyme activity versus inhibitor concentration using GraphPad Prism software or other similar software. A typical inhibition plot is demonstrated in **Fig. 2**, which shows inhibition of CYP3A4 by test compound A. However, partial inhibition is occasionally observed, as shown by test compound B (*see* **Note 11**).

Alternatively, IC_{50} values can be estimated by linear extrapolation using the following equation:

$$IC_{50} = \frac{(50\% - \text{low percentage}) * (\text{high conc.} - \text{low conc.})}{(\text{high percentage} - \text{low percentage})} = (\text{low conc.}),$$

where low percentage = highest percent inhibition less than 50%, high percentage = lowest percent inhibition greater than 50%, low concentration = concentration of test compound corresponding to the low percentage inhibition, and high concentration = concentration of test compound corresponding to the high

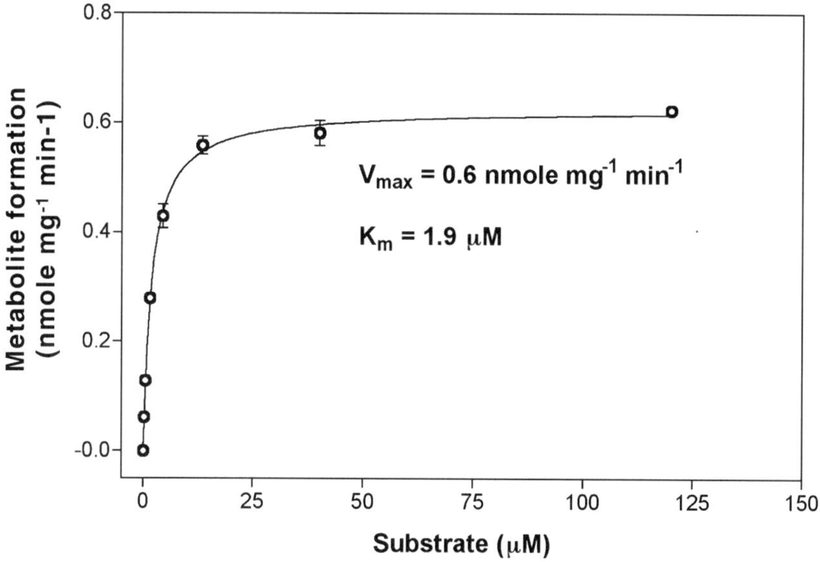

Fig. 1. Michaelis-Menten plot of a CYP probe substrate.

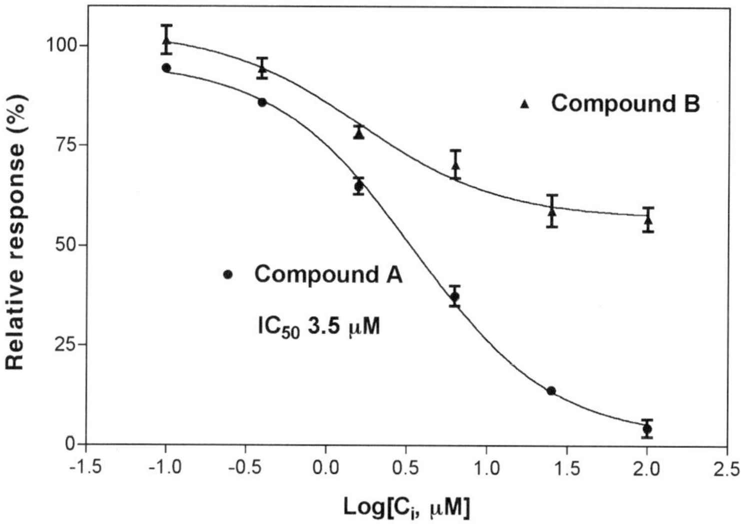

Fig. 2. Inhibition of CYP3A4 by two test compounds, A and B.

percentage inhibition. Furthermore, the inhibition constant (K_i) can be estimated from IC_{50} values by assuming test compounds as competitive inhibitors (*see* **Note 12**). Practically, an irreversible CYP inhibitor is less favorable in drug development. It is of great importance to experimentally distinguish different inhibition patterns. A significant decrease in the IC_{50} value resulting from preincubation is initial evidence for irreversible inhibition (*see* **Note 13**), and more detailed studies are required to further confirm the conclusion *(12,13)*.

4. Notes

1. Many drugs have been studied for the specificity of CYP enzymes. Ideally, a CYP probe substrate should be metabolized predominantly by a single CYP enzyme through a simple metabolic scheme *(5)*. Therefore, the production rate of a metabolite specifically reflects the activity of a particular CYP enzyme. In addition, the metabolite should be commercially available and is readily to be detected by available instruments. It is current consensus *(11)* that two distinct substrates such as testosterone and midazolam should be used to evaluate CYP3A4 inhibition because this enzyme probably possesses different substrate-binding domains, and inhibition of CYP3A4 is substrate dependent.
2. Use 0.5 *M* K_2HPO_4 if the pH is below 7.4 or KH_2PO_4 if the pH is above 7.4.
3. As an internal standard for LC-MS/MS analysis, the compound must be highly stable under experimental conditions and show good sensitivity in MS analysis and minimal loss in the sample preparation process.
4. Because the Michaelis-Menten equation is valid only under initial kinetic conditions, several factors should be considered in the experiment, including nonspecific binding, protein concentration, and incubation time. The low protein concentration should be helpful to minimize protein binding, especially with basic lipophilic compounds. In addition, substrate depletion can be avoided at low protein concentrations. Prolonged incubation can lead to the depletion of both substrates and test compounds. In general, consumption of substrates should be limited within 20% of the initial amount after incubation. If the sensitivity of analytical methods is high enough, 0.25 mg/mL of microsomal proteins in incubation is recommended.
5. Substrate concentrations should span a range of $1/4 \times K_m$ to $4 \times K_m$, with at least six concentrations. K_m values given in **Table 1** are very helpful to initially determine the substrate concentration range.
6. A total volume of 2.5 mL HLM-substrate mixture is required for every CYP probe substrate. For CYP3A4, two probe substrates should be included in kinetic studies, such as testosterone and midazolam.
7. Effective concentrations of CYP-selective inhibitors should be experimentally determined by running a normal inhibition assay over a concentration range.
8. Organic solvents at certain concentrations often inhibit CYP activity *(14)*. It is desired to dissolve test compounds at highest concentrations, so that the final concentration of solvents can be lower and the solvent effect minimized. Deionized water, methanol, and acetonitrile are solvents commonly used in P450 inhibition assays. Knowledge about the structure of test compounds would be very

helpful. Occasionally, acidified, basified, or mixed solvents can be tested, depending on the property of compounds.

9. Incubation samples generated from all different CYP substrates at each test compound concentration are pooled in duplicate.
10. Non-Michaelis-Menten kinetics refers to nonhyperbolic velocity with respect to probe substrate-concentration relationships that are caused by substrate inhibition and activation.
11. Abnormal inhibition curves include two types: (1) activation of CYP activity by test compounds and (2) partial inhibition of CYP activity in which CYP activity is not completely inhibited by test compounds at high concentrations. Clinical implications of CYP activation by a drug are unclear at present. In the cases of partial inhibition, IC_{50} values are less reliable, regardless of calculation methods.
12. The inhibition mechanism is often unknown in the early stage of drug discovery. More detailed inhibition studies are required to determine the inhibition pattern before a test compound is finally selected for further development. When substrate concentration used in the inhibition assay is at the K_m value, K_i equals $0.5 \times IC_{50}$ for a competitive or uncompetitive inhibitor, whereas K_i equals $2 \times IC_{50}$ for a noncompetitive inhibitor.
13. A significant change is defined as a twofold decrease in IC_{50}. For an irreversible inhibitor, inhibition percentages decreased over the entire concentration range after preincubation.

References

1. Yan, Z. and Caldwell, G. W. (2001) Metabolism profiling, and cytochrome P450 inhibition and induction in drug discovery. *Curr. Top. Med. Chem.* **1,** 403–425.
2. Crespi, C. L. and Stresser, D. M. (2001) Fluorometric screening for metabolism-based drug-drug interactions. *J. Pharm. Toxicol. Methods* **44,** 325–331.
3. Chu, I., Favreau, L., Soares, T., Lin, C. C., and Nomeir, A. A. (2000) Validation of higher-throughput high-performance liquid chromatography/atmospheric pressure chemical ionization tandem mass spectrometry assays to conduct cytochrome P450s CYP2D6 and CYP3A4 enzyme inhibition studies in human liver microsomes. *Rapid Comm. Mass Spectr.* **14,** 207–214.
4. Prueksaritanont, T., Tang, C., Qiu, Y., Mu, L., Subramanian, R., and Lin, J. H. (2002) Effects of fibrates on metabolism of statins in human hepatocytes. *Drug Metab. Dispos.* **30,** 1280–1287.
5. Yuan, R., Madani, S., Wei, X. X., Reynolds, K., and Huang, S. M. (2002) Evaluation of cytochrome P450 probe substrates commonly used by the pharmaceutical industry to study in vitro drug interactions. *Drug Metab. Dispos.* **30,** 1311–1319.
6. Dierks, E. A., Stams, K. R., Lim, H.-K., Cornelius, G., Zhang, H., and Ball, S. E. (2001) A method for the simultaneous evaluation of the activities of seven major human drug-metabolizing cytochrome P450s using an in vitro cocktail of probe substrates and fast gradient liquid chromatography tandem mass spectrometry. *Drug Metab. Dispos.* **29,** 23–29.

7. Peng, S. X., Barbone, A. G., and Ritchie, D. M. (2003) High-throughput cytochrome P450 inhibition assays by ultrafast gradient liquid chromatography with tandem mass spectrometry using monolithic columns. *Rapid Comm. Mass Spectr.* **17,** 509–518.
8. Bu, H. Z., Knuth, K., Magis, L., and Teitelbaum, P. (2000) High-throughput cytochrome P450 inhibition screening via cassette probe-dosing strategy: IV. Validation of a direct injection on-line guard cartridge extraction/tandem mass spectrometry method for simultaneous CYP3A4, 2D6 and 2E1 inhibition assessment. *Rapid Comm. Mass Spectr.* **14,** 1943–1948.
9. Yin, H., Racha, J., Li, S. Y., Olejnik, N., Saton, H., and Moore, D. (2000) Automated high throughput human CYP isoform activity assay using SPE-LC/MS method: application in CYP inhibition evaluation. *Xenobiotica* **30,** 141–154.
10. Tucker, G. T., Houston, J. B., and Huang, S. M. (2001) Optimizing drug development: strategies to assess drug metabolism/transporter interaction potential-toward a consensus. *Pharm. Res.* **18,** 1071–1080.
11. Bjornsson, T. D., Callaghan, J. T., Einolf, H. J., Fischer, V., Gan, L., Grimm, S., et al. (2003) The conduct of in vitro and in vivo drug-drug interaction studies: a Pharmaceutical Research and Manufacturers of America (PhRMA) perspective. *Drug Metab. Dispos.* **31,** 815–832.
12. Ha-Duong, N.-T., Dijols, S., Macherey, A.-C., Goldstein, J. A., Dansette, P. M., and Mansuy, D. (2001) Ticlopidine as a selective mechanism-based inhibitor of human cytochrome P450 2C19. *Biochemistry* **40,** 12,112–12,122.
13. Palamanda, J. R., Casciano, C. N., Norton, L. A., Clement, R. P., Favreau, L. V., Lin, C.-C., et al. (2001) Mechanism-based inactivation of CYP2D6 by 5-fluoro-2-[4-[(2-phenyl-1H-imidazol-5-yl)methyl]-1-piperazinyl]pyrimidine. *Drug Metab. Dispos.* **29,** 863–867.
14. Busby, W. F., Jr., Ackermann, J. M., and Crespi, C. L. (1999) Effect of methanol, ethanol, dimethyl sulfoxide, and acetonitrile on in vitro activities of CDNA-expressed human cytochromes P-450. *Drug Metab. Dispos.* **27,** 246–249.

16

Identification of CYP Mechanism-Based Inhibitors

Amin A. Nomeir, Jairam R. Palamanda, and Leonard Favreau

Summary

Metabolic drug–drug interactions occur when a drug A alters the pharmacokinetics of a coadministered drug B by either inhibiting, activating, or inducing the activity of the enzyme(s) that metabolize drug B. Inhibitory drug–drug interactions could result in serious adverse effects, including fatalities in patients receiving multiple medications. Cytochrome P450 superfamily (CYPs) are the major oxidative enzymes that participate in the metabolism of commercially available drugs. In addition to direct inhibition (reversible), these enzymes could be subjected to metabolism- or mechanism-based inhibition. Metabolism-based inhibition results from a metabolic product of the drug that is a more potent reversible inhibitor, whereas mechanism-based inhibition results from a metabolic product that binds irreversibly to the enzyme, rendering it inactive. Potent CYP inhibitors, including metabolism- and mechanism-based inhibition, are usually excluded from further consideration for development. The potential of new chemical entities (NCEs) to inhibit human CYPs, including metabolism- and mechanism-based inhibition, is assessed during the discovery stage in major pharmaceutical companies using in vitro screens. Metabolism- and mechanism-based inhibition is differentiated from direct inhibition primarily by being time dependent and involves catalytic steps. Metabolism- and mechanism-based inhibitors are differentiated by extensive dialysis, which would result in the recovery of enzyme activity for metabolism-based inhibition but not for mechanism-based inhibition. This chapter discusses the importance of identifying metabolism- and mechanism-based inhibitors and provides detailed experimental procedures for their identification early in drug discovery.

Key Words: CYP; cytochrome P450; mechanism-based inhibition; drug–drug interactions; mechanism-based inactivation; human CYP.

From: *Methods in Pharmacology and Toxicology*
Optimization in Drug Discovery: In Vitro Methods
Edited by: Z. Yan and G. W. Caldwell © Humana Press Inc., Totowa, NJ

1. Introduction

Inhibition of drug-metabolizing enzymes is one of the major determinants of drug–drug interactions, which could lead to adverse drug reactions in patients receiving multiple medications. Inhibition of one enzyme by a drug (and/or its metabolite) that metabolizes a coadministered drug would result in the alteration of the pharmacokinetics of the coadministered drug by increasing its plasma concentration and/or its duration in the body. This increase in plasma concentration could be substantial (as much as 20-fold and higher based on the area under the plasma concentration vs time curve [AUC]), and if the second drug has a narrow therapeutic index, this could result in serious adverse drug reactions, including fatalities ***(1)***.

Cytochrome P450 superfamily (CYPs) are the major oxidative enzymes that participate in the metabolism of commercially available drugs. With the completion of the sequencing of the human genome, the number of human CYPs seems to be approx 53 ***(2)***; however, only 6 enzymes are known thus far to play a major role in xenobiotic metabolism. In particular, CYPs 1A2, 2B6, 2C9, 2C19, 2D6, and 3A4 are the major isoforms that catalyze drug metabolism reactions, of which CYPs 3A4 and 2D6 participate in the metabolism of approx 80% of commercially available drugs ***(3)***. Inhibition of CYPs has been implicated in the majority of reported clinically relevant drug–drug interactions.

Inhibition of CYPs could be classified into direct and metabolism- or mechanism-based inhibition ***(4)***. Direct inhibition is reversible, whereby the drug itself binds (noncovalently) to the enzyme, resulting in the alteration of the Michaelis-Menten kinetic parameters (K_m and V_{max}). This interaction could be competitive, noncompetitive, mixed, or uncompetitive inhibition. Metabolism- or mechanism-based inhibition results from the binding of a metabolic product to the enzyme. Metabolism- and mechanism-based inhibitions are further differentiated; the first results from the direct inhibition of CYP by a metabolic product of the drug that is a more potent reversible inhibitor ***(4)***. Mechanism-based inhibition results from irreversible covalent or noncovalent tight binding of a chemically reactive metabolic product to the enzyme, resulting in the inactivation of the enzyme (i.e., removing it from participating in metabolic reactions). Mechanism-based inhibitor are also called suicide substrates (also referred to as Trojan horses) as the compound is "metabolized" by the enzyme to the reactive intermediate. Another nomenclature is enzyme-activated irreversible inhibitors ***(5)***.

Mechanism-based inactivation can also be considered as an activation reaction, in that the drug substrate (mechanism-based inhibitor) is metabolically activated to a reactive intermediate that inactivates the CYP by binding to the heme, apoprotein, or both. Compounds that bind to the heme do so after oxidative metabolism into reactive intermediates that form a complex with the CYP heme. A stable ferrous–heme complex is formed, rendering the enzyme catalytically nonfunctional. Alkyl amines such as orphenadrine, macrolide antibiotics such as troleandomycin (TAO), and tricyclic antidepressants such as imipramine and desipramine are examples ***(6)***. A mechanism-based inhibitor presents itself to the active site of the enzyme as an innocuous molecule, but the catalytic action of the enzyme activates it to a reactive intermediate that binds to the enzyme. Thus, the reactive intermediate would have a high specificity to the enzyme catalyzing its formation and is therefore likely to react primarily with the target enzyme. Usually, this results in the covalent incorporation of a part or all of the modified inhibitor into the enzyme molecule or a noncovalent tight binding complex with the enzyme.

Because drug-metabolizing enzymes are inhibited in mechanism-based inactivation, as is the case with direct inhibitors, drug–drug interactions may result, which is one of the adverse effects of mechanism-based inactivation. Another aspect of mechanism-based inactivation, which does not apply to direct inhibitors, is that the modified CYP may produce a toxic response by itself. An example is the case with the *N*-alkyl heme products "green pigments," which could disrupt porphyrin synthesis ***(7)***. Furthermore, CYPs that are covalently modified by chemically reactive intermediates may act as antigens and elicit autoimmune responses ***(8,9)***, which have been implicated in some drug idiosyncratic effects. This has been correlated with some types of hepatitis, although a cause–effect relationship has not been established ***(2)***.

In mechanism-based inactivation reactions, usually there is competition between inactivation of the enzyme and turnover of the inhibitor, so conversion of the inhibitor to products could occur (partitioning). The degree of partitioning (partition ratio) depends on the efficiency of the inhibitor molecule to inactivate the enzyme. Compounds with low-partition ratios are more efficient inactivators and vice versa ***(5)***. Partition ratios are experimentally measured by determining the ratio of metabolite released vs the amount of the inactivated enzyme.

General characteristics of mechanism-based inactivation of CYPs are as follows:

1. Catalytic step(s) are involved in the inactivation process (reflecting the formation of reactive intermediate).
2. There is a time- and nicotinamide adenine dinucleotide phosphate (NADPH)–dependent loss of enzyme activity.
3. Rate of inactivation is dependent on the inhibitor concentration at low but not at high concentrations (reflecting the formation of an enzyme-reactive intermediate complex).

4. Rate of inactivation is slower in the presence of a substrate or a competitive inhibitor (substrates or competitive inhibitors protect the enzyme by competing for the active site of the enzyme).
5. Catalytic activity is not recovered after dialysis (reflecting that the inhibitor becomes irreversibly bound to the enzyme).

Mechanism-based inhibition of human CYPs has been well documented. Examples include furafylline inhibition of CYP1A2 ***(10)***; menthofuran inhibition of CYP2A6 ***(11)***; tienilic acid inhibition of CYP2C9 ***(12,13)***, SCH 66712 (5-fluoro-2-[4-[(2-phenyl-1H-imidazol-5-yl)methyl]-1-piperazinyl] pyrimidine) ***(14)***, (–)-chloroephedrine ***(15)*** and paroxetine ***(16)*** inhibition of CYP2D6; halothane inhibition of CYP2E1 ***(17)***; and gestodene inhibition of CYP3A4 ***(18)***. Mechanism-based inactivators of animal CYPs have also been well documented ***(19–23)***.

Because of the potential health implications of CYP inhibition in humans, it is important to screen out potent CYP inhibitors as early as possible in the discovery process. A compound could be a potent direct inhibitor and a potent metabolism- or mechanism-based inhibitor. However, it is not uncommon for a compound to be a weak direct inhibitor but a potent metabolism- or mechanism-based inhibitor. Therefore, performing the inhibition assays must include the assessment of metabolism- or mechanism-based inactivation by the performance of co- and preincubation experiments (explained later). In vitro models for screening for CYP inhibition are available. The utility of these models is based on the belief that metabolic drug–drug interactions involving CYP can be forecast using in vitro methods. This assumption has been proven true in many cases; however, it must be kept in mind that the situation in vivo is far more complex than the in vitro systems. Many factors, in addition to the potency of the compound as an inhibitor (K_i, K_{intact}, and partition ratio; explained later), must be considered. Among these are the concentration at the inhibition site, protein binding, relative contribution of various enzymes at different metabolic sites to the overall metabolism of the compound, and the formation of various metabolites, which could be inhibitors as well. Furthermore, CYP inhibitors and/or their metabolites could be inducers or activators of various enzymes, making the situation far more complex. Therefore, in vitro data could only determine what might happen in humans, and only clinical drug–drug interaction studies provide conclusive data.

Most pharmaceutical companies routinely evaluate the potential of new chemical entities (NCEs) to produce drug–drug interaction using in vitro models. The most common experimental systems are human liver microsomes and recombinant CYP isoforms isolated from cell cultures overexpressing individual CYPs ***(24)***. Other less common systems such as human hepatocytes and cryopreserved human hepatocytes have been used. Our laboratory had evaluated the recombinant CYP and human liver microsomes and decided to use the latter in all of our screenings *(25)*. Advances in mass spectrometry and robotics have made these assays fast, simple, and amenable to high-throughput screening, which made it possible to meet the increasing demands for such screens in early discovery. CYPs 2C9, 2C19, 2D6, and 3A4 are routinely evaluated during the discovery stage *(4,26–28)*. Significant inhibition of CYP, including metabolism- or mechanism-based inhibition, may preclude the compound from further consideration for development, unless for life-threatening, previously untreatable disease.

2. Materials

2.1. CYP Inhibition Assays

2.1.1. Probe Substrates and Metabolites for Human CYP Reactions

1. Testosterone (Sigma, St. Louis, MO).
2. 6β-Hydroxytestosterone (Sigma, St. Louis, MO).
3. Dextromethorphan (Sigma, St. Louis, MO).
4. Dextrorphan (Sigma, St. Louis, MO).
5. Phenacetin (Sigma, St. Louis, MO).
6. 4-Acetamidophenol (Sigma, St. Louis, MO).
7. Tolbutamide (ICN Pharmaceuticals, Costa Mesa, CA).
8. Hydroxytolbutamide (Ultrafine Chemicals, Manchester, England).
9. *S*-(+)-Mephenytoin (Ultrafine Chemicals, Manchester, England).
10. Hydroxymephenytoin (Ultrafine Chemicals, Manchester, England).

2.1.2. Selective Inhibitors for CYP Reactions

1. Troleandomycin (TAO; Sigma, St. Louis, MO).
2. Ketoconazole (ICN Pharmaceuticals, Costa Mesa, CA).
3. Quinidine (Sigma, St. Louis, MO).
4. Sulfaphenazole (Sigma, St. Louis, MO).
5. Ticlopidine (Sigma, St. Louis, MO).
6. Furafylline (Ultrafine Chemicals, Manchester, England).
7. SCH 66712 (5-fluoro-2-[4-[(2-phenyl-1H-imidazol-5-yl)methyl]-1-piperazinyl] pyrimidine) was synthesized at Schering-Plough Research Institute (Kenilworth, NJ).

2.1.3. Materials for Microsomal Incubation

1. Tris base (Sigma, St. Louis, MO).
2. Glacial acetic acid (Sigma, St. Louis, MO).
3. Potassium chloride (Sigma, St. Louis, MO).
4. Human liver microsomes (a pool of ≥25 male and female donors; Tissue Transplantation Technologies, Edison, NJ).
5. Genesis Workstation 150 (TECAN US, Research Triangle Park, NC).

6. Microplate incubator capable of accommodating 37°C (part of the Genesis Workstation 150).
7. Perchloric acid, 70% (Fisher, Pittsburgh, PA).
8. β-Nicotinamide adenine dinucleotide phosphate (NADPH; Sigma, St. Louis, MO).

2.1.4. New Chemical Entities Preparation

1. NCEs (Schering-Plough Research Institute, Kenilworth, NJ).
2. High-performance liquid chromatography (HPLC)-grade methanol, dimethylsulfoxide, and acetonitrile (Fisher, Pittsburgh, PA).

2.1.5. Sample Preparation for Liquid Chromatography/Tandem Mass Spectrometry (LC-MS/MS) Analysis

1. Corticosterone (Sigma, St. Louis, MO).
2. Levallorphan (Sigma, St. Louis, MO).
3. Refrigerated centrifuge capable of accommodating 96-well plates at 1800*g* such as the Allegra 25R (Beckman Coulter, Fullerton, CA).
4. Clear sealing film for microplates (ABgene, Epsom, Surrey, UK).

2.1.6. LC-MS/MS Analysis

1. API 3000 Mass Spectrometer (Applied Biosystems Sciex, Toronto, Ontario, Canada).
2. Shimadzu LC-10ADvp pumps and SCL-10A controller (Shimadzu, Columbia, MD).
3. Leap PAL autosampler (Leap Technologies, Carrboro, NC).
4. HPLC and mass spectrometer interfaced through a Sciex-heated nebulizer (an atmospheric pressure chemical ionization interface; Applied Biosystems Sciex, Toronto, Ontario, Canada).
5. Develosil Combi-RP5, 3.5 × 20-mm column (Phenomenex, Torrance, CA).

2.2. Specific Materials for the Dialysis Experiment (see Subheading 3.3.)

1. Spectra/por® cellulose ester sterile dispodialyzer with a molecular weight cutoff of 10,000 Da (Spectrum Laboratory, Rancho Dominguez, CA).
2. Maxirotator (Barnstead International, Dubuque, IA).

2.3. Specific Materials for the Effect of Trapping Agents and Free Radical Scavengers Experiments (see Subheading 3.5.)

1. Shaking waterbath (Precision Scientific, Winchester, VA).
2. Glutathione (Sigma, St. Louis, MO).
3. Superoxide dismutase (Sigma, St. Louis, MO).
4. Mannitol (Sigma, St. Louis, MO).

3. Methods

3.1. High-Throughput Screening for Direct and Metabolism- and Mechanism-Based Inhibition

The high-throughput protocol was designed to evaluate the potential of NCEs to inhibit human CYPs, including metabolism- and mechanism-based inhibition, in the early stage of drug discovery. In practice, CYP inhibition screening involves four processes: (1) in vitro incubation, (2) metabolite quantification, (3) data analysis, and (4) data reporting, as the generation of a large amount of data requires that the data be entered into an easily searchable database.

These assays are typically performed in 96-well microplates in triplicate in an incubation volume of 200 μL, using a Genesis Workstation liquid handler, which automates the dilution, pipetting, and the incubation steps. With each assay, prototype direct and mechanism-based inhibitors (if available) are usually used to ensure that the system works properly (*see* **Table 1**).

The selection of the probe substrate and its concentration is important to ensure that only one CYP is generating the metabolite in human liver microsomes. Thus, the substrate concentration should be at or below the *Km* for the reaction. Under these conditions, the IC_{50} determined is usually within twofold of the K_i for direct inhibitors. **Table 1** shows a list of the five major CYPs, their probe substrates, and their inhibitors and concentrations commonly used.

Probe substrates are initially dissolved in an organic solvent and diluted with water to yield solutions that can be stored at –20°C without precipitation. These solutions are typically stored for 2 to 4 mo. The substrate stock solutions are prepared as follows: 8 m*M* dextromethorphan in 20% dimethylsulfoxide (DMSO), 8 m*M* tolbutamide in 50% acetonitrile, 8 m*M* *S*-mephenytoin in 30% acetonitrile, and 5 m*M* phenacetin in 10% DMSO. Testosterone is prepared as a 20-m*M* solution in 100% acetonitrile. Prior to each assay, this solution is diluted fivefold in 50% aqueous acetonitrile to produce a 4-m*M* solution in 60% acetonitrile. For high-throughput assays, testosterone (a CYP3A4 marker substrate) and dextromethorphan (a CYP2D6 marker substrate under the conditions used in this assay) are combined in one assay. Similarly, tolbutamide (a CYP2C9 marker) and *S*-mephenytoin (a CYP2C19 marker) are combined in a separate assay. This approach has been validated by determining the IC_{50} values for a large number of compounds using both the single and combined assays. The phenacetin assay (for CYP1A2) is only occasionally done and is performed separately.

Table 1
Major Human CYPs Involved in Drug Metabolism, Their Probe Substrates, Metabolites, and Direct and Mechanism-Based Inhibitors Used

CYP	Substrate (concentration used)	Metabolite	Direct inhibitor	Mechanism-based inhibitor
CYP1A2	Phenacetin (100 μ*M*)	Acetaminophen	α-Naphthoflavone (0.1–1 μ*M*)	Furafylline
CYP2C9	Tolbutamide (200 μ*M*)	Hydroxytolbutamide	Sulfaphenazole (30 μ*M*)	Tienilic acid
CYP2C19	*S*-(+)-Mephenytoin (125 μ*M*)	4'-Hydroxymephenytoin	Tranylcypromine (50 μ*M*)	Ticlopidine
CYP2D6	Dextromethorphan (16 μ*M*)	Dextrorphan	Quinidine (5 μ*M*)	SCH 66712
CYP3A4	Testosterone (100 μ*M*)	6β-Hydroxytestosterone	Ketoconazole (1 μ*M*)	Troleandomycin (TAO)

3.1.1. Buffer Preparation

1. Dissolve 6.06 g Tris base and 11.2 g potassium chloride in 985 mL water.
2. Adjust the pH to 7.4 with glacial acetic acid.
3. Bring the volume to 1 L.
4. Filter the solution using a 0.2-μm filter and store at room temperature.

3.1.2. Substrate Preparation

1. Dissolve 100 mg testosterone in 17.3 mL acetonitrile.
2. Dissolve 148 mg dextromethorphan in 10 mL DMSO, complete the volume to 50 mL with water, and mix well.
3. Dissolve 217 mg tolbutamide in 50 mL acetonitrile, complete the volume to 100 mL with water, and mix well.
4. Dissolve 10 mg *S*-(+)-mephenytoin in 2.75 mL acetonitrile, add 6.4 mL of water, and mix well.
5. Dissolve 89.5 mg phenacetin in 10 mL DMSO, complete the volume to 100 mL with water, and mix well.

3.1.3. NCE Stock Solution Preparation

1. Samples of new chemical entities are initially dissolved in methanol to make 3-m*M* solutions. Gentle sonication may occasionally be necessary to completely dissolve the compound.
2. The 3-m*M* solution containing the compound is then serially diluted to 300 and 30 μ*M* in methanol.
3. These three solutions are then diluted 2.5-fold with water to make 1200-, 120-, and 12-μ*M* solutions in 40% methanol.

3.1.4. Preparation of Selective Inhibitor Controls

Inhibitor controls are dissolved in minimal amounts of methanol and diluted to produce solutions that are in approx 40% aqueous methanol. Whenever possible, known mechanism-based inhibitors are also used as standards. The solutions are made as follows:

1. Make an 8-m*M* solution of TAO in 40% aqueous methanol by dissolving 1 mg in 61 μL methanol, add 92 μL water, and mix well. Dilute 10-fold with 40% aqueous methanol to make an 800-μ*M* solution.
2. Make a 2-mg/mL solution of SCH 66712 in 20% aqueous methanol by dissolving 2 mg in 200 μL methanol followed by the addition of 800 μL of water and mixing. Dilute to 40 μg/mL with 40% aqueous methanol.
3. Make a 15-m*M* solution of sulfaphenazole by dissolving 1 mg in 212 μL methanol. Dilute to 1.2 m*M* by adding 40 μL of the methanol solution to 60 μL of water and complete the volume to 500 μL with 40% aqueous methanol. Dilute 10-fold in 40% aqueous methanol to make a 120-μ*M* solution.

4. Make a 5-m*M* solution of ticlopidine by dissolving 1 mg in 666 μL methanol. Dilute 60 μL of the methanol solution with 90 μL of water and add 100 μL of 40% aqueous methanol to make a 1.2-m*M* solution. Dilute 30-fold with 40% aqueous methanol to obtain a 40-μ*M* solution.
5. Make a 5-m*M* solution of furafylline by dissolving 1 mg in 769 μL methanol. Dilute 120 μL of the methanol solution with 180 μL of water and add 200 μL of 40% aqueous methanol to make a 1.2-m*M* solution. Dilute 10-fold with 40% aqueous methanol to obtain a 120-μ*M* solution.
6. Make a 2-m*M* solution of ketoconazole by dissolving 1 mg in 941 μL methanol. Dilute 50-fold with 40% methanol to obtain a 40-μ*M* solution.
7. Make a 20-m*M* solution of quinidine by dissolving 7.6 mg in 400 μL methanol, add 600 μL water, and mix well. Dilute 100-fold with 40% aqueous methanol to obtain a 200-μ*M* solution.

3.1.5. Preparation of Internal Standard Solutions for LC-MS/MS Analysis

1. Make a 15-m*M* solution of levallorphan by dissolving 5 mg in 769 μL water. Dilute 1000-fold with water to make a 15-μ*M* solution.
2. Make a 1-mg/mL solution of corticosterone by dissolving 1 mg in 1 mL methanol. Dilute 100-fold with methanol to obtain a 10-μg/mL solution.
3. Mix 7 mL levallorphan solution with 17.5 mL corticosterone solution.

3.1.6. Microsomal Incubation Procedure

The reaction mixture consists of liver microsomes at a protein concentration of 0.4 mg/mL, 1 m*M* NADPH, and probe substrate(s) at concentrations near the K_m values (*see* **Table 1**) in 50 m*M* Tris-acetate buffer, pH 7.4, containing 150 m*M* potassium chloride and NCEs at 0.3-, 3.0-, and 30-μ*M* concentrations. The NCEs are added in 40% aqueous methanol, resulting in a final methanol concentration of 1% by volume. The procedure outlined below is for an experiment in which 15 NCEs are simultaneously analyzed for CYP3A4 and CYP2D6 inhibition under both the co- and preincubation conditions. Adjustments are made if the number of NCEs to be evaluated is different. A similar protocol is followed for the combined CYP2C9 and CYP2C19 assay and for the individual CYP1A2 assay with the appropriate changes.

3.1.6.1. Coincubation

The coincubation experiment is carried out as follows:

1. In a 50-mL tube, add 31.5 mL buffer, 76 μL 8 m*M* dextromethorphan, 950 μL 4 m*M* testosterone, and 760 μL microsomal protein (20 mg/mL); mix well; and store on ice.
2. Dissolve 50 mg NADPH in a 6-mL buffer and store on ice.
3. Add 5 μL buffer, 40% aqueous methanol, 40 μ*M* ketoconazole solution, 200 μ*M* quinidine solution, 1 μg/mL SCH 66712 or 800 μ*M* TAO solution to separate wells (in triplicate) of a 96-well microplate.

4. Add 5 μL of each dilution of the NCEs (in triplicate) to separate wells of the 96-well plate.
5. Add 175 μL of the microsomes-substrate mixture (prepared in **step 1**) to each well.
6. Warm at 37°C for 5 min.
7. Add 20 μL of the NADPH solution, mix, and incubate for 13 min at 37°C.
8. Stop the reaction by the addition of 30 μL of 35% perchloric acid solution and mixing.
9. Add 70 μL of the internal standard solution that contains both levallorphan and corticosterone and mix well.
10. Centrifuge for 20 min at 1800*g* in a refrigerated centrifuge.
11. Seal the plates with a clear sealing film for LC-MS/MS analysis.

3.1.6.2. Preincubation

To identify metabolism- and mechanism-based inhibitors, a "preincubation" step is employed. The NCE at the same concentrations as above is allowed to react with the microsomes in the presence of the cofactor NADPH for 30 min before the substrate is added. The probe substrates are then added, and the reaction is allowed to proceed for an additional 13 min. The procedure outlined below is designed to complement that outline in **SubSubheading 3.1.6.1.** so that potential metabolism- and mechanism-based inhibitors can be identified.

1. Dissolve 50 mg NADPH in a 6-mL buffer and store on ice.
2. In a 50-mL tube, add 28.7 mL buffer, 3.8 mL NADPH, and 760 μL microsomal protein (20 mg/mL); mix well; and store on ice.
3. Prepare a 96-well microplate as described in **Subheading 3.1.6.1., steps 3** and **4**.
4. Prepare the substrate solution by adding 200 μL of 8 m*M* dextromethorphan and 2.5 mL of 4 m*M* testosterone to 7.3 mL buffer, mix well, and store at room temperature.
5. Add 175 μL of the microsomes-cofactor mixture (prepared in **step 2**) to each well.
6. Incubate at 37°C for 30 min.
7. Add 20 μL of the substrate solution to each well, mix, and incubate for 13 min at 37°C.
8. Stop the reaction by the addition of 30 μL of 35% perchloric acid solution and mixing.
9. Add 70 μL of the internal standard solution and mix well.
10. Centrifuge for 20 min at 1800*g* in a refrigerated centrifuge.
11. Seal the plates with clear sealing film for LC-MS/MS analysis.

3.1.7. LC-MS/MS Analysis

The quantification of the metabolites of the probe substrates is carried out using a SCIEX API 3000, running in the single-reaction monitoring (SRM) mode. Supernatants are injected into the Develosil Combi-RP5 HPLC column, and the earlier eluting salts are diverted to waste using a Valco two-position valve. The analytes are separated from the salts using a gradient elution with a mobile phase consisting of 65% solution A (0.1% formic acid in 5% aqueous methanol) and 35% solution B (0.1% formic acid in 95% aqueous methanol) for the first 0.2 min after injection. For the next 0.2 min, the mobile phase is changed to 100% solution B, and then the mobile phase is changed to the initial conditions. The cycle time for this assay is approx 1.3 min. Each metabolite of the probe substrate is quantified by linear regression using a calibration curve that is composed of the analyte at a concentration range that accommodates those found in the incubation mixture. The IC_{50} is calculated as the concentration that inhibits 50% of the metabolite formation compared to solvent alone under each incubation condition.

The potential for a test compound to be classified as a metabolism- or mechanism-based inhibitor is assessed using both sets of data from preincubation and coincubation experiments. If the IC_{50} values under both conditions are similar (within one- to threefold), it is unlikely that the compound is a metabolism- or mechanism-based inhibitor. If there is a greater inhibition after preincubation ($IC_{50} \leq$ fivefold after preincubation), the compound is likely to be a metabolism- or mechanism-based inhibitor.

Unlike direct inhibition, metabolism- and mechanism-based inhibition is time dependent; therefore, the IC_{50} determined after preincubation would be dependent on the preincubation time. In our system, we use a 30-min preincubation time to provide sufficient time for inhibitory metabolite(s) to be formed. Also, because of the time dependency of metabolism- and mechanism-based inhibition, the IC_{50} value determined after preincubation should not be used in the absolute sense as a measure of potency of the compound; rather, it should be used for comparison to the IC_{50} generated after coincubation to ascertain if the compound is likely to be a metabolism- or mechanism-based inhibitor. However, to confirm the initial findings and to differentiate between mechanism- and metabolism-based inhibitors, additional experiments are required. These experiments are usually carried out on rare occasions, as metabolism- and mechanism-based inhibitors are eliminated from further consideration for development. Nevertheless, if mechanism- or metabolism-based inhibition is a problem with an entire chemical series, or there is still an interest in a metabolism- or mechanism-based inhibitor, further characterization of the inhibition is in order.

3.2. Evaluation of NADPH Dependency

One of the major characteristics that differentiate direct from metabolism- and mechanism-based inhibition is that in the latter, catalytic steps are involved to form the reactive metabolite, and therefore NADPH is required. The effect of NADPH on the inhibition of the enzymatic activity is determined as follows:

1. NCE at a range of concentrations (3–4) is incubated with human liver microsomes at a protein concentration of 0.4 mg/mL for 30 min at 37°C in the presence and absence of 1 m*M* NADPH.
2. The activity of the enzyme is determined by the addition of the appropriate marker probe substrate at concentrations as previously.
3. The IC_{50} values are determined in the presence and absence of NADPH.
4. A requirement for NADPH for the inhibition is ascertained if the activity of the enzyme is diminished to a greater extent in the presence of NADPH during preincubation; therefore, this would result in increased inhibition of CYP (lower IC_{50}), suggesting metabolism- or mechanism-based inhibition. However, this would not differentiate between metabolism- and mechanism-based inhibitions.

3.3. Dialysis

A dialysis experiment is carried out to differentiate between metabolism- and mechanism-based inhibitors. The effect of dialysis on the enzyme activity is evaluated as follows:

1. NCE is preincubated (in the absence of substrate) with human liver microsomes for 30 min at 37°C in the presence of 1 m*M* NADPH at a protein concentration of approx 10-fold higher than that required for activity assays (4 mg/mL).
2. Following preincubation, 20-μL aliquots are removed and immediately assayed for enzyme activity after 10-fold dilution (total volume is 200 μL) with the addition of NADPH (1 m*M*) as indicated above.
3. Additional samples of the incubation mixture are subjected to dialysis against the same buffer (100-fold volume) for 3 to 6 h at 4°C with three buffer changes using Spectra/por® cellulose ester sterile dispodialyzer with a molecular weight cutoff of 10,000 Dalton samples are rotated using a Maxirotator.
4. After dialysis, the enzyme activity is determined in 20-μL aliquots after the 10-fold dilution with the addition of 1 m*M* NADPH as mentioned above. Dialysis is expected to remove the majority of test compound and/or its metabolites that are reversibly bound to the microsomal enzyme, and only metabolites that are irreversibly bound to the enzyme would remain, hence inhibiting the enzyme. Diluting the reaction mixture by 10-fold in the activity assay would minimize the direct contribution of the test compound still remaining after dialysis to the inhibition.
5. If the activity of the enzyme following dialysis is not restored to levels that are near control levels, it can be concluded that the compound is likely to be a mechanism-based inhibitor. If the activity of the enzyme is restored to near control values, it is likely that a more potent reversible inhibitor is formed during the preincubation stage; hence, it is metabolism-based, not mechanism-based, inhibition.
6. Control incubations from the same microsomal pool without the test compound are carried out and subjected to dialysis with the sample for the same period and are used for basal activity, as dialysis might affect the absolute enzyme activity.

3.4. Determination of Inactivation Rate Constants

These experiments are carried out to evaluate the potency of a compound as a mechanism-based inactivator, which allows for the determination of both the time-dependent (K_{intact}) and the concentration-dependent (K_i) inactivation constants. These are time-consuming studies and seldom carried out in drug discovery, as potential metabolism- and mechanism-based inactivators are identified early and eliminated from further consideration. However, on rare occasions when a mechanism-based inactivator is considered for development (e.g., a first-in-class compound for life-threatening, previously untreatable disease), it is prudent to characterize the inactivation potency of the compound. These experiments are carried out as follows:

1. Several concentrations (usually 4–5) of test compound are preincubated at 37°C with 1 m*M* NADPH and human liver microsomes at a protein concentration of 4 mg/mL.
2. At selected time intervals (0–15 min), 20-µL aliquots of the preincubation mixture are transferred to tubes containing buffer, pH 7.4, and a marker probe substrate. NADPH (1 m*M*) is added to initiate the turnover of the substrate (activity assay). The final reaction mixture is diluted 10-fold compared to that of the preincubation assay (total volume is 200 µL). Dilution quenches the inactivation reaction at the desired time point. The probe substrate concentration for the activity assay should be that which produces maximal velocity for transformation (V_{max}) to minimize competitive inhibition. The activity assay is carried out for 13 to 20 min, depending on the enzyme, and the reaction is terminated by the addition of perchloric acid for protein precipitation followed by centrifugation and LC-MS/MS analysis as mentioned above.
3. The slopes obtained from linear regression of the log percentage remaining activity vs time plots at each concentration of the test compound are determined.
4. The first-order inactivation rate constant (k) at each concentration is obtained by multiplying 2.303 by the slope.
5. The $t_{1/2}$ values of the inactivation reaction are determined ($t_{1/2} = 0.693/k$) for each concentration and plotted on the *y*-axis vs the reciprocal of the concentration of the test compound on the *x*-axis (Kitz-Wilson plots).
6. The K_{intact}, which has a unit of time^{-1} (rate constant for maximal inactivation), and K_i, which has a unit of concentration, are determined from the *y*- and the *x*-intercepts of the Kitz-Wilson plots, respectively. Other methods for the determination of K_{intact} and K_i have also been reported *(5)*.

3.5. Effect of Trapping Agents and Free Radical Scavengers

Two additional experiments can be carried out to confirm that mechanism-based inactivation is a result of a chemically reactive intermediate that is formed from test compound rather than from artifacts of the assay. First is the evaluation of the effect of a trapping agent such as glutathione (GSH at 1–2 m*M*) on the inactivation of the enzyme. GSH would be expected to trap reactive electrophilic species that may leave the enzyme during the inactivation reaction. A GSH adduct of the reactive metabolite can be monitored using LC-MS/MS. On the other hand, if the electrophilic species is bound instantly to the enzyme, no such adduct is detected. Protection of the enzyme from inactivation by GSH and the detection of the GSH adduct are indicative of a test compound that forms a reactive electrophilic species that is not instantly bound to the enzyme. This experiment is carried out as follows:

1. NCE is preincubated at 37°C with 1 m*M* NADPH and microsomal protein (0.4 mg/mL) in the presence and absence of 1 to 2 m*M* GSH.
2. The probe substrate is added, and the enzyme activity is determined.

The second experiment is based on the fact that during the catalytic cycle of CYP, reactive oxygen species such as the superoxide ion and hydroxy radical may be generated *(2)*. These species have the potential to inactivate the enzyme; therefore, it may be prudent to rule out the contribution of reactive oxygen species to the inactivation process as follows:

1. NCE is preincubated at 37°C with 1 m*M* NADPH and 0.4 mg/mL microsomal protein in the presence and absence of scavengers of reactive oxygen species, such as superoxide dismutase (1000 U/mL) and mannitol (1 m*M*), which are added individually.
2. The probe substrate is added, and the enzyme activity is determined.

Protection of the enzyme by free radical scavengers would suggest that the inactivation of the enzyme might be proceeding via the generation of reactive oxygen species during preincubation.

4. Conclusion

This chapter discussed the identification of CYP metabolism- and mechanism-based inhibitors in drug discovery. The importance of screening new chemical entities for the potential inhibition, including metabolism- and mechanism-based inhibition, is discussed as well as various experimental procedures to confirm the initial findings. These assays are very effective drug metabolism and pharmacokinetics (DMPK) screens; they are simple, fast, well validated, and could be performed in a high-throughput format. Therefore, they are used extensively in a discovery screening paradigm by the major pharmaceutical companies. Detailed experimental protocols and notes are included. The cutoff point for the acceptable level of direct inhibition of a drug candidate is variable, and other considerations such as the intended therapy, the stage of the discovery program, and the pharmacological potency of the compound as well as its pharmacokinetics must be taken into account. However, because of a greater risk, potent metabolism- and mechanism-based inhibitors are usually excluded from consideration for development.

5. Notes

1. It is important to recognize that microsomal CYP reactions are sensitive to the type and concentration of the solvent used even at concentrations as low as 1%.
2. In cases when a test compound is not soluble in the incubation mixture, the concentration of methanol may be increased to up to 3% by volume, or DMSO at 1% final concentration could be used. The drawback is that the basal enzyme activity might decrease considerably. However, under these conditions, an approximate assessment of the inhibition potential of the compound can be made.
3. One caveat in the dialysis experiment is that dialysis may not always remove reversibly bound material that has partitioned with high affinity to the microsomal lipid membrane (usually with high molecular weight, highly lipophilic compounds). In such cases, the dialysis experiment may not be able to differentiate between mechanism- and metabolism-based inhibition.
4. Prototype mechanism-based inhibitors are added at one concentration at which a large decrease in the enzymatic activity can be observed after the 30-min preincubation.
5. The inhibition data are entered into Excel spreadsheets, and the IC_{50} values are estimated from the three concentrations using linear regression. If there is less than 50% inhibition at the highest concentration, the IC_{50} value is reported as >30 μ*M*. If there is more than 50% inhibition at the 0.3 μ*M* concentration, the IC_{50} value is reported as <0.3 μ*M*. Data analysis is performed using Activity Base software, which results in direct data entry into the database. Once the results are entered, they become available for searches, and the entire discovery research community has access to it. Under these conditions, approx 30 to 45 compounds can be assayed for multiple CYPs for both direct and metabolism- and mechanism-based inhibition per day with an overnight analysis using the mass spectrometer. The next morning, data analysis and database entry can be accomplished within 1 to 2 h.
6. One important consideration in assessing the potential of a test compound to be a metabolism- or mechanism-based inhibitor is its solubility. It is possible that a compound with a limited solubility in the incubation mixture (common in discovery) may be dissolved to a greater extent during preincubation for 30 min at 37°C, resulting in a greater inhibition after preincubation compared to coincubation. This would lead to the erroneous conclusion that the compound is a metabolism- or mechanism-based inhibitor. To guard against this, the solubility of the compound in the incubation buffer needs to be determined. However, this may not be feasible in the high-throughput discovery mode.

References

1. Honig, P. K., Wortham, D. C., Zamani, K., Conner, D. P., Mullin, J. C., and Cantilena, L. R. (1993) Terfenadine-ketoconazole interaction, pharmacokinetics and electrocardiographic consequences. *JAMA* **269,** 1513–1518.
2. Guengerich, F. P. (2001) Common and uncommon cytochrome P450 reactions related to metabolism and chemical toxicity. *Chem. Res. Toxicol.* **14,** 611–650.
3. Guengerich, F. P. (1996) In vitro techniques for studying drug metabolism. *J. Pharmacokin. Biopharmaceut.* **44,** 521–533.
4. White, R. E. (2000) High-throughput screening in drug metabolism and pharmacokinetic support of drug discovery. *Ann. Rev. Pharmacol. Toxicol.* **40,** 133–157.
5. Silverman, R. B. (1988) *Mechanism-Based Enzyme Inactivation: Chemistry and Enzymology*. CRC Press, Boca Raton, FL.
6. Sinal, C. J. and Bend, J. R. (1995) Isozyme-selective metabolic intermediate complex formation of guinea pig hepatic cytochrome P450 by N-aralkylated derivatives of 1-aminobenzotriazole. *Chem. Res. Toxicol.* **8,** 82–91.
7. Ortiz de Montellano, P. R. and Correia, M. A. (1983) Suicidal destruction of cytochrome P-450 during oxidative drug metabolism. *Annu. Rev. Pharmacol. Toxicol.* **23,** 481–503.
8. Beaune, P., Dansette, P. M., Mansuy, D., Kiffel, L., Finck, M., Amar, C., et al. (1987) Human anti-endoplasmic reticulum autoantibodies appearing in a drug-induced hepatitis are directed against a human liver cytochrome P-450 that hydroxylates the drug. *Proc. Natl. Acad. Sci. USA* **84,** 551–555.
9. Beaune, P., Pessayre, D., Dansette, P., Mansuy, D., and Manns, M. (1994) Autoantibodies against cytochromes P450: role in human diseases. *Adv. Pharmacol.* **30,** 199–245.
10. Kunze, K. L. and Trager, W. F. (1993) Isoform selective mechanism based inhibition of human cytochrome P4501A2 by furafylline. *Chem. Res. Toxicol.* **6,** 649–656.
11. Khojasteh-Bakht, S. C., Koenigs, L. L., Peter, R. M., Trager, W. F., and Nelson S. D. (1998) (R)-(+)-Menthofuran is a potent, mechanism-based inactivator of human liver cytochrome P4502A6. *Drug Metab. Dispos.* **26,** 701–704.
12. Lopez-Garcia, M. P., Dansette, P. M., and Mansuy, D. (1994) Thiophene derivatives as new mechanism-based inhibitors of cytochromes P-450: inactivation of yeast-expressed human liver cytochrome P-450 2C9 by tienilic acid. *Biochemistry* **33,** 166–175.
13. Jean, P., Lopez-Garcia, P., Dansette, P., Mansuy, D., and Goldstein, J. L. (1996) Oxidation of tienilic acid by human yeast-expressed cytochromes P-450 2C8, 2C9, 2C18 and 2C19: evidence that this drug is a mechanism-based inhibitor specific for cytochrome P-450 2C9. *Eur. J. Biochem.* **241,** 797–804.
14. Palamanda, J. R., Casciano, C., Norton, L., Clement, R., Favreau, L., Lin, C. C., et al. (2001) Mechanism-based inactivation of CYP2D6 by 5-fluoro-2-[4-[(2-phenyl-1H-imidazol-5-yl)methyl]-1-piperazinyl]pyrimidine. *Drug Metab. Dispos.* **29,** 863–867.

15. Rege, B., Carter, K. M., Sarker, M. A., Kellogg, G. E., and Soine, W. H. (2002) Irreversible inhibition of CYP2D6 by (–)-chloroephedrine, a possible impurity of methamphetamine. *Drug Metab. Dispos.* **30,** 1337–1343.
16. Bertelsen, K. M., Venkatakrishnan, K., Von Moltke, L. L., Obach, S., and Greenblatt, D. J. (2003) Apparent mechanism-based inhibition of human CYP2D6 in vitro by paroxetine: comparison with fluoxetine and quinidine. *Drug Metab. Dispos.* **31,** 289–293.
17. Madan, A. and Parkinson, A. (1996) Characterization of the NADPH-dependent covalent binding of [^{14}C]halothane to human liver microsomes: a role for cytochrome P4502E1 at low substrate concentrations. *Drug Metab. Dispos.* **24,** 1307–1313.
18. Guengerich, F. P. (1990) Mechanism-based inactivation of human liver microsomal cytochrome P-450 IIIA4 by gestodene. *Chem. Res. Toxicol.* **3,** 363–371.
19. Hopkins, N. E., Foroozesh, M. K., and Alworth, W. L. (1992) Suicide inhibitors of cytochrome P4501A1 and P4502B1. *Biochem. Pharmacol.* **44,** 787–796.
20. Crowley, J. R. and Hollenberg, P. F. (1995) Mechanism-based inactivation of rat liver cytochrome P4502B1 by phencyclidine and its oxidative product, the iminium ion. *Drug Metab. Dispos.* **23,** 786–793.
21. Roberts, E. S., Hopkins, N. E., Zaluzec, E. J., Gage, D. A., Alworth, W. L., and Hollenberg, P. F. (1995) Mechanism-based inactivation of cytochrome P4502B1 by 9-ethynylphenanthrene. *Arch. Biochem. Biophys.* **323,** 295–302.
22. Sharma, U., Roberts, E. S., Kent, U. M., Owens, S. M., and Hollenberg, P. F. (1996) Metabolic inactivation of cytochrome P4502B1 by phencyclidine: immunochemical and radiochemical analysis of the protective effects of glutathione. *Drug Metab. Dispos.* **25,** 243–250.
23. Foroozesh, M., Primrose, G., Guo, Z., Bell, L. C., Alworth, W. L., and Guengerich, F. P. (1997) Aryl acetylenes as mechanism-based inhibitors of cytochrome P450-dependent monooxygenase enzymes. *Chem. Res. Toxicol.* **10,** 91–102.
24. Crespi, C. L., Miller, V. P., and Penman, B. W. (1997) Microtiter plate assays for inhibition of human drug-metabolizing cytochromes P-450. *Anal. Biochem.* **248,** 188–190.
25. Nomeir, A. A., Ruegg, C., Shoemaker, M., Favreau, L., Palamanda, J. R., Silber, P., et al. (2001) Inhibition of CYP3A4 in a rapid microtiter plate assay using recombinant enzyme and in human liver microsomes using conventional substrates. *Drug Metab. Dispos.* **29,** 748–753.
26. Lin, J. H. and Lu, A. H. (1997) Role of pharmacokinetics and metabolism in drug discovery and development. *Pharmacol. Rev.* **49,** 403–449.
27. Palamanda, J. R., Favreau, L., Lin, C. C., and Nomeir, A. A. (1998) Validation of a rapid microtiter plate assay to conduct cytochrome P4502D6 enzyme inhibition studies. *Drug Discovery Today* **10,** 466–470.
28. Chu, I., Favreau, L. V., Soares, T., Lin, C.-C., and Nomeir, A. A. (2000) Validation of a higher-throughput high-performance liquid chromatographic/atmospheric pressure chemical ionization tandem mass spectrometry assays to conduct cytochrome P450s CYP2D6 and CYP3A4 enzyme inhibition studies in human liver microsomes. *Rapid Commun. Mass Spectrom.* **14,** 207–214.

17

Detection of DNA Adducts by ^{32}P-Postlabeling Analysis

Naomi Suzuki, Padmaja M. Prabhu, and Shinya Shibutani

Summary

^{32}P-Postlabeling analysis is a powerful technique for the detection, quantification, and identification of DNA adducts induced by mutagens or carcinogens, including large numbers of drugs and their metabolites. The method includes enzymatic digestion of a deoxyribonucleic acid (DNA) sample to the adducted nucleoside 3'-monophosphates and partial purification of the adducted nucleotides, followed by the 5'-labeling with ^{32}P. For analysis of DNA adducts, polyethyleneimine-cellulose thin-layer chromatography (TLC) plates were generally used to resolve ^{32}P-labeled DNA adducts (^{32}P-postlabeling/TLC analysis). However, the procedure detecting DNA adducts using the TLC plate is time-consuming and labor intensive. To expedite analyses, nondenaturing polyacrylamide gel electrophoresis (PAGE) has recently been adapted for the ^{32}P-postlabeling analysis (^{32}P-postlabeling/PAGE analysis); the detection limit for 5 μg DNA is approx 7 adducts/10^9 nucleotides, which is similar to that for ^{32}P-postlabeling/TLC. HPLC on-lined with a radioisotope detector system (^{32}P-postlabeling/high-performance liquid chromatography [HPLC] analysis) is also used to increase the resolution and detection limit (approx 3 adducts/10^{10} nucleotides) of DNA adducts. These three ^{32}P-postlabeling techniques are described for the analysis of DNA adducts.

Key Words: ^{32}P-postlabeling; DNA adduct; DNA damage; TLC; gel electrophoresis; HPLC.

1. Introduction

^{32}P-Postlabeling analysis has been widely used for the detection of a variety of deoxyribonucleic acid (DNA) adducts induced by endogenous and exogenous mutagens or carcinogens ***(1–3)***. This technique has also been applied to

From: *Methods in Pharmacology and Toxicology*
Optimization in Drug Discovery: In Vitro Methods
Edited by: Z. Yan and G. W. Caldwell © Humana Press Inc., Totowa, NJ

explore the genotoxic events of large numbers of drugs that relate to anticancer treatment ***(4)***, antibiotics ***(5)***, estrogens ***(6–9)***, and antiestrogens ***(10,11)*** and to identify the carcinogenic substance contained in Chinese herbs ***(12)***. The methods, including enzymatic digestion of the DNA sample and labeling the adducted nucleotides with ^{32}P, have not significantly changed in past two decades. Polyethyleneimine (PEI)–cellulose thin-layer chromatography (TLC) plates are generally used to resolve ^{32}P-labeled DNA adducts two-dimensionally using several different buffer conditions (^{32}P-postlabeling/TLC analysis) ***(1,13,14)***; however, using this technique, only one ^{32}P-labeled sample can be analyzed per TLC plate, and the migration of DNA adducts on a TLC plate is variable on each TLC plate. Separation by TLC is time-consuming and labor intensive. To expedite analyses, nondenaturing 30% polyacrylamide gel electrophoresis (PAGE) has been adapted for the ^{32}P-postlabeling analysis (^{32}P-postlabeling/PAGE analysis) ***(15)***. The major advantages of this technique are (1) many DNA samples can be loaded concomitantly on the PAGE along with standard markers, (2) DNA adducts can be resolved in only a few hours, and (3) exposure to ^{32}P during the handling can be minimized. The detection limit for both ^{32}P-postlabeling/TLC and ^{32}P-postlabeling/PAGE analyses is approx 7 adducts/10^9 nt. To increase the resolution and detection limit (approx 3 adducts/10^{10} nt) of DNA adducts, high-performance liquid chromatography (HPLC) on-lined with a radioisotope detector is also used (^{32}P-postlabeling/HPLC analysis) ***(2,11,16)***. Although many modified procedures have been published, we introduce the general methods of three different ^{32}P-postlabeling techniques applied for the analysis of DNA adducts. A flow diagram for the procedures used for ^{32}P-postlabeling analyses is presented in **Fig. 1**.

2. Materials

2.1. Isolation of DNA From Cultured Cells and Animal and Human Tissues

1. 1.0% Sodium dodecyl sulfate (SDS)/10 m*M* ethylenediaminetetraacetic acid (EDTA)/20 m*M* Tris-HCl, pH 7.4, at 4°C.
2. Ribonuclease (RNase) A (Worthington Biochemical Corp., Freehold, NJ) (*see* **Note 1**).
3. RNase T1 (Worthington Biochemical Corp., Freehold, NJ).
4. Proteinase K (Sigma-Aldrich, St. Louis, MO).
5. Tris-saturated phenol (Roche Molecular Biochemicals, Indianapolis, IN) at 4°C (*see* **Note 2**).
6. Chloroform (molecular biology grade).
7. Absolute ethanol (100% pure).
8. 1X SSC: 0.15 *M* NaCl/1 m*M* EDTA/0.015 *M* sodium citrate, pH 7.2, at 4°C.
9. Polytoron homogenizer.

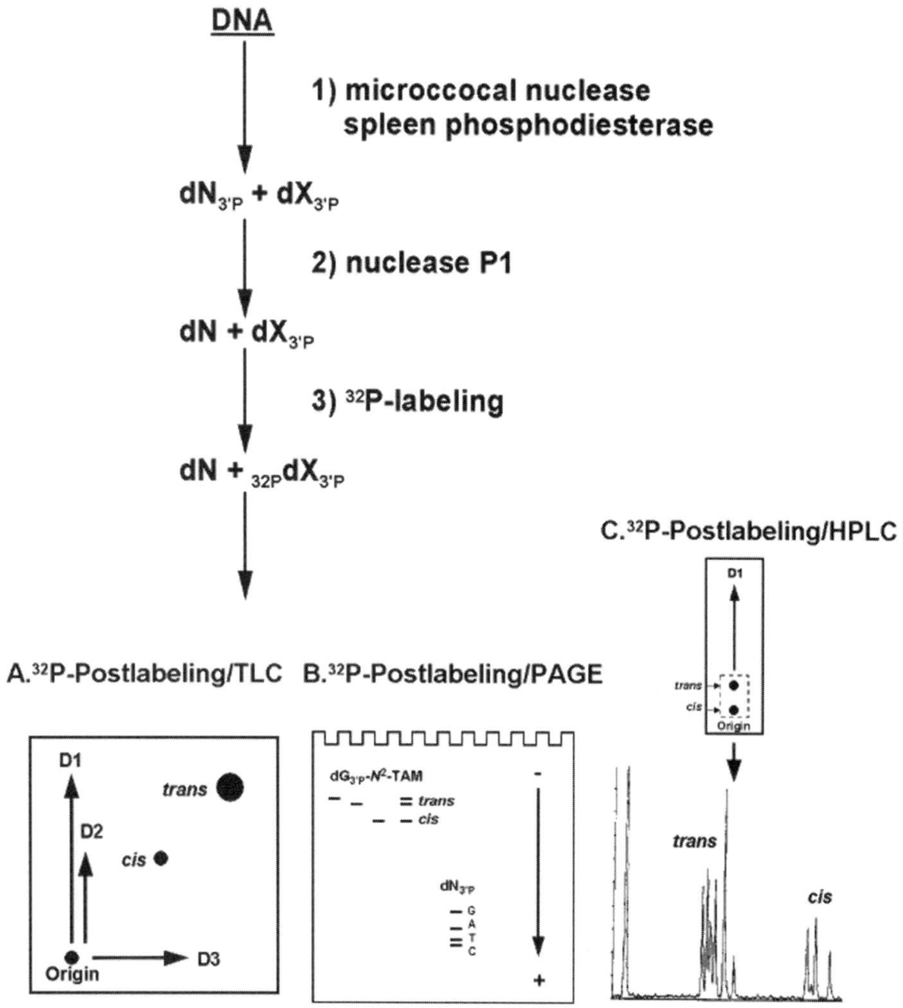

Fig. 1. A flow diagram for the procedures used for ^{32}P-postlabeling analyses.

2.2. Enzymatic Digestion of DNA Sample

1. Buffer: 8 m*M* $CaCl_2$/17 m*M* sodium succinate buffer, pH 6.0, at 4°C.
2. Micrococcal nuclease (Worthington Biochemical Corp., Freehold, NJ).
3. Spleen phosphodiesterase II (Worthington Biochemical Corp., Freehold, NJ) (*see* **Note 3**).
4. Nuclease P1 (Roche Molecular Biochemicals, Indianapolis, IN).
5. 1-Butanol (molecular biology grade).

2.3. Labeling Adducted Nucleotides With ^{32}P

1. [γ-^{32}P]–adenosine triphosphate (ATP) (specific activity, >6000 Ci/mmol) at –20°C (*see* **Note 4**).
2. 3'-Phosphatase-free T4 polynucleotide kinase (Roche Molecular Biochemicals, Indianapolis, IN) at –20°C (*see* **Note 5**).
3. Potato apyrase (Sigma-Aldrich, St. Louis, MO).
4. 10 m*M* Spermidine aqueous solution at –20°C.
5. 50 m*M* Dithiothreitol (DTT) aqueous solution at –20°C.
6. 10X linker-kinase buffer: 100 m*M* $MgCl_2$/700 m*M* Tris-HCl buffer, pH 7.6, at 4°C.
7. 10X formamide dye: 10 mg bromophenol blue and 10 mg xylene cyanol in 10 mL formamide.

2.4. ^{32}P-Postlabeling/TLC Analysis

1. PEI-cellulose thin-layer plate (Machery-Nagel, Duren, Germany).
2. Chromatography paper (Whatman Grade 3MM Chr.).
3. D1 buffer: 1.7 *M* sodium phosphate buffer, pH 6.0.
4. D2 buffer: 1.1 *M* lithium formate/2.7*M* urea, pH 3.5.
5. D3 buffer: 0.48 *M* LiCl/0.3*M* Tris-HCl/5.1 *M* urea, pH 8.0.
6. 4 *M* Pyrimidinium formate, pH 4.3. 7. β-Phosphorimager.

2.5. ^{32}P-Postlabeling/PAGE Analysis

1. 40% Acrylamide solution: 38 g acrylamide and 2 g *N,N'*-methylene bisacrylamide in final volume 100 mL of distilled water at 4°C.
2. 10X Tris borate (TBE) buffer: 2.24 *M* boric acid/25.5 m*M* EDTA/1 *M* Tris-base, pH 7.0.
3. 10% Ammonium persulfate aqueous solution. Make fresh and store for weeks at 4°C.
4. *N,N,N',N'*-tetramethylethylenediamine (TEMED) at 4°C.
5. Electrophoresis apparatus.

2.6. Measurement of ^{32}P-Labeled DNA Adducts

1. β-Phosphorimager.
2. X-ray film.
3. X-ray film developer.
4. Scintillation liquid.
5. Scintillation vials.
6. β-Liquid scintillation counter.

2.7. Determination of ^{32}P-Labeled-DNA Adducts by HPLC

1. 4 *M* Pyrimidinium formate, pH 4.3.
2. 0.2 *M* Ammonium formate, pH 4.0.
3. Acetonitrile/methanol (6:1, v/v).
4. Thermo Hypersil BDS C_{18} analytical column (0.46 × 25 cm, 5 μm, Thermo Hypersil, Bellefonte, PA).

5. HPLC.
6. Radioisotope detector.

3. Methods

3.1. Isolation of DNA From Cultured Cells or Tissues

When cultured cells or animals are exposed to a drug or its metabolite, the DNA can be extracted from the cells or tissues by using **steps 1–4**. When the DNA is directly incubated with a drug or its metabolite using cytosol, microsome, or a purified enzyme, the DNA should be extracted, following **steps 3–4**.

1. Suspend the cells (10^7–10^8) or tissue (10–100 mg) in ice-cold 1.5 mL of 1.0% SDS/10 m*M* EDTA/20 m*M* Tris-HCl, pH 7.4, in a polypropylene tube and homogenize for 30 s at 0°C using a Polytron homogenizer.
2. Incubate the homogenate at 37°C for 30 min with RNase (300 µg) and RNase T1 (50 U), followed by incubation in 750 µg proteinase K for 30 min.
3. Add an equal volume of Tris-saturated phenol to the reaction mixture, mix well for 30 s at room temperature using vortex, and centrifuge at 1600*g* for 10 min. If the organic (lower) and aqueous (upper) phases are not well separated, centrifuge again at a higher speed and/or for a longer time. Transfer the aqueous phase carefully in a fresh tube; discard the interface and organic phases. Add an equal volume of Tris-saturated phenol/chloroform (1:1, v/v), mix for 30 s, and centrifuge. Transfer again the aqueous phase in a fresh tube. Add an equal volume of chloroform, mix for 30 s, and centrifuge. Transfer the aqueous phase in a fresh tube.
4. To extract the DNA, add 3 volumes of ice-cold absolute ethanol, mix well for 30 s, centrifuge at 14,000*g* for 10 min, and remove the supernatant. Dissolve the precipitate in 100 µL distilled water, add 500 µL of ice-cold absolute ethanol, mix well, and centrifuge; repeat this process once.

To avoid contamination by the RNA, **steps 2** and **3** should be repeated. The purified DNA should be dissolved in 1 mL of 0.01X SSC. Estimate concentration of the DNA using a UV spectrophotometer (50 µg = 1.0 OD at 260 nm). Approximately 100 µg DNA can be extracted from 10^8 cells or 100 mg of the tissue; the recovery of DNA varies depending on the cell type and organs used. Store the DNA sample at –70°C.

3.2. Enzymatic Digestion of DNA Sample

This process enriches the adducted nucleotides that result from enzymatic digestion of the DNA. DNA is digested using micrococcal nuclease and spleen phosphodiesterase to produce normal deoxynucleoside 3'-monophosphate ($dN_{3'P}$) and adducted deoxynucleoside 3'-monophosphate ($dX_{3'P}$). By incubating with nuclease P1, $dN_{3'P}$ is 3'-dephosphorylated to form the deoxynucleosides (dN), whereas $dX_{3'P}$ is generally resistant to the enzyme. Therefore, adducted nucleotides are enriched during this process (nuclease P1 enrichment) (*see* **Note 6**).

1. Incubate 5 μg of DNA at 37°C overnight (approx 16 h) with 1 μL of micrococcal nuclease (1.5 U) and 1 μL of spleen phosphodiesterase (0.1 U) in 50 μL of 17 m*M* sodium succinate buffer, pH 6.0, containing 8 m*M* $CaCl_2$ (*see* **Note 7**).
2. Add 1 μL of nuclease P1 (1.0 U) into the reaction mixture and incubate at 37°C for 1 h.
3. Evaporate the sample to dryness using a Speedvac.

If adducted nucleotides such as tamoxifen-derived DNA adducts ***(10,11)*** are efficiently extracted by 1-butanol, the following butanol fractionation can be used to minimize the contamination of $dN_{3'P}$ and to enrich the $dX_{3'P}$ in the DNA digest. This additional procedure minimizes the background of $dN_{3'P}$ during ^{32}P-postlabeling analysis, which in turn increases the detection limit.

4. To enrich $dX_{3'P}$, dissolve the digested DNA in 100 μL distilled water, and extract twice with 200 μL butanol. Centrifuge at 14,000*g* for 5 min at room temperature and transfer the top layer (butanol phase) to a fresh tube. Back-extract the butanol fraction with 50 μL distilled water, centrifuge, and remove the bottom layer (aqueous phase). Evaporate the remaining butanol fractions to dryness and use for the adduct analysis.

3.3. Labeling Adducted Nucleotides With ^{32}P

Wild-type T4 polynucleotide kinase is used to label the $dX_{3'P}$ with ^{32}P. However, the wild-type enzyme has 3'-phosphatase activity, which may remove the 3'-monophosphate from the $dX_{3'P}$, resulting in an inefficient labeling with ^{32}P. To avoid this, 3'-phosphatase-free T4 polynucleotide kinase is used for labeling the 5'-site of $dX_{3'P}$. When authentic $dX_{3'P}$ is available, label the standard with ^{32}P and use as a marker.

1. Dissolve the digested DNA or authentic standard in 16 μL of distilled water, 3 μL of 10X linker-kinase buffer, pH 7.6, 3 μL 50 m*M* DTT, and 3 μL 10 m*M* spermidine in an Eppendorf tube and incubate at 37°C for 40 min with 3 μL of [γ-^{32}P]-ATP (10 μCi/μL) and 2 μL of 3'-phosphatase-free T4 polynucleotide kinase (10 U/μL).
2. To decompose nonreacted [γ-^{32}p]-ATP, dd 1 μL of potato apyrase (50 mU/μL) and incubate at 37°C for additional 30 min.
3. Evaporate the reaction mixture to dryness under vacuum.

While handing with [γ-^{32}P]-ATP, minimize the exposure to ^{32}P by wearing protective clothing and gloves, using Plexiglas shielding and body dosimeters, and monitoring the work area with a Geiger counter. ^{32}P-labeled waste materials should be discarded following the appropriate safety procedures.

3.4. ^{32}P-Postlabeling/TLC Analysis

To separate the ^{32}P-labeled adduct in two dimensions on a PEI-cellulose TLC plate, several buffers are required that depend on the individual adducts (*see* **Note 8**). We describe here the typical example used for the separation of tamoxifen-DNA adducts *(12)*.

1. Cut the PEI-cellulose TLC plate (20 × 20 cm) into four plates (10 × 10 cm). Wash the plates using distilled water (approx 500 mL) for 30 min at room temperature with shaking and dry.
2. Staple a paper wick (10 × 15 cm) at the top of the TLC plate.
3. Dissolve the ^{32}P-labeled nucleotides in 5 μL distilled water and apply the sample at the corner 2 cm from the bottom and 2 cm from the left side of the TLC plate (10 × 10 cm) using a capillary tube and a air dryer (*see* **Note 9**). Rinse the sample tube with 3 μL of distilled water and apply onto the TLC plate. Discard the sample tube after testing for radioactivity using a Geiger counter.
4. TLC plates are developed using D1 buffer in a glass chamber overnight (approx 16 h) at room temperature (*see* **Note 10**). Remove the paper wick and staples, wash the TLC plate twice using 500 mL of distilled water with shaking, and dry the plate.
5. Staple a new paper wick (10 × 10 cm) at the top of the TLC plate and subsequently develop in the same direction with D2 buffer in a glass chamber for approx 3 h at room temperature. After that, remove the paper wick, wash the TLC plate twice using 500 mL of distilled water with shaking, and dry the plate.
6. Staple a new paper wick (10 × 10 cm) to the right side of the TLC plate and develop further at a right angle to the previous direction of development in a D3 buffer in a glass chamber for approx 3 h at room temperature. After that, remove the paper wick, wash the TLC plate twice using 500 mL of distilled water with shaking, and dry the plate.
7. The position of adducts on the TLC plate can be established by exposing to a β-phosphorimage screen or by autoradiography. The time of exposure for the β-phosphorimager or X-ray film varies depending on the radioactivity of the targeted adducts; lower radioactivity needs overnight exposure.

3.5. ^{32}P-Postlabeling/PAGE Analysis

^{32}P-Postlabeling/PAGE analysis can be applied to any DNA adducts using nondenaturing 30% polyacrylamide gel under the following experimental condition. The detection limit of DNA adducts is approx 7 adducts/10^9 bases. A typical ^{32}P-postlabeling/PAGE used for analysis of tamoxifen-induced DNA adduct is presented in **Fig. 2**.

3.5.1. Preparation of Polyacrylamide Gel

1. Mix 60 mL 40% polyacrylamide solution, 10 mL of distilled water, and 10 mL of 10X TBE buffer, pH 7.0.

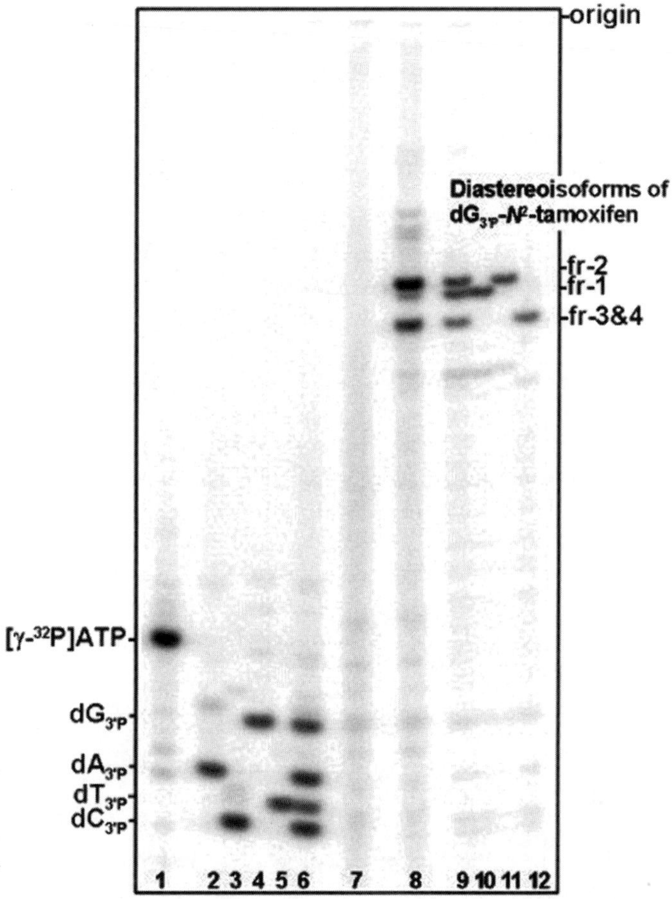

Fig. 2. ^{32}P-Postlabeling/PAGE analysis of antiestrogen-derived DNA adducts. Standard markers: 1, [γ-^{32}P]-ATP (approx 0.1 μCi/33 fmol); 2, $dA_{3'P}$; 3, $dC_{3'P}$; 4, $dG_{3'P}$; 5, $dT_{3'P}$; 6, a mixture of four $dN_{3'P}$; 9, a mixture of *trans*- and *cis*-isoforms of dG-N^2-tamoxifen; 10, a *trans*-isoform of dG-N^2-tamoxifen (fr-2); 11, a *trans*-isoform of dG-N^2-tamoxifen (fr-1); 12, a mixture of *cis*-isoforms of dG-N^2-tamoxifen (fr-3 and 4); 7, untreated DNA; 8, DNA treated with tamoxifen α-sulfate.

2. Before pouring the gel, add 1.0 mL of 10% ammonium persulfate and 35 μL TEMED.
3. Pour the solution between the glass plates (35 × 42 × 0.04 cm), which have been taped together. Then put the comb in the top.
4. When the gel has polymerized, remove the comb and tape carefully from the glass plates.

5. Set the glass plates/gel sandwich into the gel apparatus and fill the upper and bottom tanks with 1X TBE buffer and clean the wells by a modified spacer.
6. Run the gel by electrophoresis for at least 30 min at 1200–1400 V/20–50 mA before subjecting the ^{32}P-labeled samples.

Unpolymerized acrylamide is a neurotoxin. Wear gloves when preparing polyacrylamide gel and handling polymerized acrylamide gel.

3.5.2. Performance of Gel Electrophoresis

1. Dissolve the ^{32}P-labeled sample in 3 µL distilled water and 2 µL of 10X formamide dye. Dilute 1 µL of [γ-^{32}P]-ATP (10 µCi/µL) with 198 µL of distilled water. Take 2 µL of the diluted [γ-^{32}P]-ATP and mix well with 3 µL of 10X formamide dye.
2. Apply the ^{32}P-labeled samples or the 1/100th amounts of [γ-^{32}P]-ATP using a 10- to 20-µL pipet for electrophoresis for approx 5 h with 1200–1800 V/20–50 mA. Stop running the gel when xylene cyanol (upper dye) is approx 14 cm from the top of the gel; the position of ^{32}P-labeled $dC_{3'p}$ is approx 5 cm from the bottom.
3. Wrap the gel in plastic wrap. Determine the position of ^{32}P-labeled adducts by a β-phosphorimager analysis or by autoradiography.

3.6. Measurement of Level of ^{32}P-Labeled DNA Adducts

The level of DNA adducts resolved on the TLC plate or nondenaturing polyacrylamide gel can be estimated by the following procedures.

3.6.1. Level of DNA Adducts on PEI-Cellulose TLC Plate

1. Mark the adduct positions by placing the TLC plate on top of the developed X-ray film. When the origin spot on the TLC plate is adjusted to that of the X-ray film, the adduct positions on the TLC plate are easily determined.
2. Scrape the radioactive adducts from the TLC plate, put them into the scintillation vials, and mix well with 4 mL of scintillation liquid.
3. Measure the radioactivity by a β-liquid scintillation counter and compare with a known amount of [γ-^{32}P]-ATP used.

Relative adduct levels (RAL) are calculated using the following:

$$\text{RAL} = \frac{\text{adducted nucleotides (dpm or cpm)}}{\text{dN}_{3'\text{P}}\text{ constuted DNA (pmol)} \times \text{specific activity of } [\gamma\text{-}^{32}\text{P}]\text{ATP (dpm or cpm/pmol)}}.$$

For example, (total dpm in adducts)/2.02 × 10^{11} dpm, assuming that 5 µg of DNA represented 1.52 × 10^4 pmol of $dN_{3'p}$ and the specific activity of the [γ-^{32}P]-ATP is 1.33 × 10^7 dpm/pmol. The specific activity of [γ-^{32}P]-ATP is corrected according to the extent of decay (the half-life of ^{32}P is 14.29 d).

3.6.2. Level of DNA Adducts on Nondenaturing Polyacrylamide Gel

1. Subject ^{32}P-labeled samples to the nondenaturing gel with comigration of the 1/100th amounts of [γ-^{32}P]-ATP (10 μCi/μL), as described in **step 1** in **Subheading 3.5.2.**
2. After completion of PAGE, measure the integrated values of adducts using the β-phosphorimager and compare with that of the 1/100th amounts of [γ-^{32}P]-ATP used. When the integrated values are beyond the linear response range, the shorter exposure of ^{32}P-labeled products should be used to determine the radioactivity. RAL can be determined by the equation shown in **Subheading 3.6.1.**

3.7. Determination of ^{32}P-Labeled DNA Adducts by HPLC

To increase the resolution and the detection limit of DNA adducts, HPLC connected in line to a radioisotope detector system can be used for ^{32}P-postlabeling analysis (*see* **Note 11**). Prior to subjecting ^{32}P-labeled samples to HPLC, ^{32}P-labeled adducts should be partially purified by one of the following procedures using either PEI-cellulose TLC or nondenaturing polyacrylamide gel electrophoresis.

3.7.1. Partial Purification of Adducts by PEI-Cellulose TLC

1. Develop ^{32}P-labeled samples on a TLC plate, following **steps 1–4** in **Subheading 3.4.**
2. Following **steps 1** and **2** in **Subheading 3.6.1.**, scrape the ^{32}P-labeled adducts remaining on the TLC plate.
3. Extract ^{32}P-labeled adducts using 0.5 mL of 4 *M* pyrimidinium formate, pH 4.3, overnight at room temperature. After centrifugation (14,000*g* for 5 min), evaporate the supernatant to dryness.

3.7.2. Partial Purification of Adducts by Nondenaturing Polyacrylamide Gel Electrophoresis

1. Electrophorese ^{32}P-labeled samples, as described the protocol in **Subheading 3.5.**
2. Put the wrapped gel on a solid support (eq. used X-ray film) and tape together.
3. Staple the wrapped gel and unexposed X-ray film together in a dark room and place in a cassette. The exposure time depends on the radioactivity of ^{32}P-labeled adducts.
4. Develop the film using X-ray film developer.
5. Line up the staple holes on the wrapped gel and developed X-ray film with pins. Mark the adduct positions.
6. Cut the ^{32}P-labeled material from the gel, put in a fresh tube, and extract (no need to crush the gel) using 1 mL of distilled water with shaking overnight at room temperature.
7. Centrifuge the sample at 14,000*g* for 5 min, transfer the supernatant in a fresh tube, and evaporate to dryness.

Extraction efficiency of DNA adduct from the TLC or PAGE can be estimated as follows: for example, the radioactivity of the 1/20 volume of the supernatant fraction (S) or the whole precipitate (P) is mixed with scintillation liquid (4 mL) in a scintillation vial and measured using a β-liquid scintillation counter. The extraction efficiency of DNA adducts is estimated using the following equation:

$$\text{Recovery} = \frac{S \times 20 \text{ (dpm)}}{S \times 20 + P \text{ (dpm)}}.$$

3.7.3. ^{32}P-Postlabeling/HPLC

To resolve DNA adducts such as tamoxifen-derived DNA adducts ***(16)***, partially purified ^{32}P-labeled products are injected into a Hypersil BDS C_{18} analytical column (0.46 × 25 cm, 5 μm) and eluted at a flow rate of 1.0 mL/min using a linear gradient of 0.2 *M* ammonium formate and 20 m*M* H_3PO_4, pH 4.0, containing 20% to 30% acetonitrile/methanol (6:1, v/v) for 40 min and 30% to 50% acetonitrile/methanol (6:1, v/v) for 5 min, followed by an isocratic condition of 50% acetonitrile/methanol (6:1, v/v) for 15 min. The radioactivity is monitored using a radioisotope detector connected to an HPLC instrument (*see* **Note 12**). A typical ^{32}P-postlabeling/HPLC chromatogram for the analysis of tamoxifen-derived DNA adducts is presented in **Fig. 3**.

3.8. Quantification of DNA Adducts

The relative adduct levels are calculated by using the specific radioactivity of [γ-^{32}P]-ATP-labeled adducted nucleotides, as described in **Subheading 3.6.** In most cases, the adduct level is underestimated as a result of incomplete DNA digestion, inefficiency of adduct labeling by T4 polynucleotide kinase, and loss of adducted nucleotides during the enrichment procedure ***(17)***. When site specifically modified oligodeoxynucleotides containing a target DNA adduct are available, such an oligomer can be used as an internal standard to determine the accurate level of DNA adducts. For example, oligodeoxynucleotides containing a single tamoxifen-derived DNA adduct ($^{5'}$TCCTCCTCXCCTCTC, where X is the adduct site) can be prepared by postsynthetic methods ***(18)*** or by phosphoramidite chemical synthesis ***(19)***. The concentration of oligomer can be determined, based on the extinction coefficient at 260 nm ***(20)***. When 0.152 to 152 fmol (0.743–743 pg) of this oligomer is mixed with 5 μg of purified calf thymus DNA (15,200 pmol of $dN_{3'p}$), the actual level of tamoxifen adducts in the mixture is 1 adduct/10^8 nucleotides to 1 adduct/105 nucleotides. Such standard DNA can be used to determine the recovery of adducts and to quantify adducts using ^{32}P-postlabeling analyses. A typical standard curve is

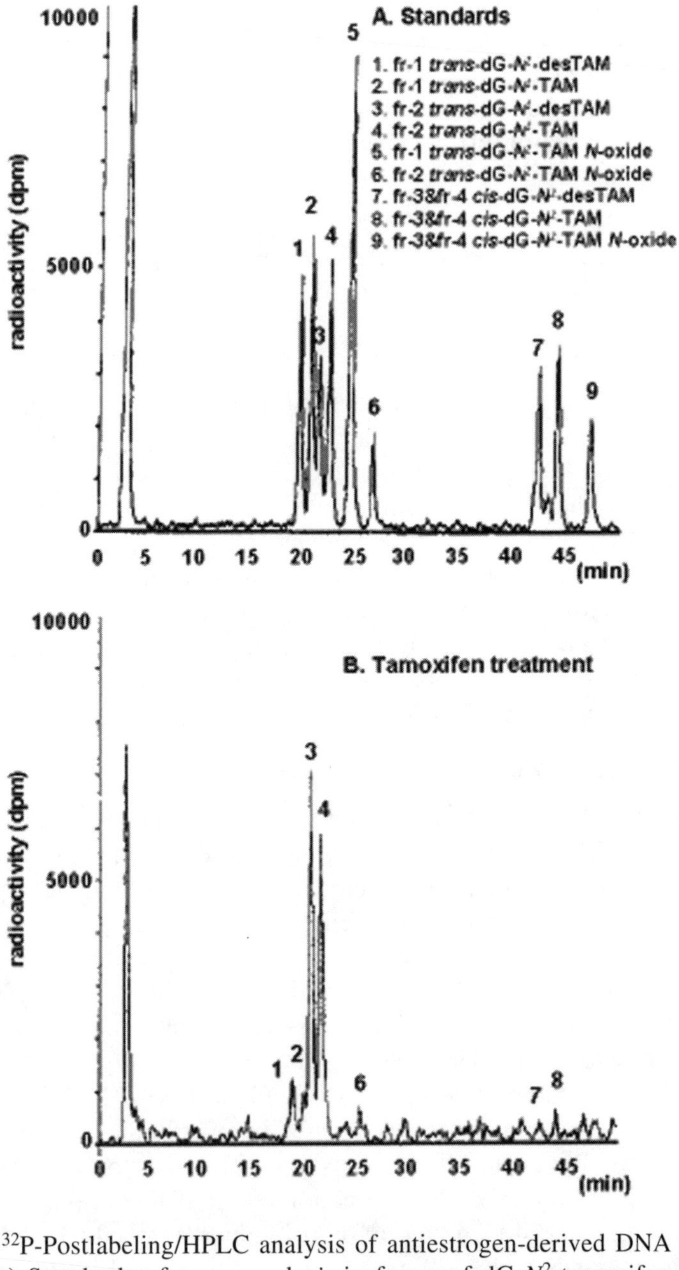

Fig. 3. ^{32}P-Postlabeling/HPLC analysis of antiestrogen-derived DNA adducts in animal. **(A)** Standards of *trans*- and *cis*-isoforms of dG-N^2-tamoxifen, dG-N^2-*N*-desmethyltamoxifen, and dG-N^2-tamoxifen *N*-oxide adducts. **(B)** Hepatic DNA from rats treated with tamoxifen.

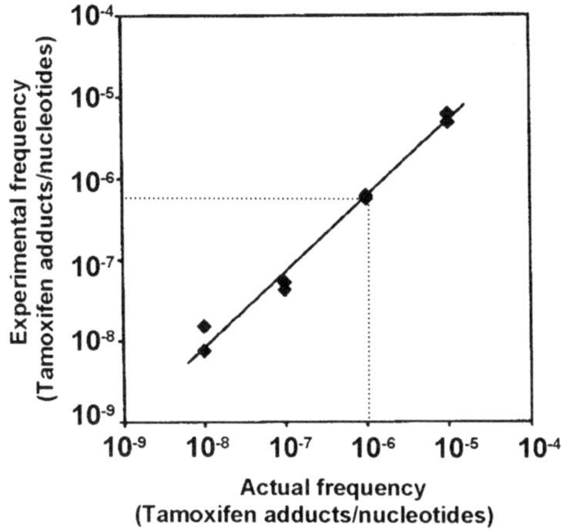

Fig. 4. Comparison of experimental and actual frequencies of antiestrogen-derived DNA adducts.

presented in **Fig. 4**. The amount of adducts detected increases linearly depending on the amount of the oligomer used. The recovery of adducts is 56% of the actual amount present; therefore, the actual level of adducts can be estimated by dividing the experimental values by 56% (*see* **Note 13**).

4. Notes

1. Commercially available RNase often contains deoxyribonuclease (DNase). Decontamination can be achieved by heating RNase solution at 95°C for 10 min.
2. The pH of Tris-saturated phenol should be 7.8–8.0 because the DNA partitions into the phenol phase under acidic conditions.
3. Some of the commercially available spleen phosphodiesterases contain 3'-phosphatase activity. Therefore, we use a spleen phosphodiesterase II from Worthington Biochemical Corp.
4. Highly radioactive [γ-^{32}P]-ATP (approx 6000 Ci/mmol) can be purchased from several companies (Amersham Biosciences, NEN Life Science Products, ICN Biomedicals, etc.); however, the concentration of ATP is not always accurate. To determine the accurate level of DNA adduct, [γ-^{32}P]-ATP should be obtained from companies that routinely determine the ATP concentration before each shipment.
5. The 3'-phosphatase activity of wild-type T4 polynucleotide kinase depends on the company and their lots. It is preferred to use 3'-phosphatase-free T4 polynucleotide kinase (Roche Molecular Biochemicals).
6. When the adduct ($dX_{3'p}$) is not resistant to nuclease P1, $dX_{3'p}$ should be isolated from the mixture of $dN_{3'p}$s in the DNA digest using HPLC or TLC *(21)*.

7. Generally, 5 μg DNA is used for the analysis. When the level of DNA adducts is expected to be low, the amounts of DNA analyzed can be increased to 50 μg. In such cases, 10-fold higher amounts of micrococcal nuclease (15 U) and spleen phosphodiesterase (1.0 U) should be used for DNA digestion using the same volume (50 μL) of sodium succinate buffer. The same amounts of nuclease P1 (1.0 U) can be applied even though amounts of DNA have been increased.
8. Extra precaution should be taken to select the appropriate buffer depending on the DNA adduct to be analyzed. Publications should be searched that describe ^{32}P-postlabeling analyses used for the related compounds and drugs to find the best buffer conditions.
9. To have the highest separation of ^{32}P-labeled adducts, the applied spot should be as small as possible.
10. The level of the buffer in the glass chamber should be less than 0.3 cm to avoid diffusion of ^{32}P-labeled adducts into the buffer. To check if ^{32}P-labeled adducts were lost in the buffer, measure the radioactivity of the buffer using a Geiger counter.
11. ^{32}P-labeled sample may be applied directly to HPLC without partial purification. However, the high background from free ^{32}P may reduce the resolution and detection limit of DNA adducts.
12. To adapt the HPLC system to resolve other DNA adducts, the gradient of acetonitrile/methanol (6:1, v/v) and/or pH of 0.2 *M* ammonium formate/20 m*M* H_3PO_4 may be modified.
13. Simply, known amounts of standard DNA (1 adduct/10^7 nucleotides or 1 adduct/10^6 nucleotides, respectively) are prepared by mixing 1.52 or 15.2 fmol of oligomer with 5 μg of purified calf thymus DNA (15,200 pmol of dNs) and are analyzed by ^{32}P-postlabeling analyses together with samples containing a known amount of adduct. When compared with the standards, the accurate level of adducts in the samples can be determined.

Acknowledgments

This work was supported by grants ES09418 and ES04068 from the National Institute of Environmental Health Sciences.

References

1. Randerath, K. and Randerath, E. (1993) Postlabeling methods—an historical review. *IARC Scientific Publications (Lyon)* **124,** 3–9.
2. Anonymous (1993) Postlabeling methods for detection of DNA adducts. *IARC Scientific Publications (Lyon)* **124,** 1–379.
3. Anonymous (1994) DNA adducts: identification and biological significance. *IARC Scientific Publications (Lyon)* **125,** 1–478.
4. Pluim, D., Maliepaard, M., van Waardenburg, R. C., Beijnen, J. H., and Schellens, J. H. (1999) ^{32}P-postlabeling assay for the quantification of the major platinum-DNA adducts. *Anal. Biochem.* **275,** 30–38.

5. Reddy, M. V. and Randerath, K. (1987) ^{32}P-analysis of DNA adducts in somatic and reproductive tissues of rats treated with the anticancer antibiotic, mitomycin C. *Mutat. Res.* **179,** 75–88.
6. Gladek, A. and Liehr, J. G. (1989) Mechanism of genotoxicity of diethylstilbestrol in vivo. *J. Biol. Chem.* **264,** 16847–16852.
7. Han, X., Liehr, J. G., and Bosland, M. C. (1995) Induction of a DNA adduct detectable by ^{32}P-postlabeling in the dorsolateral prostate of NBL/Cr rats treated with estradiol-17 beta and testosterone. *Carcinogenesis* **16,** 951–954.
8. Seraj, M. J., Umemoto, A., Tanaka, M., Kajikawa, A., Hamada, K., and Monden, Y. (1996) DNA adduct formation by hormonal steroids in vitro. *Mutat. Res.* **370,** 49–59.
9. Yasui, M., Matsui, S., Santosh Laxmi, Y. R., Suzuki, N., Kim, S. Y., Shibutani, S., et al. (2003) Mutagenic events induced by 4-hydroxyequilin in *supF* shuttle vector plasmid propagated in human cells. *Carcinogenesis* **24,** 911–917.
10. Shibutani, S., Suzuki, N., Terashima, I., Sugarman, S. M., Grollman, A. P., and Pearl, M. L. (1999) Tamoxifen-DNA adducts detected in the endometrium of women treated with tamoxifen. *Chem. Res. Toxicol.* **12,** 646–653.
11. Shibutani, S., Ravindernath, A., Suzuki, N., Terashima, I., Sugarman, S. M., Grollman, A. P., et al. (2000) Identification of tamoxifen-DNA adducts in the endometrium of women treated with tamoxifen. *Carcinogenesis* **21,** 1461–1467.
12. Stiborová, M., Fernando, R. C., Schmeiser, H. H., Frei, E., Pfau, W., and Wiessler, M. (1994) Characterization of DNA adducts formed by aristolochic acids in the target organ (forestomach) of rats by ^{32}P-postlabeling analysis using different chromatographic procedure. *Carcinogenesis* **15,** 1187–1192.
13. Randerath, K., Reddy, M. V., and Gupta, R. C. (1981) ^{32}P-labeling test for DNA damage. *Proc. Natl. Acad. Sci. USA* **78,** 6126–6129.
14. Reddy, M. V. and Randerath, K. (1986) Nuclease P1-mediated enhancement of sensitivity of ^{32}P-postlabeling test for structurally diverse DNA adducts. *Carcinogenesis* **7,** 1543–1551.
15. Terashima, I., Suzuki, N., and Shibutani, S. (2002) ^{32}P-Postlabeling/polyacrylamide gel electrophoresis analysis: application to the detection of DNA adducts. *Chem. Res. Toxicol.* **15,** 305–311.
16. Shibutani, S., Suzuki, N., Santosh Laxmi, Y. R., Schild, L. J., Divi, R. L., Grollman, A. P., et al. (2003) Identification of tamoxifen-DNA adducts in monkeys treated with tamoxifen. *Cancer Res.* **60,** 2607–2610.
17. Phillips, D. H., Farmer, P. B., Beland, F. A., Nath, R. G., Poirier, M. C., Reddy, M. V., et al. (2000) Methods of DNA adduct determination and their application to testing compounds for genotoxicity. *Environ. Mol. Mutagen.* **35,** 222–233.
18. Terashima, I., Suzuki, N., and Shibutani, S. (1999) Mutagenic potential of α-(N^2-deoxyguanosinyl)tamoxifen lesions, the major DNA adducts detected in endometrial tissues of patients treated with tamoxifen. *Cancer Res.* **59,** 2091–2095.
19. Santosh Laxmi, Y. R., Suzuki, N., Dasaradhi, L., Johnson, F., and Shibutani, S. (2002) Preparation of oligodeoxynucleotides containing a diastereoisomers of

α-(N^2-2'-deoxyguanosinyl)tamoxifen by phosphoramidite chemical synthesis. *Chem. Res. Toxicol.* **15,** 218–225.

20. Cantor, C. R., Warshaw, M. M., and Shapiro, H. (1970) Oligonucleotide interactions: 3. Circular dichroism studies of the conformation of deoxyoligonucleotides. *Biopolymers* **9,** 1059–1077.
21. Zeisig, M., Hofer, T., Cadet, J., and Möller, L. (1999) ^{32}P-postlabeling high-performance liquid chromatography (^{32}P-HPLC) adapted for analysis of 8-hydroxy-2'-deoxyguanosine. *Carcinogenesis* **20,** 1241–1245.

18

Covalent DNA Adduct Formation Mediated by Cytochrome P450

Marie Stiborová

Summary

In this chapter, the experimental details are described for the utilization of cytochrome P450-mediated reactions to examine the potential of chemicals (drugs) to be activated to reactive species, leading to the formation of covalent deoxyribonucleic acid (DNA) adducts. Methods for the isolation of subcellular fractions containing activating enzymes (microsomes or cytosols containing cytochromes P450 or other activating enzymes such as reductases xanthine oxidase, DT-diaphorase, and aldehyde oxidase, respectively), those for the activation of test drugs by these enzymatic systems (incubations) and the DNA isolation procedure are shown. In addition, the suitable techniques to detect and quantify covalent DNA adducts such as two enhancement procedures of ^{32}P-postlabeling assay (nuclease P1 version and extraction of adducts into *n*-butanol) and utilization of radioactive-labeled test compounds are described in detail in the chapter.

Key Words: Drug; enzyme activation; cytochrome P450; DNA adducts; ^{32}P-postlabeling.

1. Introduction

Cytochrome P450 (CYP) (EC 1.14.14.1) is a family of hemoproteins that are the major catalysts involved in the oxidation of xenobiotic chemicals, a significant focus of scientists in the areas of drug metabolism, toxicology, and pharmacology *(1–4)*. The effects of these oxidations can be manifested in poor drug bioavailability and various acute and chronic toxicities, including adverse drug interactions, cancer susceptibility, and birth defects *(5)*. Information about which human CYP enzymes are involved in the metabolism of new drug can-

From: *Methods in Pharmacology and Toxicology*
Optimization in Drug Discovery: In Vitro Methods
Edited by: Z. Yan and G. W. Caldwell © Humana Press Inc., Totowa, NJ

didates is required for new drug approval submissions in most countries, and information about the induction of these enzymes is a part of large-scale toxicogenomics *(5)*. On the basis of sequence identity, CYP enzymes are grouped into families (1, 2, 3, etc.), subfamilies (A, B, C, etc.), and individual CYPs (1, 2, 3, etc.)—for example, 1A1, 1A2, 1B1, and so on. For more discussion, the reader is referred to the current approach to the nomenclature at the following Web site: http://drnelson.utmem.edu/CytochromeP450html. A compilation of the allelic variants of human CYP enzymes is maintained at http://wwww.imm.ki.se./CYPalleles/.

Mammals appear to use a set of CYP enzymes in that many of the functions are the catabolism of natural products, aside from the synthesis of important steroids and eicosanoids (e.g., CYP5, 8, 11, 17, 19, 21, 24, 26, and 27). Of the remainder of the mammalian CYP, a relatively small set accounts for most of the metabolism of drugs (i.e., 1A2, 2C9, 2C19, 2D6, and 3A4), and another small set is involved in the metabolism of most protoxicants and procarcinogens that are CYP substrates (i.e., 1A1, 1A2, 1B1, 2A6, 2E1, and 3A4) *(5,6)*. Similar subfamily CYP enzymes are found in experimental animals, although the catalytic selectivity may be altered *(5)*.

The majority of these enzymes are concentrated in the liver (except CYP1A1 and 1B1). However, many of these CYP enzymes are also found in some extrahepatic tissues, and the actions of these within a target tissue may be more important, particularly if a generated reactive product is not stable enough to migrate out of the cell in which it is formed *(7)*. The enzymes are located in the endoplasmic reticulum (isolated as "microsomes").

Many CYP enzymes are inducible by chemicals; the inducer may also be a substrate, but this is not necessarily the case. Many CYP enzymes play a role in chemical (drug) toxicity. If the administered drug has a direct toxicity of its own (or acts directly on a receptor to produce toxicity), then metabolism of the drug may reduce toxicity if the CYP-generated product has less inherent toxicity. Another case is the transformation of an administered drug to another that either (1) binds covalently to macromolecules (usually because of its electrophilic or other reactive nature) or (2) otherwise interacts with a target to cause toxicity. Examples 1 and 2 are (usually) distinguished by (1) their capability for genotoxic response vs (2) their tendency to act by causing increased cell proliferation, although these two phenomena are not mutually exclusive. The list of potential deoxyribonucleic acid (DNA), lipids, and protein targets with reactive electrophiles and radicals is extensive. With DNA, understanding at least some of the most relevant gene responses and their mechanisms is becoming possible.

Genetic damage that produces a heritable loss of growth control comprises a major mechanism of carcinogenesis. Exposure to drugs having genotoxic side effects results in damage to the structural integrity of DNA, which occurs primarily as covalent binding of chemicals and is referred to as drug-DNA adduct formation ***(8)***. Such DNA damage is generally considered to be causative and directly related to tumor formation ***(8–14)***. Indeed, associations have been observed between DNA adduct formation, mutagenesis ***(9–15)***, and tumorigenesis ***(10,11,13)***, whereas reductions in DNA adduct levels have been associated with chemoprevention ***(12,16)***.

Here, the experimental details are described for the utilization of CYP-mediated reactions to examine the potential of chemicals (drugs) to be activated to reactive species, leading to formation of covalent DNA adducts. Because not only the oxidative reactions are important to activate several drugs to these reactive species, the experimental procedures employing the reduction enzymatic system are also briefly described. In addition, the suitable techniques to detect and quantify covalent DNA adducts are described in detail in this chapter.

2. Materials

2.1. Preparation of Hepatic Microsomal and Cytosolic Samples

1. 50 m*M* Tris-HCl buffer, pH 7.4, containing 150 m*M* KCl (buffer 1).
2. 100 m*M* sodium phosphate buffer, pH 7.4 (buffer 2).
3. 50 m*M* Tris-HCl buffer, pH 7.4, containing 150 m*M* KCl and 20% glycerol (buffer 3).
4. Homogenization system: Potter-Elvehjem.
5. Refrigerated centrifuge capable of generating 15,000*g* at 4°C.
6. Refrigerated ultra-(vacuum)-centrifuge capable of generating 105,000*g* at 4°C.

2.2. Incubations of Chemicals (Drugs) With DNA in the Presence of Enzymatic Systems

1. 100 m*M* sodium phosphate buffer, pH 7.4.
2. 100 m*M* Tris-HCl buffer, pH 7.4, containing 0.2% Tween-20.
3. Reaction tubes, borosilicate glass, 12 × 75 mm, with caps or plastic Eppendorf test tubes for volumes 2 mL with caps.
4. Calf-thymus DNA solution (3.3 mg/mL of distilled water).
5. Incubator (37°C).
6. Enzymatic systems: hepatic microsomal or cytosolic fractions (isolated in the laboratory or from Gentest, Woburn, MA) or Supersomes™ (Gentest, Woburn, MA), which are microsomes containing human recombinant CYP enzymes. Store all enzymes at –80°C.
7. 10 m*M* Nicotinamide adenine dinucleotide phosphate (NADPH) in distilled water

Table 1
Salt Solutions

	Concentrated solution	Final solution
Sodium acetate	2.5 *M* (pH 5.2)	0.25 *M*
Sodium chloride	5.0 *M*	0.1 *M*
Ammonium acetate	10.5 *M*	2 *M*

or the NADPH-generating system (10 m*M* $MgCl_2$, 10 m*M* D-glucose-6-phosphate, 10 m*M* nicotinamide adenine dinucleotide phosphate [$NADP^+$], 1 U/mL D-glucose-6-phosphate dehydrogenase). Store at –20°C.

8. 10 m*M* NADH. Store at –20°C.
9. 10 m*M* Hypoxanthine. Store at –20°C.
10. 10 m*M* Hydroxypyrimidine. Store at –20°C.
11. Centrifuge capable of spinning assay tubes at 2500*g*.

2.3. Isolation of DNA from Incubations

1. Tubes (Falcon tubes 50 mL, 25 mL, or borosilicate glass tubes, 12 × 75 mm, with the caps, or Eppendorf test tubes, 2 mL).
2. Phenol saturated with Tris-buffer. Store at 4°C.
3. Phenol/chloroform mixture (1:1, v/v). Store at 4°C.
4. Enzymes for the digestion of proteins and ribonucleic acid (RNA): proteinase K (20 mg/mL), ribonucleases (RNases: 2 mg RNase A and 2000 U of RNase T1/mL). Store the enzyme solutions in 1-mL aliquots at –20°C.
5. Protease buffer (200 m*M* ethylenediaminetetraacetic acid [EDTA], 400 m*M* Tris-HCl, pH 8.0). Store at 4°C.
6. Incubator (37°C).
7. Shaker.
8. Centrifuge capable of spinning tubes at 12,500*g*.
9. Ethanol absolute and 70% ethanol (ethanol/water, v/v) (both cold, –20°C).
10. Solution for extraction of drugs and their metabolites from incubations: diethyl ether, hexane, and acetone.
11. Salt solutions (*see* **Table 1**).

2.4. Procedures for Detection of DNA Adduct Formation

2.4.1. ^{32}P-Postlabeling Assay

2.4.1.1. DNA Hydrolysis

1. Micrococcal nuclease (MN) from *Staphylococcus aureus* (Sigma N3755). Store at –20°C.
2. Phosphodiesterases (SPD) from calf spleen (Boehringer [Roche] 108251). Store at –20°C. Both MN and SPD solutions must be dialyzed (MN because it contains oligonucleotides that can interfere with the analysis of normal nucleotides and

SPD because it is in solution in $(NH_4)_2SO_4$, which will inhibit the labeling). Dialysis is performed 3 × 3 h in milli-Q water or equivalent at 4°C. When dialyzing, no air should be left in the tube; otherwise, this leads to a change in volume and concentration. SPD from Roche is already not available; the enzyme from Calbiochem with the identical specific activity for the same substrate as the enzyme from Roche should be used.

3. Digestion buffer: containing sodium succinate 50 m*M* and $CaCl_2$ 12.5 m*M*, pH 6.0. Store at –20°C.
4. Incubator (37°C).
5. Vortex shaker.
6. Centrifuge capable of spinning assay tubes at 12,500*g*.
7. Speed-Vac evaporator.

2.4.1.2. Nuclease P1 Enrichment Procedure

1. 0.8 *M* Sodium acetate buffer, pH 5.0. Store at 4°C.
2. 2.0 m*M* $ZnCl_2$. Store at 4°C.
3. Nuclease P1: 4 mg/mL. Store at –20°C.
4. 0.427 *M* Tris base solution (unbuffered).
5. Incubator (37°C).
6. Vortex shaker.
7. Centrifuge capable of spinning assay tubes at 12,500*g*.
8. Speed-Vac evaporator.

2.4.1.3. *n*-Butanol Enrichment Procedure

1. 10 m*M* Tetrabutylammonium (TBA) chloride solution. Store at 4°C.
2. 11.6 m*M* Ammonium formate solution, pH 3.5. Store at 4°C.
3. 250 m*M* Tris-HCl buffer, pH 9.5. Store at 4°C.
4. *n*-Butanol (redistilled, saturated with water just before use). Store at 4°C.
5. Vortex shaker.
6. Centrifuge capable of spinning assay tubes at 12,500*g*.
7. Speed-Vac evaporator.
8. Good chemical hood.

2.4.1.4. Labeling of the Adducts

1. Polynucleotide kinase (PNK) (with or without phosphatase activity) (10 U/μL). Store at –20°C. Usually, T4 PNK from USB (Amersham) is used.
2. Buffer solution (labeling buffer): 400 m*M* bicine, 200 m*M* magnesium chloride, 300 m*M* dithiotreitol, 10 m*M* spermidine, pH 9.5 (when using PNK with phosphatase activity). Bicine buffer can be prepared in advance but stored as small aliquots (20–50 μL) at –20°C. Freezing and thawing, as well as storage at above –20°C, can cause dithiotreitol decomposition and loss of labeling efficiency.
3. 90 μ*M* Adenosine triphosphate (ATP). Store at –20°C.
4. [γ-^{32}P]-ATP (homemade or from the supplier, e.g., from the ICN Pharmaceutical, Inc.). Store at –20°C. If ATP is homemade, ^{32}Pi should be obtained in water

and not in HCl solution. When it is delivered in HCl solution, the HCl content varies from batch to batch, thus affecting the efficiency of the ATP synthesis. Whether homemade or purchased, the activity of the ATP must be verified.
5. Vortex shaker.
6. Centrifuge capable of spinning assay tubes at 12,500*g*.
7. Very effectively working chemical hood.

2.4.1.5. Test for Efficiency of NP1 or *n*-Butanol Enrichment Procedures

1. Polyethyleneimine (PEI)-cellulose thin-layer chromatography (TLC) plate.
2. A solution 280 m*M* in $(NH_4)_2SO_4$ and 50 m*M* in NaH_2PO_4, pH 6.5.

2.4.1.6. TLC Separation of Adducted Nucleotides

1. PEI-cellulose TLC plate.

For bulky adducts:

1. D1 solution: 1.0 to 1.7 *M* natrium phosphate buffer, pH 6.8.
2. D2 solution: 3.5 *M* lithium formate, 8.5 *M* urea, pH 3.5.
3. D3 solution: 0.8 LiCl, 0.5 *M* Tris-HCl, 8.5 *M* urea, pH 8.0.
4. D4 solution: 1.7 *M* sodium phosphate, pH 6.0.

For more polar adducts (e.g., adducts containing only one benzene ring):

1. D1 solution: 2.3 *M* sodium phosphate, pH 5.77.
2. D2 solution: 2.7 *M* lithium formate, 5.1 *M* urea, pH 3.5.
3. D3 solution: 0.36 *M* sodium phosphate, 0.23 *M* Tris-HCl, 3.8 *M* urea, pH 8.0.
4. D4 solution: 1.7 *M* sodium phosphate, pH 6.0.

2.4.1.7. Quantification of Normal Nucleotides After Hydrolysis

1. Reagents as in **Subheading 2.4.1.6.**.

2.4.2. Detection of Binding of Drug to DNA Using Radioactive-Labeled Drug

1. Scintillation counter with appropriate vials.
2. Scintillation solution.

3. Methods

3.1. Preparation of Hepatic Microsomal and Cytosolic Samples

Liver subcellular fractions (microsomes rich in CYP enzymes or cytosol rich in reductases) from experimental animals (usually rat, rabbit, or mice) or from human donors are prepared by simple differential centrifugation. The 105,000*g* pellet and supernatant are taken as microsomes and cytosol, respectively. All tissue fractions have to be stored at –80°C.

1. Wash the liver samples twice with buffer 1 (*see* **Subheading 2.1**) and cut the tissues into small pieces.
2. Homogenize the tissue in the presence of buffer 1 (3 vol/wt of the tissue) in a homogenizer at 4°C.
3. Discard the residual nonhomogenized pieces of the tissue by filtration.
4. Centrifuge at 600*g* for 10 min at 4°C.
5. Transfer the supernatant to another centrifugation tube.
6. Rehomogenize the pellet in a buffer 1 (1 vol/wt of the tissue) and repeat **steps 4** and **5**.
7. Discard the pellet.
8. Centrifuge pooled supernatants at 15,000*g* for 20 min at 4°C.
9. Transfer the supernatant to another centrifugation tube.
10. Centrifuge supernatant at 105,000*g* for 60 min at 4°C.
11. Collect supernatant (cytosol) and store in aliquots (1–10 mL) at –80°C.
12. Characterize cytosol for the amounts of proteins.
13. Resuspend the pellet in buffer 2 (*see* **Subheading 2.1**) (2 vol/wt of the tissue).
14. Centrifuge at 105,000*g* for 60 min at 4°C.
15. Discard the supernatant.
16. Rehomogenize the pellet (microsomes) in buffer 3 (*see* **Subheading 2.1**) (1/5 vol/wt of the tissue) in a homogenizer at 4°C.
17. Store microsomes in 0.5- to 1-mL aliquots at –80°C.
18. Characterize microsomes for the content of proteins.
19. Determine the concentration of cytochrome P450 in microsomes (*see* **Note 1**).

3.2. Incubations of Test Chemicals (Drugs) With DNA in the Presence of Enzymatic Systems

For the covalent DNA binding, the test drug should usually be activated either by oxidative or reductive reactions depending on individual drugs. Oxidative or reductive activation of drug tested is mediated by a CYP-dependent enzymatic system present in the microsomal subcellular fraction or by reduction with reductases present both in microsomes (nicotinamide adenine dinucleotide phosphate [NADPH]/CYP reductase, nicotinamide adenine dinucleotide [NADH]/cytochrome b_5 reductase, CYP enzymes) and in cellular cytosolic subcellular fractions (xanthine oxidase, DT-diaphorase, aldehyde oxidase). Reactive metabolites thereafter bind to DNA-forming DNA adducts.

3.2.1. Incubations of Test Chemicals (Drugs) With DNA in the Presence of Oxidative Enzymatic Systems Containing Cytochromes P450

1. Mix at 4°C 100 m*M* phosphate buffer, pH 7.4, (0.375 mL), 10 m*M* NADPH or NADPH-generating system (*see* **Subheading 2.2**) (75 µL), microsomes or Supersomes™ containing 50 to 100 pmol CYP enzymes (variable volume, e.g.,

10–100 μL, depending on concentrations of CYP enzymes in microsomal or supersomal preparations), 1 mg calf thymus DNA (0.3 mL of stock solution), and 0.1 to 1.0 m*M* test drug (variable volume, e.g., 1–7.5 μL of stock solution of a drug dissolved in distilled water, methanol, ethanol, or dimethylsulfoxide [DMSO], depending on solubility of the drug) and a variable amount of distilled cold water to reach a final volume of the reaction mixture of 0.75 mL. Drug labeled with ^3H or ^{14}C or (nonradioactive) one can be used, depending on the procedure for detection of DNA adducts (*see* below).

2. Prepare also two control incubations analogously but (1) without an activating enzymatic system (microsomes) or (2) with an activating system but without the test drug.
3. Shake on a vortex shaker.
4. Incubate in opened tubes at 37°C for 30 to 60 min.

3.2.2. Incubations of Test Chemicals (Drugs) With DNA in the Presence of Reductive Enzymatic Systems

1. Mix at 4°C 100 m*M* Tris-HCl buffer, pH 7.4, containing 0.2% Tween-20 (0.375 mL), 10 m*M* solution of cofactors of either reductive enzymes (NADPH or NADH for DT-diaphorase, hypoxanthine for xanthine oxidase, or hydroxypyrimidine for aldehyde oxidase) (75 μL), cytosolic fraction containing 1 mg protein (variable volume, e.g., 10–100 μL, depending on protein concentrations in cytosolic preparations), 1 mg calf thymus DNA (0.3 mL of stock solution), and 0.1 to 1.0 m*M* test drug (variable volume, e.g., 1–7.5 μL of stock solution of a drug dissolved in distilled water, methanol, ethanol, or DMSO, depending on solubility of the drug) and a variable amount of distilled water to reach a final volume of the reaction mixture of 0.75 mL. Drug labeled with ^3H or ^{14}C or cold one can be used, depending on the procedure for detection of DNA adducts (*see* below).
2. Prepare also two control incubations analogously but (1) without an activating enzymatic system (cytosolic fractions) or (2) with an activating system but without the test drug.
3. Shake on a vortex shaker.
4. Purge the reaction mixture with argon for 1 min.
5. Incubate in closed tubes at 37°C for 30 to 60 min.

3.2.3. Extraction of Incubation Mixtures With Organic Solvents to Remove the Excess of Test Drugs

To remove the excess of a test drug from the reaction mixture, extraction of incubations with organic solvent should be performed. For such purposes, ethyl acetate, diethyl ether, and/or hexane are usually used.

1. Mix the incubation mixture in a test tube with a cap with an equal volume of ethyl acetate (or diethyl ether or hexane) by adding these solvents.
2. Shake the content of the tube on a vortex shaker until an emulsion forms.

3. Centrifuge for 3 min at 1600*g* or for 15 s in an Eppendorf centrifuge at room temperature. If the organic and aqueous phases are not well separated, centrifuge again for a longer time or at a higher speed.
4. Remove the upper, organic phase, collecting with a Pasteur's pipet. For small volumes (<400 μL), use an automatic pipettor fitted with a disposable tip. Discard this organic phase.
5. Repeat **steps 1–4**.
6. Remove residual organic solvents by blowing a stream of nitrogen gas over the surface of the solution for 5 to 10 min.

3.3. Isolation of DNA From Incubations

The key step of DNA isolation from incubations, the removal of proteins, can often be carried out simply by extracting aqueous solutions of DNA with phenol and/or chloroform. However, incubation mixtures might sometimes be contaminated by traces of RNA from subcellular fractions. To remove these small amounts of RNA, digestion of incubations with RNase is usually performed.

3.3.1. Digestion of RNA With RNase

The mixture of two RNases is successfully used for RNA digestion (RNases A and T1). Both RNases digest RNA efficiently. The excess of RNases is removed by digestion with proteinase K.

1. Add 15 μL of stock solution of RNases (*see* **Subheading 2.3**).
2. Incubate at 37°C for 60 min.
3. Add 75 μL protease buffer (200 m*M* EDTA, 400 m*M* Tris-HCl, pH 8.0).
4. Add 2 μL of stock solution of proteinase K (20 mg/mL).
5. Incubate at 37°C for 60 min.

The digestion with RNases might be omitted when microsomal or cytosolic samples in the amount lower than 10 μL are used for activation of test drugs.

3.3.2. Extraction with Phenol/Chloroform and Precipitation With Ethanol

The standard way to remove proteins from nucleic acid solutions is to extract once with phenol, once with a 1:1 mixture of phenol and chloroform, and once with chloroform. This procedure takes advantage of the fact that deproteinization is more efficient when two different organic solvents are used instead of one. Furthermore, although phenol denatures proteins efficiently, it does not completely inhibit RNase activity, and it is a solvent for RNA molecules that contain long tracts of poly(dA). Both of these problems can be circumvented by using a mixture of phenol and chloroform (1:1). Also, the final extraction with chloroform removes any lingering traces of phenol from the nucleic acid preparation. The most widely used method for concentrating DNA is precipitation with ethanol. The precipitate of DNA, which is allowed to form at a low temperature (–20°C or less) in the presence of moderate concentrations of monovalent cations, is recovered by centrifugation and redissolved in an appropriate buffer at the desired concentration. The technique is rapid and quantitative even with nanogram amounts of DNA.

1. Mix the incubation with an equal volume of phenol or phenol/chloroform in a polypropylene tube (Falcon or Eppendorf tube) with a plastic cap.
2. Mix the contents of the tube until an emulsion forms.
3. Centrifuge for 3 min at 1600*g* or for 15 s in an Eppendorf centrifuge at room temperature. If the organic and aqueous phases are not well separated, centrifuge again for a longer time or at a higher speed.
4. Use a Pasteur's pipet to transfer the upper, aqueous phase to a fresh polypropylene tube. For small volumes (<400 mL), use an automatic pipettor fitted with a disposable tip. Discard the interface and lower organic phase. To achieve the best recovery, the organic phase and interface may be "back-extracted" as follows. After the first, aqueous phase has been transferred as described above, add an equal volume of distilled water to the organic phase and interface. Mix well. Separate the phases by centrifugation. Combine the second aqueous phase with the first and proceed to **step 5**.
5. Add an equal volume of a 1:1 mixture of phenol and chloroform. Repeat **steps 2–4**.
6. Add an equal volume of chloroform and repeat **steps 2–4**.
7. Recover the DNA by precipitation with ethanol.
8. Estimate the volume of the DNA solution.
9. Adjust the concentration of monovalent cations either by dilution with distilled water if the DNA solution contains a high concentration of salts or by addition of one of the salt solutions shown in **Table 1**.
10. Mix well. Add exactly 2 vol of ice-cold ethanol and mix well. Chill to –20°C.
11. Store at a low temperature to allow the DNA precipitate to form. Usually 10 to 30 min at –20°C is sufficient (*see* **Note 2**).
12. Centrifuge at 0°C. For most purposes, 10 min at 1600*g* or 1 min in an Eppendorf centrifuge at 12,000*g* is sufficient. When low concentrations of DNA or very small fragments are being processed, more extensive centrifugation (30 min) may be required.
13. Discard the supernatant. To remove any solutes (or residual traces of the test drug) that may be trapped in the precipitate, the DNA pellet should be washed with a solution of 70% ethanol, ethanol, and diethyl ether.
14. Wash the DNA pellet by adding 1 mL cold 70% ethanol (–20°C). Mix well.
15. Centrifuge at 0°C. For most purposes, 10 min at 1600*g* or 1 min in an Eppendorf centrifuge at 12,000*g* is sufficient.
16. Discard the supernatant (*see* **Note 3**).
17. Repeat the **steps 14–16**.
18. Wash the DNA pellet by adding 1 mL cold ethanol (–20°C). Mix well.
19. Centrifuge at 0°C. For most purposes, 10 min at 1600*g* or 1 min in an Eppendorf centrifuge at 12,000*g* is sufficient.

20. Discard the supernatant.
21. Repeat **steps 18–20**.
22. Stand the tube in an inverted position on a layer of absorbent paper to allow as much of the supernatant as possible to drain away. Use capillary pipets to remove any drops of fluid that adhere to the walls of the tube.
23. Wash the DNA pellet by adding 1 mL diethyl ether. Diethyl ether can be used to remove residual traces of test drug from DNA. Ether is highly volatile and extremely flammable and should be worked with and stored in an explosion-proof chemical hood.
24. Centrifuge at 0°C. For most purposes, 10 min at 1600*g* or 1 min in an Eppendorf centrifuge at 12,000*g* is sufficient.
25. Discard the supernatant. Remove traces of ether by heating the DNA to 37°C for 5 to 10 min.
26. Dissolve the DNA pellet in the desired volume (usually in 100–200 μL to achieve a DNA concentration approx 2 μg/μL) of distilled water (or in 0.15 m*M* sodium citrate and 1.5 m*M* sodium chloride). Rinse the walls of the tube well with water or scrape them with a sealed pipet to aid in the recovery of the DNA. The sample can stand at 4°C overnight or be heated to 37°C for 10 to 30 min to assist in dissolving the pellet (*see* **Note 4**).
27. Before storage, separate the DNA into small aliquots (10–20 μL) because it has been observed that repeated freezing and thawing of DNA solutions tend to lead to loss of adducts.
28. Store at –80°C or colder.

3.4. Procedures for Detection of DNA Adduct Formation

Two independent procedures to determine whether the test drug, activated by enzymatic systems, is bound to DNA are recommended: the ^{32}P-postlabeling technique and using the radioactive-labeled drug (e.g., ^{3}H or ^{14}C). For the first pilot screening, the ^{32}P-postlabeling assay is recommended the most. Determination of the DNA content in solutions, precisely evaluated, must precede both methods.

3.4.1. Spectrophotometric Determination of DNA

A simple and accurate method that is widely used to measure the amount of DNA in a preparation if the sample is pure (i.e., without significant amounts of contaminants such as protein, phenol, or other nucleic acids) is spectrophotometric measurement of the amount of DNA of ultraviolet (UV) irradiation absorbed by the bases. For quantitating the amount of DNA, readings should be taken at wavelengths at 260 nm and 280 nm. The reading at 260 nm allows calculation of the concentration of DNA in the sample. An OD of 1 corresponds to approx 50 μg/mL for double-stranded DNA and 40 μg/mL for single-stranded DNA. The ratio between the readings at 260 nm and 280 nm (OD_{260}/OD_{280}) provides an estimate for the purity of the nucleic acid. Pure preparations of DNA have an OD_{260}/OD_{280} of 1.8. If there is contamination with protein or phenol, the OD_{260}/OD_{280} will be significantly less than the value give above, and accurate quantitation of the amount of nucleic acid will not be possible. To test the purity of DNA, two complementary methods are used.

1. Before hydrolysis. A full spectrum is taken between 220 and 320 nm (using, if possible, two different spectrophotometers). The maximum absorption should be at 258 to 259 nm for DNA not contaminated with RNA. A shift of this maximum toward 250 nm indicates contamination with RNA. A shoulder at 280 nm indicates contamination with proteins. In either case, DNA must be repurified before proceeding with hydrolysis.
2. After hydrolysis (used when the ^{32}P-postlabeling technique is employed). Two methods can be used that will allow (a) quantitation of normal nucleotides and (b) a check for RNA contamination. These are labeling of an aliquot of the digest (*see* **Subheading 3.4.2.4.**) and TLC separation of normal nucleotides (*see* **Subheading 3.4.2.6.**) or high-performance liquid chromatography (HPLC) analysis of an aliquot of the digest. The former method has been selected for the following reasons:
   a. It allows checking for protein contamination (a tailing spot at the origin is an indication of protein contamination and will generate an increased background on the 2D TLC separation of the adducts).
   b. It allows for correction of the efficiency of hydrolysis.
   c. It allows for correction of batch-to-batch variability in the activity of the ATP provided by the supplier.

3.4.2. ^{32}P-Postlabeling Assay

The ^{32}P-postlabeling method is based on the enzymatic hydrolysis of nonradioactive carcinogen-modified DNA to 3'-phosphonucleosides, subsequent [^{32}P]phosphorylation at the free 5'-OH group, and chromatographic separation of carcinogen-nucleotide adducts from nonmodified (normal) nucleotides *(17)* (**Fig. 1**). In this technique, carcinogen-modified DNA is digested enzymatically to deoxyribonucleoside 3'-monophosphates with endonuclease (micrococcal nuclease) and exonuclease (spleen phosphodiesterase). Thereafter, DNA hydrolysates (normal and modified deoxyribonucleoside 3'-monophosphates) are converted to 5'-^{32}P-labeled 3',5'-bisphosphates by incubation with [γ-^{32}P]-ATP in the presence of carrier ("cold") ATP and T4-polynucleotide kinase at pH 9.5 ("standard" procedure in **Fig. 1**). This alkaline pH is used to minimize the 3'-phosphatase activity of the polynucleotide kinase. ^{32}P-Labeled adducts are separated and resolved from the excess of labeled nonmodified nucleotides in two dimensions by multidirectional anion-exchange TLC on PEI cellulose plates (**Fig. 2**). During the first elution (D1 direction) with aqueous electrolyte, labeled unmodified nucleotides and [^{32}P]phosphate are removed from the origin onto a paper wick, whereas hydrophobic adducts are retained at the origin

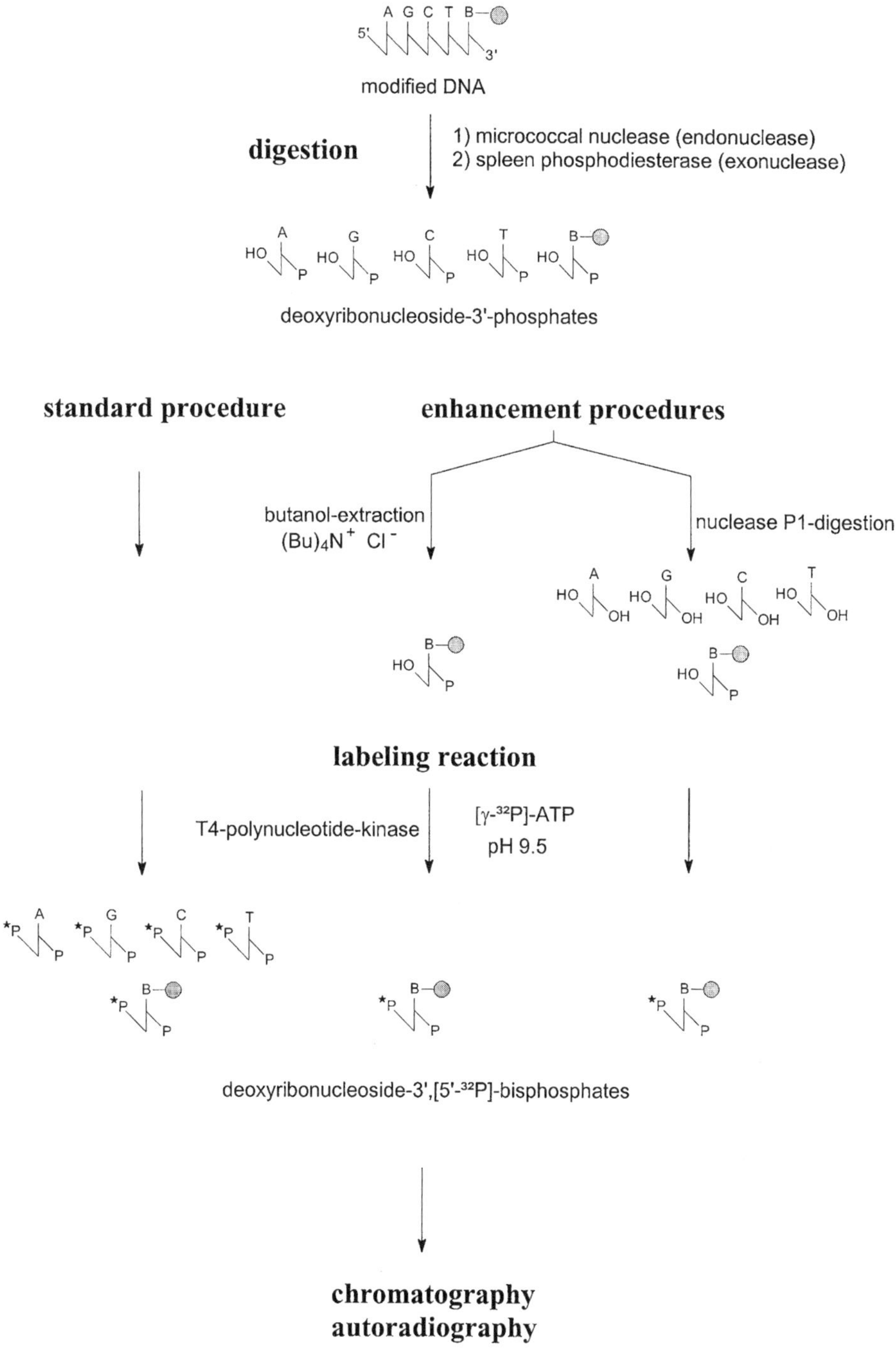

Fig. 1. Scheme of the ^{32}P-postlabeling assay.

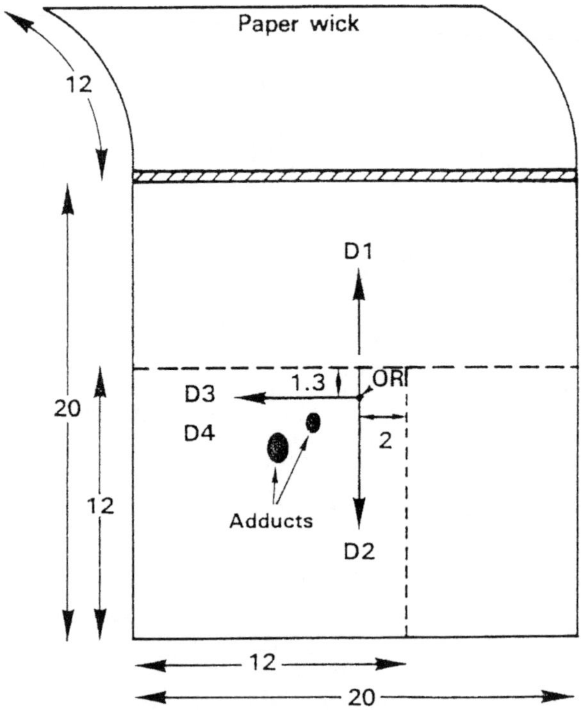

Fig. 2. Elution pattern of PEI-cellulose TLC plates.

for subsequent resolution using different solvent systems (D2, D3 directions) (**Fig. 2**). Location of the adducts is carried out by screen-enhanced autoradiography and visualized as dark distinct spots on X-ray films. These areas are then excised for quantitation by liquid scintillation or Cerenkov counting. A technique known as storage phosphor imaging was recently adapted for the mapping and quantitation of DNA adducts on chromatograms generated by the ^{32}P-postlabeling assay *(18)*. This technique yields approx 10-fold improvement in sensitivity compared to screen-enhanced autoradiography for the detection of ^{32}P *(19)*.

Adduct levels are calculated as relative adduct labeling (RAL) values according to the following:

$$\text{RAL} = \frac{\text{cpm in adduct nucleotides}}{\text{specific activity of } ^{32}\text{P-ATP (in cpm/pmol)} \times \text{pmol dNp}}$$

RAL values represent the ratio of count rates of adducted nucleotides over count rates of total (adducted and normal dNp) nucleotides ***(20,21)***. However, this calculation is based on equal labeling efficiencies of adducts and normal nucleotides ***(22)***. The "standard" protocol of the ^{32}P-postlabeling method is suitable for most DNA adducts (bulky and/or nonbulky adducts), but its sensitivity is not sufficient to detect adducts present in lower levels in DNA. Using this protocol, DNA adducts present at levels of 1 adduct in 10^7 normal nucleotides (0.3 fmol adduct/μg DNA) can be detected.

Several modifications of the standard assay have been employed to increase the sensitivity of the method. ^{32}P-labeling of adducts with limiting amounts of [γ-^{32}P]-ATP has been shown to enhance the method's sensitivity 10- to 100-fold for a number of adducts (the intensification procedure) ***(23,24)***. An additional enhancement procedure uses an enzymatic postincubation of DNA digests with nuclease P1 (from *Penicillium citrinum*) ***(21)*** (**Fig. 1**) to enrich adducts. Nuclease P1 preferentially dephosphorylates unmodified deoxyribonucleoside 3'-monophosphates to deoxyribonucleosides and, in most cases, not the adducted nucleotides. Deoxyribonucleosides do not serve as substrates for T4-polynucleotide kinase for the transfer of [^{32}P]phosphate from [γ-32P]-ATP. However, some adducted nucleotides are dephosphorylated by nuclease P1 (e.g., arylamine adducts substituted at C8 of deoxyguanosine), whereas others are not (primarily adducts substituted at N2 of deoxyguanosine). This version makes the assay significantly more sensitive (by three orders of magnitude). This adduct enrichment over normal nucleotides allows the use of larger amounts of DNA (5–10 μg) and the excess of carrier-free [γ-^{32}P]-ATP.

The additional enrichment procedure introduced by Gupta ***(25)*** exploits the properties of bulky nucleotide adducts that can be extracted into *n*-butanol in the presence of a phase transfer agent tetrabutylammonium chloride (**Fig. 1**) prior to [^{32}P]phosphate labeling, whereas normal nucleotides are extracted only to some extent. More polar adducts containing nonaromatic bulky residues or a small alkyl moiety, however, are hardly extractable into *n*-butanol and cannot be analyzed with this version of the ^{32}P-postlabeling technique. The nuclease P1 and *n*-butanol extraction enrichment methods enhance the sensitivity of detection and quantitation of DNA adducts by several orders of magnitude, enabling the detection of one adduct per 10^{9-10} normal nucleotides (0.3–3 amol/μg DNA) depending on the structures of adducts. These two methods are recommended to be used to test the drugs for their efficiency to covalently bind to DNA; therefore, they are described in this chapter in detail.

3.4.2.1. DNA Hydrolysis (*see* **Note 5**)

1. Dissolve MN in water at a concentration of approx 450 U/mL.
2. Dialyze against distilled water and adjust to 300 U/mL.
3. Dialyze spleen phosphodiesterase (SPD) solution 4 U/mL.
4. Mix MN and SPD to final concentrations 150 mU/μL MN and 2.5 mU/μL SPD (MN/SPD solution). *See* **Notes 6** and **7**.

5. Take an equivalent of 12.5 μg DNA solution and evaporate to dryness in a Speedvac evaporator. Dissolve in 6.5 μL distilled water.
6. Add 5.0 μL MN/SPD solution: the final concentration of MN is 60 mU/μL, and the final concentration of SPD is 1 mU/μL. Add 1.0 μL digestion buffer: the final concentration of sodium succinate is 20 m*M*, and the final concentration of $CaCl_2$ is 8 m*M*. The final volume of the mixture is 12.5 μL.
7. Shake on a vortex shaker to dissolve DNA and allow to react 3 h at 37°C.
8. Remove 2.5 μL (transfer to another tube) for dilution and analysis of normal nucleotides (*see* **Subheading 3.4.2.7.**). *See* **Notes 8** and **9**.

3.4.2.2. Nuclease P1 Enrichment Procedure

1. To the remaining 10.0 μL of hydrolysate, add the following: 0.65 μL sodium acetate buffer (final concentration, 40 m*M*), 0.65 μL $ZnCl_2$ solution (final concentration 0.1 m*M*), 1.25 μL NP1 solution (final concentration, 0.385 μg/μL), and 0.45 μL distilled water. Final volume of the mixture is 13 μL.
2. Allow to react 30 min at 37°C, and then stop the reaction by addition of the 3-μL Tris-HCl solution.

3.4.2.3. *n*-Butanol Enrichment Procedure

1. To the remaining 10.0 μL of DNA hydrolysate, add the following: 215 μL of 11.6 m*M* ammonium formate solution, pH 3.5, and 25 μL 10 m*M* TBA chloride solution.
2. Extract immediately with 250 μL *n*-butanol (saturated with water) by shaking on a vortex shaker (full speed) for at least 1 min.
3. Centrifuge to separate layers and collect the top layer (*n*-butanol layer).
4. Extract a second time with 250 μL *n*-butanol (saturated with water), centrifuge, collect *n*-butanol, and pool with previous extract.
5. To pooled *n*-butanol extracts, add 400 μL water (saturated with *n*-butanol) and shake for at least 1 min in a vortex shaker (full speed).
6. Centrifuge to separate layers and discard aqueous washes (bottom layer).
7. Repeat washing of the *n*-butanol phase with 400 μL water (saturated with *n*-butanol).
8. Add 3 μL of 250 m*M* Tris-HCl solution, pH 9.5, to the *n*-butanol layer.
9. Evaporate *n*-butanol to dryness in a speedvac evaporator at room temperature.
10. Take residue in 100 μL *n*-butanol by vortex shaking, evaporate to dryness again, and then take in 16.0 μL water by vortex shaking. *See* **Notes 10** and **11**.

3.4.2.4. Labeling of the Adducts

1. Add 1 μL of bicine buffer solution (labeling buffer) and 3.0 μL of a mix containing 100 μCi [γ-32P]-ATP, 45 pmol of cold ATP, and 10.0 U PNK to the 16.0-μL solution from the NP1 or butanol enrichment mix. The final concentrations of the reagents will be as follows: 20 m*M* bicine, 10 m*M* $MgCl_2$, 10 m*M* dithiotreitol, 0.5 m*M* spermidine, 0.5 U/μL PNK, and 3 μ*M* ATP. The total volume of the mixture is 20 μL. *See* **Note 12**.

2. Allow to react 30 min at room temperature. *See* **Note 13**.
3. The whole sample (i.e., 20 µL) will be applied on the PEI-cellulose TLC plate (*see* **Subheading 3.4.2.6.**).

3.4.2.5. Test for Efficiency of NP1 or *n*-Butanol Enrichment Procedures

1. Wash the bottom of the tube with 50 µL water.
2. Shake for 30 s in a vortex shaker and centrifuge to ensure no contamination of the lid.
3. Spot 5 µL on a PEI-cellulose TLC plate (20 × 20 cm).
4. Chromatograph using a solution 280 m*M* in $(NH_4)_2SO_4$ and 50 m*M* NaH_2PO_4, pH 6.8. *See* **Note 14**.

3.4.2.6. TLC Separation of Adducted Nucleotides

1. Prewashing of the TLC plates is recommended, especially from homemade plates. It may be performed to remove the yellow color from some plates, a color that will increase the background, especially at the solvent front. *See* **Note 15**.
2. Spot the entire sample on the TLC plate for chromatography (*see* **Subheading 3.4.2., step 3**) cleanup of the adducts in D1 (**Fig. 1**).
3. Develop the plate in a D1 direction (**Fig. 1**). It is recommended using a range of natrium phosphate concentrations to ensure that adducts remain at the origin. *See* **Note 16**.
4. Wash the plate in deionized water after chromatography by shaking gently for approx 5 min in two successive baths, and then allow to dry.
5. Develop the plates in the D2 and D3 (residual radioactive impurities on the plate) direction (**Fig. 1**). The solvents should be adjusted to spread the spots over the TLC plate. *See* **Note 17**.
6. To avoid the problems of front in D3 (residual radioactive impurities on the plate), after D3 development and a brief water wash, the sheets can be developed (along D3) in 1.7 *M* sodium phosphate, pH 6.0 (D4), to the top of a paper wick (12 × 11.5 cm) or to the top of the plate, followed by an additional 30- to 40-min development with the TLC tank partially opened to allow the radioactive impurities to concentrate in a band close to the top edge. *See* **Note 18**.

3.4.2.7. Quantification of Normal Nucleotides After Hydrolysis

1. Dilute an aliquot of hydrolysate (from **Subheading 3.4.2.**, which describes DNA hydrolysis) 1:1500 with distilled water (i.e., 2.5 µL of digest from **Subheading 3.4.2.** adjusted to 250 µL and 10 µL of this solution adjusted to 150 µL).
2. Take a 5-µL (10 pmol normal nucleotides) aliquot of this digest, add 2.5 µL 10 m*M* Tris-HCl buffer (pH 9.0), and label as in **Subheading 3.4.2.** (the final volume of the mixture is 10 µL).
3. Allow to react 30 min at room temperature.
4. Take a 4-µL aliquot of the mixture and dilute to 750 µL with 10 m*M* Tris-HCl, pH 9.0.
5. Shake and centrifuge to remove contamination from the lid.
6. Spot 5 µL on a PEI-cellulose TLC plate.

7. Develop the TLC plate in a solution of 280 m*M* $(NH_4)_2SO_4$ and 50 m*M* NaH_2PO_4, pH 6.5.
8. Allow to dry after TLC.
9. Perform autoradiography for approx 45 min at room temperature to locate the four normal nucleotides bis-phosphate.
10. Cut spot for quantification by either liquid scintillation or Cerenkov counting. *See* **Notes 19** and **20**.

3.4.2.8. Calculation of the Relative Adduct Labeling

1. After correcting where necessary for decay factors, you will have obtained values for the counts in the adduct spots and the counts in the aliquot of labeled normal nucleotides. The latter will have been determined on 180,000 less material than the former, and this figure is therefore the conversion factor to apply to the count of normal nucleotides for determining the RAL values of adduct levels.

3.4.3. Detection of Binding of the Test Drug to DNA Using Radioactive-Labeled Drug

The ^{3}H or ^{14}C radioactivity of modified DNA is determined by liquid scintillation counting.

1. Add a 10- to 50-µL solution of DNA to 3 mL of a scintillation solution in the scintillation vial. Mix well.
2. Measure the radioactivity using the scintillation counter (e.g., Packard Tri-Carb 200 CA). *See* **Note 21**.

4. Notes

1. The concentration of cytochrome P450 in microsomes is measured according to Omura and Sato *(26)*, who measured the absorption of the complex of reduced CYP with carbon monoxide. Carbon monoxide is extremely toxic and should be handled with care and in a good chemical hood.
2. When DNA is fragmented during the incubations (e.g., by formation of oxygen radicals during the enzymatic activation reaction) or during the isolation procedure, when the size of the DNA is small (<1 kb) or when it is present in small amounts (<0.1 mg/mL), the period of storage should be extended and the temperature lowered to –70°C.
3. After the 70% ethanol wash, the pellet does not adhere tightly to the wall of the tube, so great care must be taken when removing the supernatant.
4. The dissolution will be preferentially performed in glass tubes. Plastic tubes may result in DNA damage and adduct losses. If the latter is used, they should be washed with water and ethanol and then dried before use.
5. The hydrolysate prepared at this stage will be used for the analysis of adducts (**Subheadings 3.4.2.–3.4.2.8.**) and normal (unmodified) nucleotides (**Subheading 3.4.2.**).

6. Solutions of enzymes can be stored separately or as a ready-use mixture at approx 20°C and in small aliquots (30–50 μL) to avoid freezing and thawing problems.
7. If SPD is used beyond the expiration date (not more than 3 mo), the concentration can be increased by approx 30% to 50% by increasing the volume of SPD added and reducing the volume of water.
8. Digestion time should be adapted to the DNA sample and the type of adducts looked at. A long digestion time can lead to losses of adducts.
9. The DNA digest can be stored frozen overnight as such for subsequent butanol extraction and labeling on the following day or after treatment with nuclease P1 (NP1) and stopping of the reaction with the Tris-HCl base solution.
10. The extractions and back extractions can be performed at room temperature.
11. The samples can be labeled immediately or stored at –80°C in the butanol phase or after transfer into water.
12. Exposure to ^{32}P should be avoided by working in a confined laboratory area with protective clothing, Plexiglas shielding, Geiger counters, and body dosimeters. Waste must be discarded according to appropriate safety procedures.
13. No apyrase (used previously to remove the excess of ATP, *see* **ref. *17***) should be added to stop the experiment.
14. The phosphate content of the chromatography solvent can be adjusted for batch-to-batch variability of the TLC plates to allow separation of dTbisphosphate and ^{32}Pi. Poor efficiency of NP1 treatment or *n*-butanol enrichment will be demonstrated by spots of the four normal nucleotides that appear on the autoradiogram after approx 20- to 30-min exposures. If the ATP spot is absent, the sample must be discarded.
15. Two types of washes are currently performed: (1) overnight chromatography with deionized water either in an open TLC tank or in a closed tank overnight, followed by at least 1 h with the lid removed, and (2) washes with water, then with methanol, in a shaking bath.
16. For bulky adducts, 1.0 to 1.7 *M* natrium phosphate buffer, pH 6.8, will be enough. For smaller adducts, >2 *M* may be necessary. Up to 2.8 *M* can be used to retain polar adducts (pH lowering to 6.0 will be necessary). For information on a possible approach, *see* solutions described for the resolution of polar adducts (*see* **Subheading 2.4.1.6.** or *see* **refs. *27,28***). Performing an autoradiography after D1 is recommended to ensure the quality of the cleanup. The presence of a tailing peak at the origin indicates contamination of the sample with proteins, which will increase the background in D2 to D3 directions.
17. When using Li formate in D2, it should be prepared as follows. For example, for 3 *M* Li formate, pH 3.5, use 3 *M* formic acid and adjust to pH 3.5 with lithium hydroxide.
18. The D4 direction can also be omitted. In this case, the lid needs to be removed from the TLC tank when the solvent has reached the top of the TLC, allowing it to run for 30 to 60 min. This method is even better than adding a wick (the method frequently used in many laboratories to avoid the problems of front in D3 [residual radioactive impurities on the plate]; *see* above).

19. If the four spots of nucleotides are double (i.e., looks as if there are eight spots), this implies a contamination with RNA, and the samples must be discarded.
20. It has been proven by two different techniques that blank labeling (i.e., no DNA) contains a small amount of normal nucleotides. A blank must be performed and the counts from the spots in the area of the normal nucleotides subtracted from those from the normal nucleotides.
21. Exposure to radioactive elements should be avoided by working in a confined laboratory area with protective clothing, Plexiglas shielding, Geiger counters, and body dosimeters. Waste must be discarded according to appropriate safety procedures.

References

1. Guengerich, F. P. and Shimada, T. (1991) Oxidation of toxic and carcinogenic chemicals by human cytochrome P-450 enzymes. *Chem. Res. Toxicol.* **4,** 391–407.
2. Gonzalez, F. J. and Gelboin, H. V. (1992) Human cytochromes P-450: evolution and cDNA-directed expression. *Environ. Health Perspect.* **98,** 81–85.
3. Guengerich, F. P. (2000) Pharmacogenomics of cytochrome P450 and other enzymes involved in the biotransformation of xenobiotics. *Drug. Dev. Res.* **49,** 4–16.
4. Nuwaysir, E. F., Bittner, M., Trent, J., Barrett, J. C., and Afshari, C. A. (1999) Microarrays and toxicology: the advent of toxicogenomics. *Mol. Carcinogen.* **24,** 153–159.
5. Guengerich, F. P. (2001) Common and uncommon cytochrome P450 reactions related to metabolism and chemical toxicity. *Chem. Res. Toxicol.* **14,** 612–650.
6. Wrighton, S. A. and Stevens, J. C. (1992) The human hepatic cytochromes P450 involved in drug metabolism. *Crit. Rev. Toxicol.* **22,** 1–21.
7. Guengerich, F. P. and Liebler, D. C. (1985) Enzymatic activation of chemicals to toxic metabolites. *Crit. Rev. Toxicol.* **14,** 259–307.
8. Hemminki, K., Dipple, A., Shuker, D. E. G., Kadlubar, F. F., Segerback, D., and Bartsch, H. (eds) (1994) *DNA Adducts: Identification and Biological Significance.* IARC Scientific Publications No. 125, IARC, Lyon.
9. Hemminki, K. (1993) DNA adducts, mutations and cancer. *Carcinogenesis* **14,** 2007–2012.
10. Lutz, W. K. (1986) Qantitative evaluation of DNA binding data for risk estimation and for classification of direct and indirect carcinogens. *J. Cancer Res. Clin. Oncol.* **112,** 85–91.
11. Otteneder, M. and Lutz, W. K. (1999) Correlation of DNA adduct levels with tumour incidence: carcinogenic potency of DNA adducts. *Mutat. Res.* **424,** 237–247.
12. Poirier, M. C. (1996) Concepts and mechanism in carcinogen-DNA interactions, in *Control Mechanisms of Carcinogenesis* (Hengstler, J. G. and Oesch, F., eds.), Druckerei Thieme, Meissen, pp. 193–220.
13. Poirier, M. C., Santella, R. M., and Weston, A. (2000) Carcinogen macromolecular adducts and their measurement. *Carcinogenesis* **21,** 353–359.
14. Wiencke, J. K. (2002) DNA adduct burden and tobacco carcinogenesis. *Oncogene* **21,** 7376–7391.

15. Verna, L., Whysner, J., and Williams, G. M. (1996) 2-Acetylaminofluorene mechanistic data and risk assessment: DNA reactivity, enhanced cell proliferation and tumour initiation. *Pharmacol. Ther.* **71,** 83–105.
16. Kensler, T. W., Groopman, I. D., and Wogan, G. N. (1996) Use of carcinogen-DNA and carcinogen-protein adduct biomarkers for cohort selection and as modifiable and points in chemoprevention trials, in *Principles of Chemoprevention* (Steward, B. W., McGregor, D., and Kleihues, P., eds.), IARC, Lyon, pp. 237–248.
17. Randerath, K., Reddy, M. V., and Gupta, R. C. (1981) ^{32}P-labeling test for DNA damage. *Proc. Natl. Acad. Sci. USA* **78,** 6128–6129.
18. Reichert, W. L., Stein, J. E., French, B., Goodwin, P., and Vanarasi, U. (1992) Storage phosphor imaging technique for detection and quantitation of DNA adducts measured by the ^{32}P-postlabeling assay. *Carcinogenesis* **13,** 1475–1479.
19. Chang, L. W., Hsia, S. M. T., Chang, P. C., and Hsieh, L. L. (1994) Macromolecular adducts: biomarkers for toxicity and carcinogenesis. *Annu. Rev. Pharmacol. Toxicol.* **34,** 41–67.
20. Gupta, R. C., Reddy, M. V., and Randerath, K. (1982) ^{32}P-Post-labeling analysis of nonradioactive aromatic carcinogen DNA adducts. *Carcinogenesis* **3,** 1081–1092.
21. Reddy, M. V. and Randerath, K. (1986) Nuclease-P1-mediated enhancement of sensitivity of ^{32}P-postlabeling test for structurally diverse DNA adducts. *Carcinogenesis* **7,** 1543–1551.
22. Mourato, L. L. G., Beland, F. A., and Marques, M. M. (1999) ^{32}P-Postlabeling of N-(deoxyguanosin-8-yl)arylamine adducts: a comparative study of labeling efficiencies. *Chem. Res. Toxicol.* **12,** 661–669.
23. Randerath, E., Agrawal, H. P., Weaver, J. A., Bordelon, C. B., and Randerath, K. (1985) ^{32}P-Postlabeling analysis of DNA adducts persisting for up to 42 weeks in the skin, epidermis and dermis of mice treated topically with 7,2-dimethylbez[a]anthracene. *Carcinogenesis* **6,** 1117–1126.
24. Everson, R. B., Randerath, E., Santella, R. M., Cefalo, R. C., Avits, T. A., and Randerath, K. (1986) Detection of smoking-related covalent DNA adducts in human placenta. *Science* **231,** 57–65.
25. Gupta, R. C. (1985) Enhanced sensitivity of ^{32}P-postlabeling analysis of aromatic carcinogen-DNA adducts. *Cancer Res.* **45,** 5656–5662.
26. Omura, T. and Sato R. (1964) The carbon monoxide-binding pigment of liver microsomes: I. Evidence for its hemoprotein nature. *J. Biol. Chem.* **239,** 2370–2378.
27. Laws, G. M., Adams, S. P., Nichols, W. W., and Selde, J. R. (1994) Detection of DNA-adducts by ^{32}P-postlabeling and multifraction contanct-transfer thin-layer chromatography. *Fund. Appl. Toxicol.* **23,** 308–312.
28. Stiborová, M., Asfaw, B., Frei, E., Schmeiser, H. H., and Wiessler, M. (1995) Benzenediazonium ion derived from Sudan I forms an 8-(phenylazo)guanine adduct in DNA. *Chem. Res. Toxicol.* **8,** 489–498.

19

Application of In Vitro Comet Assay for Genotoxicity Testing

Bojana Žegura and Metka Filipič

Summary

The comet assay, also called the single-cell gel electrophoresis (SCGE) assay, is a simple, rapid, and sensitive technique for detecting deoxyribonucleic acid (DNA) damage at the level of individual eukaryotic cells. The types of DNA damage that can be observed with this method are DNA double-strand breaks (DSB) and single-strand breaks (SSB), alkali labile sites (ALS) such as apurinic/apyrimidinic (AP) sites, DNA–DNA and DNA–protein cross-links, and SSB associated with incomplete excision repair. To carry out the assay, the cells are embedded in agarose gel on microscope slides and lysed under mild alkaline conditions to remove cellular proteins. The slides are then exposed to alkaline conditions to cause the DNA to unwind and electrophorese. During the electrophoresis, undamaged supercoiled DNA migrates slowly and close to the nucleoid, whereas broken DNA fragments and relaxed chromatin migrate faster and further away from the nucleoid toward the anode, giving the appearance of a "comet tail." The DNA is stained with a fluorescent dye, and the DNA damage is quantified under a fluorescence microscope by visual scoring or by computerized image analysis.

Key Words: Comet assay; single-cell gel electrophoresis; genotoxicity; strand breaks; DNA damage.

1. Introduction

The single-cell gel electrophoresis (SCGE) assay, known as the comet assay, was first developed by Ostling and Johanson in 1984 *(1)*. DNA liberated from single cells embedded in agarose was electrophoresed for a short time under neutral conditions, enabling DNA double-strand breaks (DSB) to be detected.

From: *Methods in Pharmacology and Toxicology*
Optimization in Drug Discovery: In Vitro Methods
Edited by: Z. Yan and G. W. Caldwell © Humana Press Inc., Totowa, NJ

In 1988, Singh et al. *(2)* modified the assay using electrophoresis at pH >13.0, under which alkaline conditions both single-strand breaks (SSB) and alkali labile sites (ALS) could also be detected *(3)*. Later on, Olive et al. *(4)* described another version of the assay with electrophoresis carried out under mild alkaline conditions, pH 12.3, in which ALS are not expressed as SSB.

In the comet assay, a single-cell suspension is embedded in agarose on a microscope slide, lysed by detergent and a high salt concentration at pH 10.0, and then electrophoresed for a short time under alkaline conditions, pH >13.0. During lysis, the cell contents, except the nucleoids with highly supercoiled deoxyribonucleic acid (DNA), are removed. When placed in alkali, DNA starts to unwind from sites of strand breaks so that cells with more DNA damage display increased migration of DNA from nucleoids toward the anode, giving the appearance of a "comet tail" (**Fig. 1**). The nucleoids are stained with a fluorescent DNA binding dye, visualized by fluorescence microscopy, and the DNA damage quantified by image analysis or visual scoring *(5)*. The types of DNA damage detected by the alkaline comet assay are SSB and DSB, together with the transient SSB and ALS, which occur as intermediates during base and nuclear excision repair. The assay thus enables the activity of genotoxic agents to be assessed, both qualitatively and quantitatively. A high level of breaks detected by the comet assay indicates either major DNA damage or efficient repair of DNA damage *(6)*. At pH 12.6 and higher, ALS are quickly transformed to SSB and, because almost all genotoxic agents induce orders of magnitude more SSB and ALS than DSB, the alkaline (pH >13.0) version is recommended as optimal for identifying such agents *(3)*.

To improve the sensitivity and specificity of the method, one can apply several modifications. The sensitivity can be increased by using DNA repair inhibitors, which lead to the accumulation of DNA strand breaks. Specific classes of DNA adducts can be detected by incubating the lysed cells with lesion-specific DNA repair enzymes. Collins et al. used endonuclease III *(7)* and formamidopyrimidine-DNA glycosylase *(8)*, which convert oxidized pyrimidines and purines, respectively, to strand breaks. The major applications of the comet assay are in genetic toxicology for identifying genotoxic agents, DNA repair studies, eco-toxicology and environmental biomonitoring, nutrition toxicology, clinical applications, and biomonitoring in human population studies, cell cycle analysis, and free radical biology. During drug development, the comet assay can be the test of choice for genotoxicity screening of drug candidates. Its main advantages, relative to other genotoxicity tests, are high sensitivity for detecting low levels of DNA damage, flexibility, low cost, ease of application, the need for relatively small amounts of test substance, and a short period needed to complete the experiment *(3)*.

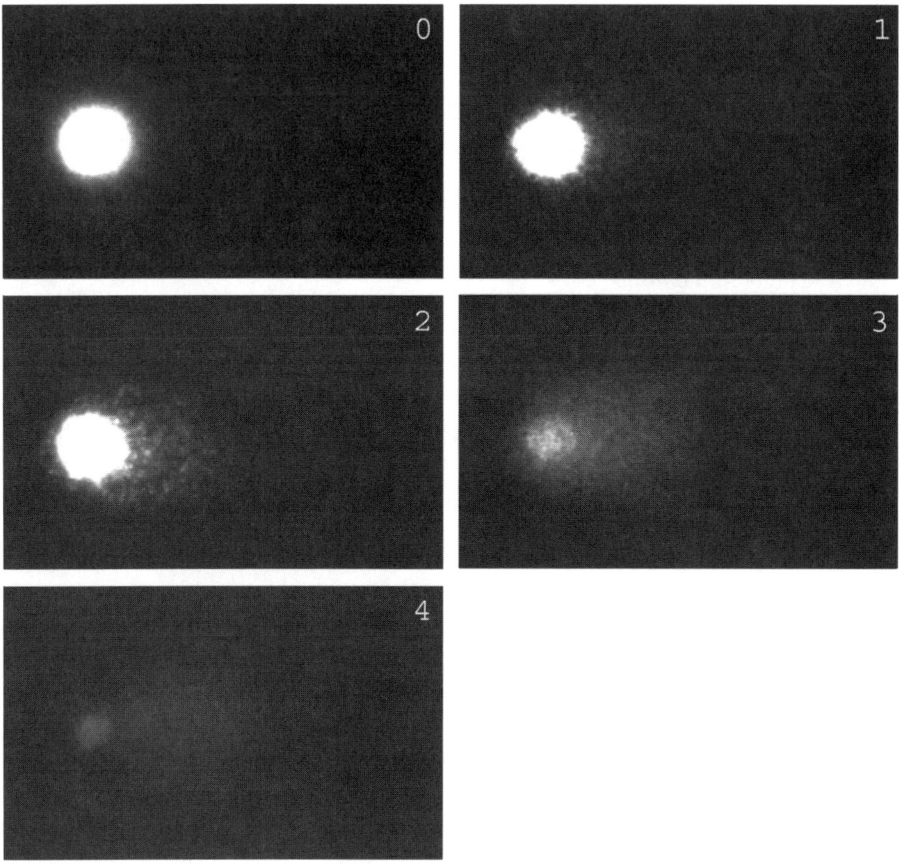

Fig. 1. Comet images of HepG2 cells after comet assay, which illustrate categories for visual scoring. In class 0, almost no tail is visible, which means no DNA damage is observed; in class 4, almost all the DNA is in the tail, and the head is very small and hardly visible.

We describe here the alkaline comet assay version, based on the method described by Singh et al. *(2)*, with minor modifications introduced in our laboratory.

2. Materials

2.1. Equipment

1. Horizontal electrophoresis apparatus (preferable with recirculating unit).
2. Power supply.
3. Fluorescence microscope: ×40 or ×60 objective.

4. Digital camera (optional).
5. Image analysis system (optional).

2.2. Chemicals

1. Phosphate-buffered saline (PBS), Ca^{2+} and Mg^{2+} free.
2. Low melting point (LMP) agarose (e.g., Gibco BRL, 15517-022).
3. Normal melting point (NMP) agarose (e.g., Gibco BRL, 15510-027).
4. NaOH (sodium hydroxide).
5. NaCl (sodium chloride).
6. Na_2EDTA (ethylenediaminetetraacetic acid).
7. Tris-HCl (Tris (hydroxymethyl) aminomethane).
8. Triton X-100 (*t*-octylphenoxypoly-ethoxyethanol).
9. DMSO (dimethylsulfoxide).
10. Fluorescent dye (4'6-diamidino-2-phenylindote [DAPI]/ethidium bromide/propidium iodide, etc.).

The chemicals should be of analytical grade.

2.3. Slides

Slides used in the comet assay can be either fully frosted or clear (with a frosted end). Fully frosted slides are more expensive but give better anchorage for the agarose. When using clear slides, they should be soaked in methanol overnight and then precoated with a thin layer of 0.5% NMP (100 mg per 20 mL 1X PBS) agarose by dipping the slides in hot agarose. The excess agarose on the underside of the slide should be wiped off and the slides air-dried. Slides can then be stored until use. This precoating with NMP agarose ensures better attachment of the second layer of NMP agarose. Fully frosted slides should only be soaked in methanol overnight.

2.4. Preparation of Reagents

2.4.1. Agarose: High-Resolution Agarose

1. 1% NMP.
2. 1% LMP.

NMP (100 mg per 10 mL) and LMP (100 mg per 10 mL) are dissolved in serum-free medium or 1X PBS by mixing and heated (in a microwave oven) to boiling. Dissolved agarose can be reheated during the experiment when necessary.

2.4.2. Lysis Solution

1. 2.5 *M* NaCl.
2. 0.1 *M* Na_2EDTA.
3. 10 m*M* Tris-HCl.

The lysis solution should be prepared freshly prior to use. For 1 L of lysis solution, add 146.1 g NaCl, 37.2 g Na_2EDTA, and 1.21 g Tris-HCl to 750 mL distilled water (dH_2O). To dissolve the reagents, stir and heat slightly. Adjust the volume to 990 mL with dH_2O and adjust the pH to 10.0 with either concentrated NaOH solution (10 *M*) or HCl. Keep at 4°C until use. Immediately before use for lysis, add Triton X-100 (1 mL per 100 mL of lysis solution) and mix gently for at least 15 min to dissolve. If using blood or animal tissues that contain heme, then 10% DMSO *(3)*, a free radical scavenger, should be added to the lysis solution to prevent free radical–induced DNA damage. Some types of cells may need the presence of a second detergent (1% sodium *N*-lauryl sarcosine) to complete the lysis *(2)*.

Because of the high pH, wear gloves when preparing the solution.

2.4.3. Electrophoresis Buffer

1. 0.3 *M* NaOH.
2. 1 m*M* EDTA.

The electrophoresis buffer should be prepared immediately prior to use. Stock solutions of 10 *M* NaOH and 0.2 *M* EDTA can be prepared in advance and should be stored at room temperature and 4°C, respectively. Add 30 mL NaOH (10 m*M*) and 5 mL EDTA (0.2 *M*) to 900 mL dH_2O and adjust the volume to 1 L. The pH should be >13.0. Because of the high pH, wear gloves when preparing the solution.

2.4.4. Neutralizing Buffer

1. 0.4 *M* Tris-HCl.

Neutralizing buffer should be prepared fresh just prior to use. For 1 L, add 48.88 g to dH_2O. Adjust the pH to 7.5 with HCl. Keep at 4°C.

2.4.5. Stains

The stains are dissolved in 1X PBS at the following concentrations:

1. Ethidium bromide = 2 µg/mL, with an excitation and emission of 518/605 nm.
2. Propidium iodide = 2.5 µg/mL, with an excitation and emission of 535/617 nm.
3. DAPI = 1 µg/mL, with an excitation and emission of 358/461 nm.

Wear gloves; the stains are toxic.

3. Methods

The following protocol describes the basic procedures (**Fig. 2**) of the comet assay and presents the alkaline unwinding conditions (pH >13.0) *(2)* for detecting single- and double-strand breaks and alkali labile sites, including AP sites.

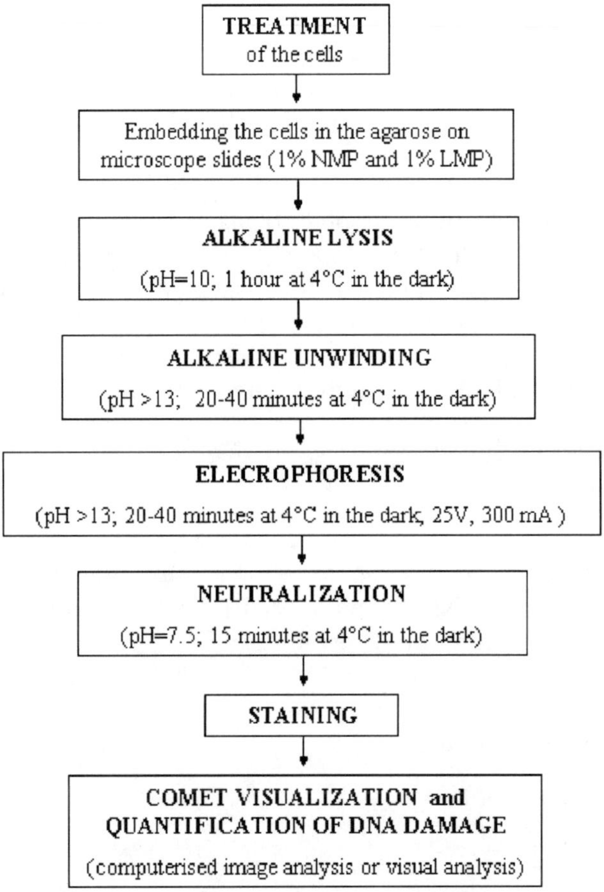

Fig. 2. Schematic representation of steps in alkaline comet assay.

3.1. Alkaline Comet Assay

3.1.1. Preparation of Cell Suspension

When using monolayer cell cultures, the cells are washed with PBS and harvested by trypsinization or by scraping. The cell suspension is then centrifuged, the supernatant is removed, and the pellet is resuspended in PBS or medium. The cells are counted and diluted to a density of approx 3×10^5 cells/mL. When the test is performed on cells in suspension, the cells are centrifuged, washed with PBS, resuspended in medium or PBS, counted, and diluted to the appropriate density.

3.1.2. Embedding the Cells in Agarose

On each precoated clear slide or fully frosted slide, place 80 µL of 1% NMP agarose and, while still liquid, cover the agarose with a coverglass. On each slide, you can set two gels using two coverglasses (18 × 18 or 22 × 22 mm). Leave the slides at 4°C (refrigerator) for at least 5 min to allow the agarose to solidify. Gently remove the coverglasses from the slide. Mix 30 µL of cell suspension (~3 × 10^5 cells/mL) with 70 µL of 1% LMP agarose (approx 37°C) and place 70 µL on the NMP agarose layer. Cover with the coverglass to spread the cell suspension. Leave the slides at 4°C for at least 5 min and then gently remove the coverglass.

3.1.3. Lysis

Immerse the slides in cold (4°C) lysis solution for at least 1 h at 4°C in the dark. After lysing the cells, rinse the slides carefully in distilled water to remove excess lysis solution. The slides should be handled with care to avoid the gels slipping from the slides.

3.1.4. Alkaline Unwinding

Place the slides side by side in the horizontal electrophoresis tank. To ensure constant electrophoresis current, fill free spaces in the electrophoresis tank with blank slides. Fill the tank with freshly prepared precooled (4°C) alkaline electrophoresis buffer (pH >13.0) until the level covers the slides (2–3 mm above the slides) and leave for 20 min at 4°C in the dark to allow unwinding of DNA and expression of ALS.

3.1.5. Electrophoresis

Samples are electrophoresed in the same buffer as for the alkaline unwinding for 20 min at 4°C in the dark at 25 V (0.7–1 V/cm). The current should be adjusted to 300 mA by raising or lowering the level of the electrophoresis buffer. For each run, fresh electrophoresis buffer should be used. After electrophoresis, remove the slides from the electrophoresis tank and wash them in distilled water to remove excess alkaline buffer.

3.1.6. Neutralization

Place the slides horizontally in a tray, immerse them in three lots of neutralizing solution, and leave for 5 min each or once for 15 min at 4°C in the dark. *Note:* Lysis, unwinding, electrophoresis, and neutralization should be performed in the dark or under yellow light at 4°C.

3.1.7. Storing Slides

Slides can be kept for several days in moist chambers in the dark at 4°C prior to analysis. If not analyzed within a few days, the slides can be dehydrated (only clear slides, but not fully frosted) by immersing twice in absolute ethanol or methanol for 5 min, drying at room temperature, and storing in a low-humidity environment until analyzed. The other way to dehydrate slides is to wash them in distilled water and dry at room temperature *(3)*. Dried slides have the advantage that they can be rescored at any time.

3.1.8. Staining

The slides are stained with a fluorescent DNA intercalating dye. Place 20 μL of dye solution (e.g., ethidium bromide: 2 μg/mL) on each slide and cover it with the coverglass. Use the least concentration of the stain to avoid high background fluorescence. The most used alternative stains are propidium iodide, DAPI, and YOYO-1.

3.1.9. Comet Visualization

All slides, including those of the positive and negative controls, should be coded independently before microscopic analysis and scored without knowledge of the code. Fifty randomly selected nuclei per culture (25 per each of the two replicate slides) are analyzed per sample. The comets are visualized under ×400 (×200 or ×600 can be used, depending on the cell type being evaluated) magnification using a fluorescence microscope with an excitation filter of 510 to 560 nm and a barrier filter of 590 nm when using ethidium bromide as a dye. Comets should be scored from the center of the gel and not near the edges of the gel. Also avoid analyzing the comets around air bubbles trapped in the agarose.

3.1.10. Quantification of DNA Damage

DNA damage can be quantified by computerized image analysis or by visual scoring.

3.1.10.1. Computerized Image Analysis

There are several commercially available software programs for image analysis. The fluorescence microscope should be equipped with a digital camera to capture comet images. These are then analyzed with a software program, which quantitates and calculates different parameters according to differentiation between the comet head and the tail. The most commonly used parameters to express DNA damage are the percentage of migrated DNA in the comet (from the head to the tail), the tail length (distance of migrated DNA from the head to the last DNA fragment in the tail, expressed in microns), olive tail moment (percent DNA in the tail × distance of the center of gravity of the tail DNA from the center of gravity of head DNA), and the extended tail moment (percent DNA in the tail × tail length). When using tail moments, data on the percentage of tail DNA or tail length should also be provided. From our experience, the percentage of tail DNA is a reliable indicator of DNA damage.

3.1.10.2. Visual Analysis

Comets can be analyzed without image analysis software by visual classification into several categories (usually five), according to tail intensity from *undamaged* (0) to *highly damaged* (4) cells (**Fig. 1**). The intensity of each comet is assessed visually and given a numerical value (for each migration category from 0, 1, 2, 3, or 4). Usually, 100 randomly selected comets are scored. The total score for 100 comets could range from 0 (all undamaged) to 400 (all highly damaged). The results are presented in arbitrary units. This visual scoring was suggested and described by Collins et al. *(5)* and was confirmed by computerized image analysis to be as effective as software-based scoring.

4.1. Cells and Cell Treatment

4.1.1. Cell Types and Culture Conditions

In principle, any eukaryotic cell can be used for genotoxicity testing in the comet assay. For in vitro testing, well-characterized cell lines or primary cells are used. The cells are cultured in the appropriate culture media and incubation conditions (culture vessels, CO_2 concentration, temperature, and humidity). Most of the cell lines are metabolically noncompetent and should be exposed to the test compound in the presence and absence of an appropriate exogenous metabolic activation system. The most commonly used system is a cofactor-supplemented postmitochondrial fraction (S9) prepared from male rats treated with enzyme-inducing agents *(3)*. The advantage of using metabolically competent cells is that they have the potential for endogenous activation of chemicals. The most frequently used metabolically competent cells for genotoxicity studies are primary cultured rat liver cells. A good alternative is the use of the metabolically competent human hepatoma cell line, HepG2, which has retained the activities of phase I and phase II enzymes that play a key role in the activation and detoxification of DNA reactive carcinogens. The use of cell lines also reduces the use of laboratory animals in genetic toxicology *(9)*.

4.1.2. Test Conditions

The test substance should be dissolved or suspended in solvents or vehicles that are compatible with the survival of the cells and do not react with the test chemical. The cells to be exposed to the test substance can be in the form of monolayers or in suspension. The duration of exposure should be from 3 to 6 h *(3)*, and at least three nontoxic concentrations should be tested. Concurrently, with each comet assay experiment, cytotoxicity should be evaluated using standard cytotoxicity assays. In general, comet assays should be performed at concentrations of agents that do not reduce the cell viability by more than 25%. Appropriate positive and negative (solvent or vehicle) controls should be included in each experiment. Examples of positive control substances that do not require metabolic activation are methyl methanesulfonate, ethyl methanesulfonate, and 4-nitroquinoline-oxide. Those requiring metabolic activation include benzo(a)pyrene, 7,12-dimethylbenzanthracene, and cyclophosphamide. At least two cultures, each resulting in successful assays, should be tested at each concentration, including negative and positive control groups.

4.1.3. Analysis and Treatment of Results

The experimental unit of exposure is the culture, and the statistical analysis is based on the individual culture response. The mean or median of extent of DNA damage with the associated error is calculated for each dose group, as well as for each culture within a dose group. When the data are not normally distributed, the median is preferred. The results of each experiment should be verified in an independent experiment.

The criteria for positive response are a dose-related increase in DNA damage and a significant corresponding increase in DNA damage at one or more dose groups. Statistical analysis should be used as an aid in evaluating test results but should not be the only determining factor for positive response. A pairwise comparison of each dose group against the concurrent control can be used to identify significant effects at individual doses and trend tests to determine the dose-response relationship. As an example, **Fig. 3** shows the result of the treatment of human hepatoma cells HepG2 with a model mutagen benzo(a)pyrene.

5. Notes

1. Results obtained with the comet assay depend strongly on the test conditions used, so it is strongly recommended to always use the same conditions during the procedure to obtain valid and reproducible results. It is most important to control the temperature during unwinding and electrophoresis. All steps from lysis onward should be performed at 4°C in the dark or under yellow light to prevent the occurrence of additional DNA damage during the assay.
2. The method should be adjusted to optimal conditions for every cell type. The duration of alkaline unwinding and of electrophoresis affects the sensitivity and specificity of the test and varies between cell lines. In general, 20 min for unwinding and 20 min for electrophoresis are considered adequate for most pur-

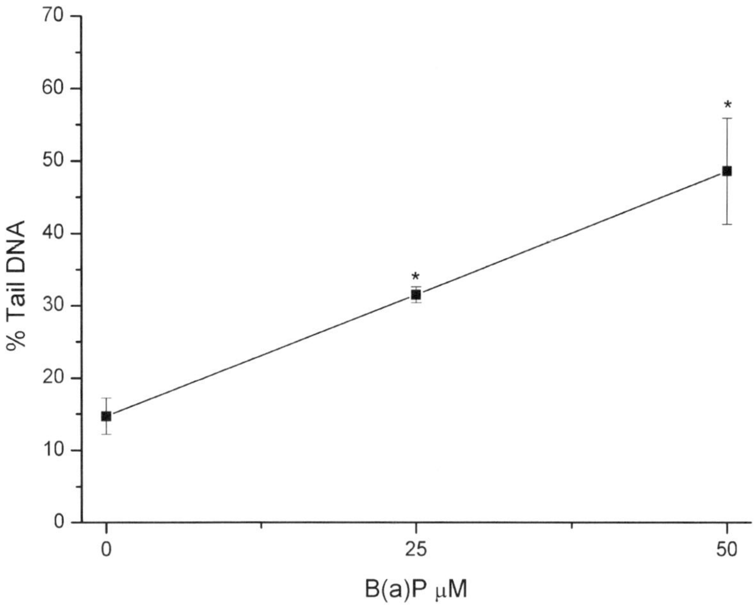

Fig. 3. Benzo(a)pyrene (BaP)–induced DNA damage in HepG2 cells. Two parallel cultures of cells were each treated with 25 or 50 μ*M* benzo(a)pyrene for 4 h. Fifty randomly selected nuclei (25 per each of the two replicate slides) were analyzed per experimental point per each of the two cultures. The results are presented as mean values of percent tail DNA of two parallel cell cultures ±SE. Differences between untreated control cells and those exposed to BaP were evaluated by application of the nonparametric Mann-Whitney *U*-test. *Significantly different from untreated control culture ($p < 0.0001$).

poses. The duration of each step may be extended up to 40 min to enhance the sensitivity and to detect smaller amounts of DNA damage, but beyond a 40-min electrophoresis, a major increase of comets may be observed in the control population. Higher sensitivity can also be obtained by using a higher voltage.

3. The concentration and amount of agarose is an important parameter because too high a concentration of agarose can decrease DNA migration. Using frosted slides can contribute to background fluorescence noise, which may obscure details of the comets. Also, a cell density that is too high should be avoided because of the overlapping comets, especially when expecting high degrees of DNA damage.
4. It is possible that the results of the comet assay are false-positive results that do not reflect genotoxicity but may arise from DNA damage associated with cytotoxicity; cell viability should therefore be tested before performing the comet assay.
5. Positive results from an in vitro comet assay indicate that the test substance induces DNA damage in cultured mammalian cells. Negative results indicate that, under the test conditions, the test substance does not induce DNA damage in

cultured cells *(3)*. To confirm negative results, one should perform additional tests using different test conditions or modified versions of the comet assay.

6. Several versions of the comet assay have been described for detecting different types of DNA damage, expressed under different unwinding and electrophoresis pH conditions. Nuclear DNA can be unwound under neutral conditions, pH 7.0–8.0, in which double-strand breaks and crosslinks are detected with the comet assay. DNA unwinding under mild alkaline conditions, pH 12.1, expresses double- and single-strand breaks, crosslinks, and breaks formed during incomplete excision repair. By using these different versions of the comet assay, different types of DNA lesions can be discriminated.
7. Specific classes of DNA adducts can be detected by incubating the lysed cells, prior to the unwinding step, with lesion-specific DNA repair enzymes. Purified endonuclease III and formamidopyrimidine-DNA glycosylase convert oxidized pyrimidines and purines, respectively, to strand breaks *(7,8)*.
8. Certain genotoxins induce DNA SSB, which are repaired very quickly after the treatment and are not detectable unless DNA repair inhibitors are added during the procedure. Cytosine β-D-arabinoside (AraC) and hydroxyurea (HU), which act by inhibiting DNA polymerization, cause accumulation of DNA strand breaks at sites of incomplete DNA repair because excision occurs, but polymerization and ligation do not. DNA repair can easily be evaluated by comparing the level of SSB in the presence and in the absence of DNA repair inhibitors.
9. For studying the kinetics of DNA repair, the cells are exposed to a DNA damaging agent and then incubated for various periods of time to allow recovery, after which the comet assay is performed. Following the appearance and removal of DNA breaks by the comet assay, the kinetics of DNA repair in cells is revealed.

Acknowledgments

We thank Tanja Fatur, MSc, for valuable suggestions and discussion and Prof. Roger Pain for critical reading of the manuscript.

References

1. Östling, O. and Johanson, K. J. (1984) Microelectrophoretic study of radiation-induced DNA damage in individual mammalian cells. *Biochem. Biophys. Res. Commun.* **123,** 291–298.
2. Singh, N. P., McCoy, M. T., Tice, R. R., and Schneider E. L. (1988) A simple technique for quantitation of low levels of DNA damage in individual cells. *Exp. Cell. Res.* **175,** 184–191.
3. Tice, R. R., Agurell, E., Anderson, D., Burlinson, B., Hartmann, A., Kobayashi, H., et al. (2000) Single cell gel/comet assay: guidelines for in vitro and vivo genetic toxicology testing. *Environ. Mol. Mutagen.* **35,** 206–221.
4. Olive, P. L., Banath, J. P., and Durand, R. E. (1990) Detection of etoposide resistance by measuring DNA damage in individual Chinese hamster cells. *J. Natl. Cancer Inst.* **82,** 779–783.

5. Collins, A. R., Ai-guo, M., and Duthie, S. J. (1995) The kinetics of repair of oxidative DNA damage (strand breaks and oxidised pyrimidines) in human cells. *Mutat. Res.* **336,** 69–77.
6. Collins, A. R., Dobson, V. L., Dusinská, M., Kennedy, G., and Stetina, R. (1997) The comet assay: what can it really tell us? *Mutat. Res.* **375,** 183–193.
7. Collins, A. R., Duthie, S. J., and Dobson, V. L. (1993) Direct enzymic detection of endogenous oxidative base damage in human lymphocyte DNA. *Carcinogenesis* **14,** 1733–1735.
8. Collins, A. R., Dusinská, M., Gedik, C. M., and Stetina, R. (1996) Oxidative damage to DNA: do we have a reliable biomarker? *Environ. Health Perspect.* **104,** 465–469.
9. Uhl, M., Helma, C., and Knasmüller, S. (2000) Evaluation of single cell gel electrophoresis assay with human hepatoma (HepG2) cells. *Mutat. Res.* **468,** 213–225.

20

Assessing DNA Damage Using a Reporter Gene System

Xuming Jia and Wei Xiao

Summary

Assessment of genotoxicity remains an important aspect of developing and approving pharmaceutical products. The authors describe a newly developed genotoxicity testing system using deoxyribonucleic acid (DNA) damage-inducible gene expression in a lower eukaryotic microorganism as a reporter. This method is able to detect a broad range of DNA-damaging agents that are highly correlated with rodent carcinogens. The protocol is rapid, sensitive, easy to perform, reliable, and, most importantly, safe to the user and environment.

Key Words: Genotoxicity test; gene expression; budding yeast; *RNR3-lacZ*.

1. Introduction

Assessing genotoxic potential is one of the key procedures for developing and marketing new compounds for pharmaceutical applications. For instance, an ideal anticancer drug aimed at selective killing of tumor cells is expected to be more toxic to growing cells than nondividing cells and to have minimal mutagenic potential, whereas most other pharmaceutical products are expected to have little genotoxic effect. Several bacterial reporter gene systems have been developed *(1–3)* initially for the purpose of detecting environmental toxins and carcinogens. A genotoxicity testing system based on deoxyribonucleic acid (DNA) damage-induced gene expression in yeast was reported recently *(4)* and found useful in assessing pharmaceutical compounds as well. There are at least four major reasons to choose yeast instead of bacterial and mammalian cells for such tests. First, yeast, as a unicellular eukaryote, shares with bacteria the advantages of rapid growth, easy manipulation, and growth on a variety of carbon sources. Second, because it is an eukaryotic organism, the metabolism

From: *Methods in Pharmacology and Toxicology*
Optimization in Drug Discovery: In Vitro Methods
Edited by: Z. Yan and G. W. Caldwell © Humana Press Inc., Totowa, NJ

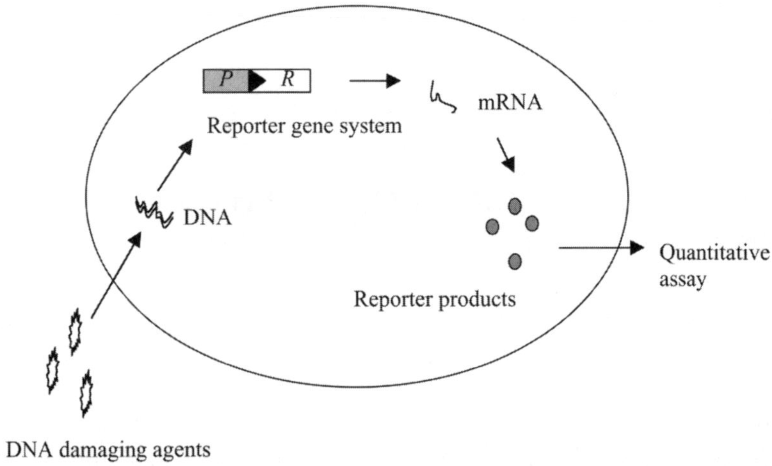

Fig. 1. A schematic illustration of a reporter gene assay based on assessing the induction of gene expression in response to DNA damage and replication blocks. Environmental DNA-damaging agents modify DNA and cause replication blocks, leading to the induction of a sensing promoter and the expression of its fused reporter gene. This reporter gene is then transcribed and translated into a measurable protein product. *P*, inducible promoter; *R*, reporter gene.

and DNA damage-induced responses closely resemble those of human cells. This is very important when using a biosensor to reveal potential hazards to higher eukaryotes such as humans. Third, the budding yeast *Saccharomyces cerevisiae* is one of the best-understood and most readily manipulated organisms. It is the first eukaryotic organism whose entire genome sequence has been determined. Finally, budding yeast has been used in food and beverage industries and is known to be safe and environmentally friendly.

For a reporter gene system to detect DNA damage, two elements are required: a sensing element and a reporter element coupled to the sensing element. The former responds to the presence of DNA damage and turns on the latter, which emits a detectable signal. The sensing element is often a promoter capable of inducing a gene in response to DNA damage. The reporter element is a gene coding for proteins with readily detectable and measurable activity. The fused promoter-reporter can be introduced into the host cell either as a free plasmid or integrated into the host chromosome through homologous recombination. The working mechanism of a reporter gene system is depicted in **Fig. 1**.

The reporter gene system described in this chapter is based on a fusion construct between a yeast *RNR3* promoter (P_{RNR3}) and a bacterial *lacZ* gene. This fusion construct is then integrated into the host genome to create a stable

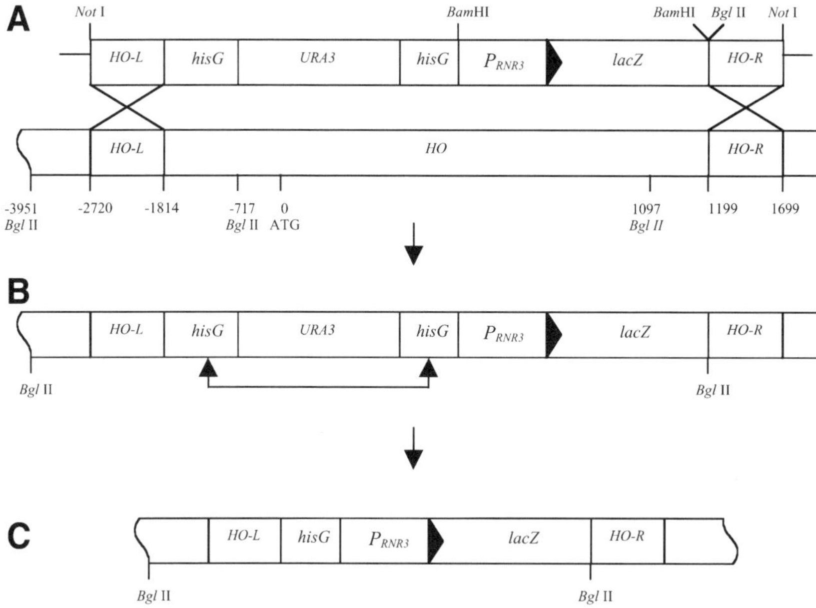

Fig. 2. Creation of a *RNR3-lacZ* fusion gene integration system. A P_{RNR3}-*lacZ* cassette was inserted into the plasmid M4366, flanked by a *hisG-URA3-hisG* cassette and a fragment from the right end of the *HO* gene. **(A)** After being released by *Not*I cleavage and transformed into host DBY747 cells, the *hisG-URA3-hisG*-P_{RNR3}-*lacZ* dual cassettes can replace the endogenous *HO* gene (defective and dispensible in DBY747) through homologous recombination at *HO-L* and *HO-R*. **(B)** The resulting chromosome structure at the *HO* locus after replacement. **(C)** Homologous recombination occurs between two *hisG* tandem repeats, resulting in the removal of *URA3*. This strain (WXY1111) becomes stable at the *HO* locus and is used for genotoxicity assays. The chromosomal structure at the *HO* locus after transformation can be confirmed by Southern hybridization using either *HO* or *lacZ* as a probe.

integrant (**Fig. 2**). *RNR3* encodes a large subunit of ribonucleotide reductase, and its expression in response to DNA damage is well characterized *(5,6)*. *lacZ* encodes a β-galactosidase whose activity can be readily measured *(7)*. Previous studies have established that the centromere-based, single-copy P_{RNR3}-*lacZ* faithfully represents the steady-state *RNR3* transcript level both in treated and untreated cells *(8)*. A stable integrant of the P_{RNR3}-*lacZ* reporter gene was created and characterized recently *(4)*, making the assay more user-friendly.

2. Materials

1. Buffer Z (60 m*M* $Na_2HPO_4 \cdot 7H_2O$, 40 m*M* $NaH_2PO_4 \cdot H_2O$, 10 m*M* KCl, 1 m*M* $MgSO_4 \cdot 7H_2O$, 40 m*M* β-mercaptoethanol, pH 7.0).

2. 1% Sodium dodecyl sulfate (SDS) solution.
3. Chloroform.
4. 4 mg/mL Orthonitrophenyl-β-galactoside (ONPG), dissolved in sterile-distilled water.
5. 1 *M* Na_2CO_3.
6. Yeast reporter strain WXY1111, a derivative of DBY747 carrying a stable integration of a P_{RNR3}-*lacZ* cassette *(4)*.
7. Yeast extract-peptone-dextrose (YPD) liquid culture medium: 1% (w/v) Bacto-yeast extract, 2% (w/v) Bacto-peptone, and 2% (w/v) glucose dissolved in distilled water, autoclaved at 121°C for 20 min, and stored at room temperature.
8. YPD agar plates: 1% (w/v) Bacto-yeast extract, 2% (w/v) Bacto-peptone, 2% (w/v) glucose, and 2% (w/v) agar, dissolved in distilled water, autoclaved at 121°C for 20 min, and poured into sterile Petri dishes. Plates with solidified medium can be stored at 4°C for up to 3 mo.
9. Spectrophotometer with visible wavelengths at optical density (OD) = 600 nm and OD = 420 nm.
10. 30°C Incubator and shaker.
11. Centrifuges and other standard laboratory equipment.

3. Methods

The method described below outlines the (1) strain creation, (2) yeast cell culture, (3) optimization of drug dose, (4) β-galactosidase assay, and (5) data analysis.

3.1. Creation of Yeast Reporter Strain WXY1111

The WXY1111 strain was created by integrating a P_{RNR3}-*lacZ* cassette into the host yeast genome. A fragment containing the 0.88-kb *RNR3* promoter and the full length of *lacZ* was isolated by digesting plasmid pZZ2 *(8)* with *Nsi*I and *Eco*RI. This fragment was then inserted into *Pst*I and *Eco*RI sites of pBluescript (Strategene, CA), resulting in the P_{RNR3}-*lacZ* fusion gene flanked by two *Bam*HI sites. After insertion of the fusion gene into plasmid M4366 at the *Bam*HI site *(9)*, the P_{RNR3}-*lacZ* cassette is placed adjacent to a *hisG-URA3-hisG* cassette, and both cassettes are flanked by 5' and 3' HO sequences with a *Not*I site on each side (**Fig. 2A**). The resulting plasmid was digested with *Not*I and transformed into yeast cells. Through homologous recombination between the *HO-hisG-URA3-hisG-*P_{RNR3}*-lacZ-HO* cassette and the yeast genome at the *HO* locus, the *hisG-URA3-hisG* and P_{RNR3}-*lacZ* dual cassettes were integrated into and replaced the host *HO* gene (**Fig. 2B**). A stable integrant strain was subsequently obtained by selecting *hisG-URA3* pop-outs derived from homologous recombination between the tandem *hisG* repeats (**Fig. 2C**) on a plate containing 5-fluoroorotic acid, in which only *ura*3 mutant cells are able to grow *(10)*.

3.2. Yeast Cell Culture and Storage

WXY1111 cells are grown at 30°C either in YPD liquid medium or on a YPD plate. For liquid culture, cells are inoculated and incubated overnight with shaking and subcultured the following morning into a fresh YPD medium with a 30-fold dilution.

For long-term storage, yeast cells are grown on a YPD plate for 2 d at 30°C. Cells are then removed from the plate with a sterile toothpick and inoculated into 1.0 mL of sterile 15% (v/v) glycerol. For yeast cells grown in a liquid culture, 0.7 mL of cells are added into 0.3 mL of 50% glycerol. The cells can then be stored at –70°C.

3.3. Optimization of Drug Dose

A preliminary experiment may be required to determine the appropriate dose range of the drug to be tested. In this case, the following protocol can be followed.

1. Dilute overnight cell culture into fresh YPD at a ratio of approx 1:30.
2. Incubate at 30°C with shaking for 2 h or until the titer reaches 1×10^7 cells/mL. Make 2-mL aliquots in test tubes.
3. Make a serial dilution of the drug to be tested and add into the cell culture at desired final concentrations. One tube contains untreated cells as a control.
4. Continue incubation for 4 h.
5. Transfer 1 mL of cells to a microcentrifuge tube.
6. Harvest cells by centrifugation at 13,000 rpm for 5 s, wash once with sterile-distilled water, and resuspend the pellet in 1 mL of sterile distilled water.
7. Make a serial cell dilution and spread 100 µL onto YPD plates.
8. Incubate the plates at 30°C for 3 d before recording colonies.

The cell survival rate is determined by comparing colony-forming units (cfu) of drug-treated and untreated cells. It is recommended that the dose range that yields between 10% and 90% survival be used for the *RNR3-lacZ* genotoxicity test.

3.4. β-Galactosidase (β-Gal) Activity Assay

This method is adapted from the β-gal assay as previously described ***(11)***.

1. Inoculate 1 mL of an overnight WXY111 cell culture to 30 mL of fresh YPD medium to a final cell density of approximately $OD_{600\ nm} = 0.1$ (the volume can be adapted according to the cell titer of the overnight culture).
2. Incubate cells at 30°C for 2 h or until the final cell titer reaches approx 1×10^7 cells/mL, equivalent to a cell density of $OD_{600\ nm} = 0.2–0.3$.
3. Dispense into a series of 3-mL cultures in sterile culture tubes.
4. Dissolve the drug to be tested in an appropriate solvent at the desired concentration and add into the above culture tubes to the predetermined final concentrations.

5. Return to incubation for another 4 h or as specified.
6. Take 1 mL of culture to determine the cell density at $OD_{600\ nm}$.
7. Collect the remaining 2 mL of culture by centrifugation at 13,000 rpm for 5 s and wash twice with distilled water to reduce the background color of the YPD medium.
8. Discard the supernatant and resuspend the cells in 1 mL of buffer Z.
9. Add 50 µL of 0.1% SDS and 50 µL of chloroform and vortex at top speed for 10 s to permeabilize cells.
10. Add 200 µL of 4 mg/mL ONPG to initiate the reaction and incubate for 20 min in a 30°C shaker.
11. Stop the reaction by adding 500 µL of 1 *M* Na_2CO_3 solution.
12. Centrifuge the tubes at 4300 rpm for 5 min and transfer the supernatant into a cuvet.
13. Measure the $OD_{420\ nm}$ value of the supernatant.
14. Determine the β-gal specific activity ($SA_{\beta\text{-gal}}$) using the following equation:

$$SA_{\beta\text{-gal}} = \frac{1000 \cdot OD_{420\ nm}}{\text{reaction time (min)} \cdot \text{culture volume (mL)} \cdot OD_{600\ nm}}.$$

The recommended reaction time is 20 min. Culture volume is the amount of the culture used in the assay. For the assay, 2 mL of culture or less may be used. The β-gal activity is expressed in Miller units ***(12)***.

3.5. Data Analysis

The induced expression of P_{RNR3}-*lacZ* is expressed as fold induction of β-gal activity, which is calculated as a ratio of β-gal activity of the cells with and without treatment in the same experiment. The results should be an average of at least three independent experiments to allow calculation of standard deviations. Typical standard deviation is within 10% as the assay is highly reproducible. A twofold induction is considered to be a significant and positive result. Hence, a test drug capable of inducing P_{RNR3}-*lacZ* expression by more than twofold is considered a candidate genotoxic agent. The P_{RNR3}-*lacZ* induction profiles after treatment with the genotoxic agent methyl methanesulfonate (MMS) and the nongenotoxic agent tetracycline are shown in **Fig. 3**.

4. Notes

1. The rationale of the *RNR3-lacZ* system is based on the induction of *RNR3* in response to DNA damage. Previous research has established that the expression of *RNR3* can only be induced when the yeast cells are facing DNA damage and replication blocks, that the maximum fold induction of *RNR3* is much higher than that of other yeast genes examined, and that it reaches maximum induction at a treatment dose lower than most other DNA damage-inducible genes ***(4)***. Thus, the *RNR3-lacZ* system can specifically respond to DNA damaging agents with high sensitivity. It has also been shown that this system can respond to a broad

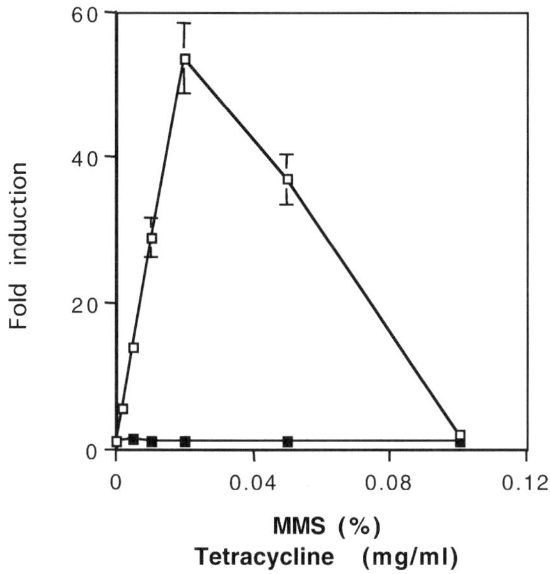

Fig. 3. The induction of the *RNR3-lacZ* reporter system by the DNA-methylating agent MMS (open squares) and the nongenotoxic agent tetracycline (solid squares). The fold induction is expressed as a ratio of β-gal-specific activity of the cells with and without treatment in the same experiment. The results are the average of three independent experiments with standard deviations.

spectrum of DNA damaging agents, including both mutagens and nonmutagenic genotoxic agents; however, it does not appear to respond to general stresses such as heat shock or cell killing by nongenotoxic agents *(4)*.

2. *RNR3-lacZ* expression responds to DNA damaging agents in a dose-dependent manner. However, after reaching maximum induction, the P_{RNR3}-*lacZ* expression often decreases with further dose increases (e.g., **Fig. 3**), probably because of excess cell killing. Hence, it is very important to predetermine an appropriate dose range for an unknown compound by assessing its cell-killing effect.
3. For each independent experiment, a control without drug treatment is necessary. If the chemical is dissolved in an organic solvent, a solvent control must be included. In this case, the fold induction is calculated as a ratio of β-gal activity of the cells with treatment and the β-gal activity of the solvent control in the same experiment.
4. The purpose of standardizing the initial subculture cell titer before drug treatment is to ensure that the cell titer at the time of β-gal assay is approx 2×10^7 cells/mL, or a cell density of $OD_{600\ nm}$ = 0.4–0.5. It has been established that DNA replication and active cell division are required for *RNR3* induction, whereas the P_{RNR3}-*lacZ* induction in stationary phase cells is severely compro-

mised *(4)*. Furthermore, cell titer appears to affect basal level β-gal activity, which in turn influences fold induction.

5. To reduce background noise for the β-gal assay, one needs to set an appropriate zero reference when measuring OD values. To measure the cell titer at $OD_{600\ nm}$, the YPD medium is used to set zero reference. To measure β-gal activity at $OD_{420\ nm}$, a parallel treatment of DBY747 cells without *RNR3-lacZ* integration is desired to set reference.
6. On certain occasions, one may wish to use special yeast strains for the *RNR3-lacZ* assay. This can be accommodated either by experimental integration of the *HO-*P_{RNR3}*-lacZ-HO* cassette into the host genome, as described with regard to the chromosomal manipulation of DBY747 *(4)*, or by simply introducing an autonomous replicating plasmid, pZZ12 *(8)*, carrying the P_{RNR3}*-lacZ* fusion gene. A standard yeast transformation protocol *(13)* can be followed. For genotoxic testing using a plasmid-based system, it is recommended to use a synthetic dextrose (SD, containing 0.67% yeast nitrogen base without amino acid and 2% glucose) minimal selective medium without uracil instead of YPD to maintain the autonomous replicating plasmid.

Acknowledgments

The authors wish to thank Dr. S. Elledge for providing the initial *RNR3-lacZ* construct and laboratory members of Wei Xiao for helpful discussion. This research was supported by the National Sciences and Engineering Research Council of Canada operating grant OPG0138338 to WX.

References

1. Quillardet, P., Huisman, O., D'Ari, R., and Hofnung, M. (1982) SOS Chromotest: a direct assay of an SOS function in *Escherichia coli* K12 to measure genotoxicity. *Proc. Natl. Acad. Sci. USA* **79,** 5971–5975.
2. Oda, Y., Nakamura, S., Oki, I., Kato, T., and Shinagawa, H. (1985) Evaluation of the new system (umu-test) for the detection of environmental mutagens and carcinogens. *Mutat. Res.* **147,** 219–229.
3. el Mzibri, M., De Meo, M. P., Laget, M., Guiraud, H., Seree, E., Barra, Y., et al. (1996) The salmonella sulA-test: a new in vitro system to detect genotoxins. *Mutat. Res.* **369,** 195–208.
4. Jia, X. M., Zhu, Y., and Xiao, W. (2002) A stable and sensitive genotoxic testing system based on DNA damage induced gene expression in *Saccharomyces cerevisiae. Mutat. Res.* **519,** 83–92.
5. Zhou, Z. and Elledge, S. J. (1993) *DUN1* encodes a protein kinase that controls the DNA damage response in yeast. *Cell* **75,** 1119–1127.
6. Huang, M., Zhou, Z., and Elledge, S. J. (1998) The DNA replication and damage checkpoint pathways induce transcription by inhibition of the Crt1 repressor. *Cell* **94,** 595–605.

7. Beck, C. F. (1979) A genetic approach to analysis of transposons. *Proc. Natl. Acad. Sci. USA* **76,** 2376–2380.
8. Zhou, Z. and Elledge, S. J. (1992) Isolation of *crt* mutants constitutive for transcription of the DNA damage inducible gene *RNR3* in *Saccharomyces cerevisiae*. *Genetics* **131,** 851–866.
9. Voth, W. P., Richards, J. D., Shaw, J. M., and Stillman, D. J. (2001) Yeast vectors for integration at the *HO* locus. *Nucleic Acids Res.* **29,** e59.
10. Boeke, J. D., Trueheart, J., Natsoulis, G., and Fink, G. R. (1987) 5-Fluoroorotic acid as a selective agent in yeast molecular genetics. *Methods Enzymol.* **154,** 164–175.
11. Xiao, W., Singh, K. K., Chen, B., and Samson, L. (1993) A common element involved in transcriptional regulation of two DNA alkylation repair genes (*MAG* and *MGT1*) of *Saccharomyces cerevisiae*. *Mol. Cell. Biol.* **13,** 7213–7221.
12. Guarente, L. (1983) Yeast promoters and *lacZ* fusions designed to study expression of cloned genes in yeast. *Methods Enzymol.* **101,** 181–191.
13. Mount, R. C., Jordan, B. E., and Hadfield, C. (1996) Transformation of lithium-treated yeast cells and the selection of auxotrophic and dominant markers, in *Methods in Molecular Biology: Vol. 53. Yeast Protocols* (Evans, I., ed.), Humana, Totowa, NJ, pp. 139–145.

21

Improvement of the Ames Test Using Human Liver S9 Preparation

Atsushi Hakura, Satoshi Suzuki, and Tetsuo Satoh

Summary

The use of the human S9 fraction in mutagenicity testing systems may be valuable for evaluating the mutagenicity of chemicals in humans. When using a crude human liver S9 fraction, which is obtained following the centrifugation of the tissue homogenate for 20 min at 9000*g*, in the Ames test, we may sometimes find contaminating bacterial colonies and/or an increasing number of His^+ revertant colonies of tester strains over the normal range on plates in a solvent control. To solve this problem, it is useful to use a purified fat- and bacteria-free human liver S9 fraction of high quality. Such a purified S9 fraction can be obtained by a simple modification to the crude S9 preparation: complete removal of fat after the centrifugation of the crude S9 fraction. This chapter states the experimental protocol for an improved Ames test using a modified human liver S9 preparation, especially highlighting our simple S9 preparation procedure for the Ames test.

Key Words: Ames test; mutagenicity; human S9; S9 preparation.

1. Introduction

The *Salmonella*/microsome bacterial mutagenicity test (Ames test) is used worldwide as a simple and rapid mutagenicity testing system for detecting mutagens and possible carcinogens *(1,2)*. Since the Ames test was originally established, some modifications have been developed. One of these includes the use of human S9 fraction in place of drug-metabolizing enzyme-induced rodent S9 fractions as a metabolic system. The reasons for this are that a large diversity in metabolism and mutagenicity of chemicals is known to exist between humans and rodents with or without treatment with phenobarbital/5,6-benzoflavone or Aroclor 1254 and, more important, that human S9 frac-

From: *Methods in Pharmacology and Toxicology*
Optimization in Drug Discovery: In Vitro Methods
Edited by: Z. Yan and G. W. Caldwell © Humana Press Inc., Totowa, NJ

tion more accurately reflects the former than the latter in the mode of metabolism. Until recently, the use of human liver S9 fraction in the mutagenicity tests has been limited ***(3–21)***, probably at least in part because of the difficulty in acquiring human liver samples. Because of the recent advances in acquiring human materials for research (commercially available) in addition to the value in evaluating the mutagenicity in humans, the use of human S9 fraction in the Ames test is starting to attract attention ***(22)***.

We recently found that a crude human liver S9 fraction, which was obtained following the centrifugation of the tissue homogenate for 20 min at 9000*g*, was not always sterile and was often accompanied with an increasing number of colonies over the normal range on plates in a solvent control in the Ames test, compromising the validity of the test results ***(20)***. In addition, a small amount of fat was sometimes incorporated in the crude human liver S9 preparation. We solved the issue using a purified fat- and bacteria-free S9 fraction, which is hereafter referred to as purified S9, in the Ames test. The purified S9 fraction can be obtained by a simple modification to the crude S9 preparation: complete removal of fat by the centrifugation of the crude S9 fraction. The experimental protocol for an improved Ames test using a modified human liver S9 preparation is described, especially highlighting our simple S9 preparation procedure for the Ames test (*see* **Note 1**).

2. Materials

1. 0.5 m*M* Histidine/0.5 m*M* biotin solution: *d*-biotin (122 mg) and L-histidine · HCl monohydrate (105 mg) are dissolved in purified water (1000 mL), and the solution is filtrated for sterilization. Stock solution stored in a refrigerator (4°C) can be used for at least 6 mo.
2. NaCl solution for the top agar: NaCl (5 g) is dissolved in purified water (900 mL). Stock solution stored in a refrigerator (4°C) can be used for at least 1 mo.
3. 0.1 *M* Sodium phosphate buffer, pH 7.4: solution II (3.6 g of NaH_2PO_4 in 300 mL of purified water) is gradually added to solution I (14.2 g of Na_2HPO_4 in 1000 mL of purified water) to adjust the pH to 7.4. The buffer is then distributed to bottles and autoclaved at 121°C for 15 min. Stock solution of the phosphate buffer stored in a refrigerator (4°C) can be used for at least 1 yr.
4. 0.05 m*M* Histidine/0.05 m*M* biotin-top agar: 0.5 m*M* histidine/0.5 m*M* biotin solution (20 mL) and Bacto Agar (Difco, 1.2 g) are added to the NaCl solution for the top agar (180 mL). The mixture is autoclaved at 121°C for 15 min prior to use, and then molten top agar is mixed and maintained at 45°C.
5. Nutrient broth liquid medium (NB): Oxoid Nutrient Broth No. 2 (2.5 g) is dissolved in purified water (100 mL) and autoclaved at 121°C for 15 min. NB stored at room temperature in the dark can be used for at least 1 mo.
6. Minimal-glucose agar medium (plate): the medium is commercially available, and we use CLIMEDIA AM-N (Oriental Yeast Co., Ltd., Tokyo). For prepara-

tion, solution A (minimal medium: 0.2 g of Mg $SO_4 \cdot 7H_2O$, 2 g of citrate · H_2O, 10 g of K_2HPO_4, 1.92 g of $(NH_4)_2HPO_4$, and 0.66 g of NaOH in 200 mL of purified water), solution B (20% glucose solution: 20 g of glucose in 100 mL of purified water), and solution C (agar solution: 15 g of agar in 700 mL of purified water) are separately prepared and mixed. The medium is distributed to plastic plates (diameter: 86 mm) at a volume of 30 mL. The plates are stored in sealed plastic bags at room temperature and can be used for at least 6 mo.

7. S9 mix: cofactors are commercially available, and we use cofactor I (Oriental Yeast Co., Ltd., Tokyo). One vial (for 10 mL of S9 mix) of cofactor I contains 8 μmol of $MgCl_2 \cdot 6H_2O$, 33 μmol of KCl, 5 μmol of glucose-6-phosphate, 4 μmol of nicotinamide adenine dinucleotide phosphate (NADPH), 4 μmol of nicotinamide adenine dinucleotide (NADH), and 100 μmol of Na_2HPO_4/$NaH_2PO_4 \cdot 2H_2O$ per mL solution, and it can be used for at least 1 yr when stored in a refrigerator (4°C). The cofactor solution is prepared by adding 9 mL of purified water into a vial containing cofactors, followed by filtration through a 0.45-μm millipore filter (Millex-HV). The solution is combined with thawed S9 fraction (usually 1 mL of S9 fraction to prepare 10% S9 in the S9 mix), mixed, and immediately placed on ice to maintain S9 enzyme activity.
8. Homogenizing solution (0.25 *M* sucrose, 0.1 m*M* ethylenediaminetetraacetic acid [EDTA], and 3 m*M* Tris-HCl, pH 7.4): sucrose (85.58 g), EDTA (29.2 mg), and Tris (363.3 mg) are dissolved in purified water. After adjustment of the pH to 7.4 by adding hydrochloric acid, the volume of the solution is adjusted to 1000 mL. The solution is autoclaved at 121°C for 15 min and stored at room temperature. The solution can be used for at least 3 mo.
9. Benzo[*a*]pyrene (BP) is used as a positive control article and is obtained from Tokyo Kasei Kogyo Co., Ltd. (Tokyo, Japan). BP (10.8 mg) is dissolved in 2 mL of dimethylsulfoxide (DMSO) added to a 5-mL polypropylene tube (FALCON® 352063) and sequentially diluted to prepare 0.27 mg/mL. The solution is distributed to tubes at a small volume (0.5 mL), tightly capped, and frozen (–80°C) until use. The stock solution can be used for at least 1 yr.
10. 2-Amino-3-methylimidazo[4,5-*f*]quinoline (IQ) is used as a positive control article and is obtained from Wako Pure Chemical Industries, Ltd. (Osaka, Japan). IQ (10 mg) is dissolved in 2 mL of DMSO added to a 5-mL polypropylene tube (FALCON® 352063), and sequentially diluted to prepare 50 ng/mL. Aliquots of 0.5 mL are distributed to tubes, tightly capped, and frozen (–80°C) until use. The stock solution can be used for at least 1 yr.
11. Dimethylnitrosamine (DMN) is used as a positive control article and is obtained from Tokyo Kasei Kogyo Co., Ltd. (Tokyo, Japan). DMN (10 mg) is dissolved in 2 mL of DMSO added to a 5-mL polypropylene tube (FALCON® 352063) and sequentially diluted to prepare 0.5 mg/mL. Aliquots of 0.5 mL are distributed to tubes, tightly capped, and frozen (–80°C) until use. The stock solution can be used for at least 3 mo.
12. *Salmonella* tester strains: TA100 (*hisG46/rfa/ΔuvrB*/pKM101), TA98 (*hisD3052/rfa/ΔuvrB*/pKM101), and YG7108 (*hisG46/rfa/ΔuvrB/*$\Delta ada_{ST}/\Delta ogt_{ST}$). The

TA100 and TA98 strains *(1,2)*, which detect base-pair substitution mutations and frameshift mutations, respectively, were provided by Dr. B. N. Ames of the University of California, Berkeley. The YG7108 strain sensitive to alkylating agents *(23)* was supplied by Drs. T. Nohmi and M. Yamada of the National Institute of Health Sciences.

3. Methods

The methods described below outline (1) the experimental procedure for the mutagenicity test and (2) the preparation procedure for human liver S9 fraction (*see* **Note 2**).

3.1. Mutagenicity Test

The experimental procedure for the mutagenicity test is described in **Subheadings 3.1.1.–3.1.6.** This includes (1) the preparation of frozen working cultures, (2) the preparation of bacterial cell cultures, (3) the mutagenicity testing, (4) the check for the sterility of the S9 mix, (5) acceptance criteria of the test, and (6) evaluation criteria of the test. Our experimental procedure of the mutagenicity test is based on the Ames test with the modification of preincubation at 37°C for 20 min (the preincubation method) *(1,2)*.

3.1.1. Preparation of Frozen Working Cultures

Frozen working cultures should be prepared from frozen permanent cultures that have been selected after completion of the strain check in terms of phenotypic characterization, spontaneous mutation induction, and sensitivity to positive control articles.

1. DMSO (0.7 mL) from freshly opened bottles is placed in a test tube and combined and mixed with 8 mL of bacterial culture in the early stationary phase of the tester strain (over 1×10^9 cells/mL).
2. The cell suspension is dispensed in 200-µL aliquots to γ-irradiated Assist tubes (cat. no. 72.694S). After being tightly capped, the tubes are quickly frozen in liquid nitrogen and kept frozen until required (–80°C). Freshly frozen working cultures stored in a deep freeze can be used for at least 1 yr.

3.1.2. Preparation of Bacterial Cell Cultures

1. Frozen working culture is taken from the deep freezer and allowed to thaw at room temperature.
2. The working culture (20 µL) is transferred to a conical flask (100 mL) containing 20 mL of NB (*see* **Note 3**). The remainder of the working culture should be discarded.
3. The conical flask is placed at 4°C in a shaking incubator equipped with a timer (Bio-shaker BR-40LF, Taitec). The incubator is set up for the first 6 h at 4°C,

followed by shaking (140 rpm) of the flask for 10 h at 37°C to obtain cell culture in the early stationary phase of the tester strain (*see* **Note 4**).

4. Cell culture thus obtained is diluted 10-fold with NB, and the optical density of the diluted cell suspension is measured at 660 nm by a spectrophotometer. Cell numbers should be confirmed at 1×10^9 cells/mL or over with reference to the working curves of optical density vs cell number. Unless the cell number satisfies the above criterion, the cell culture cannot be used in the following procedure.
5. The cell culture is placed on ice (*see* **Note 5**).

3.1.3. Mutagenicity Testing

We usually use phenobarbital/5,6-benzoflavone-induced rat liver S9 and human liver S9 fractions at 10% S9 concentration in the S9 mix (1 mg of S9 protein per plate) to examine the mutagenic diversity between them. However, the use of different S9 concentrations, particularly at high concentrations such as 30% (3 mg of S9 protein per plate), may be of value because 75% of chemicals showed no mutagenicity or less mutagenicity in the presence of human liver S9 fraction than the phenobarbital/5,6-benzoflavone-induced rat liver S9 fraction among 48 chemicals judged to be positive (mutagenic) with either S9 fraction at 10% S9 concentration ***(22)***.

1. S9 mix (0.5 mL) or buffer (if needed) is added to each test tube (105 × 16.5 mm) using an Eppendorf dispenser.
2. Test article solution dissolved in DMSO (0.1 mL) is added to each test tube (*see* **Note 6**) and mixed by a touch mixer for 1 s.
3. Bacterial culture (0.1 mL) is then added to each test tube and mixed by a touch mixer for 1 s.
4. After molten caps are put on the test tubes, the tubes are incubated for 20 min at 37°C in a shaking (120 rpm) water bath (water bath shaker MM-10, Taitec).
5. After shaking, 2 mL of molten 0.05 m*M* histidine/0.05 m*M* biotin-top agar maintained at 45°C (Dry Thermo Unit, DTU-1C, Taitec) is added to each test tube and mixed by a touch mixer for 1 to 2 s. The contents are immediately poured onto the surface of minimal-glucose agar plates (two plates per each dose) (*see* **Note 7**).
6. Within about 10 min after the top agar has hardened (1–2 min), plates are inverted and placed in an incubator at 37°C for about 48 h.
7. The number of revertants that appear on each plate is counted (*see* **Note 8**).

3.1.4. Check for S9 Mix Sterility

1. S9 mix (0.5 mL) and 0.05 m*M* histidine/0.05 m*M* biotin-top agar (2 mL) are added to a test tube (105 × 16.5 mm) and mixed. The contents are immediately poured onto the surface of a minimal-glucose agar plate (one plate).
2. After the top agar has hardened, the plate is inverted and placed in an incubator at 37°C for about 48 h.
3. The number of colonies that appeared on the plate is checked for S9 mix sterility.

3.1.5. Acceptance Criteria of the Test

The test is considered valid if the following criteria are satisfied:

1. No bacterial contamination is observed on a plate for the sterility check.
2. The number of revertants for the negative control is similar to the historical or reference data.
3. The number of revertants for the positive control is similar to the historical or reference data.

3.1.6. Evaluation Criteria of the Test

The test article is considered to be mutagenic if the following criteria are satisfied:

1. There is a dose-related increase in the number of revertants.
2. The number of revertants at one or more treatment doses is twofold or more over the negative control.

3.2. Human Liver S9 Preparations

S9 fractions from human liver specimens (*see* **Note 9**) can be prepared from one donor liver of interest or from a mixture of an equal weight of 12 to 15 individual human livers (pooled human liver). All materials and supplies should be sterilized before use.

1. Frozen donor liver sample(s) of interest are taken from a deep freezer, excised by a knife at an arbitrary weight, and placed in preweighed beakers.
2. After the frozen livers are allowed to thaw, thick blood vessels are removed from the tissue, and the tissue is minced with scissors. For the preparation of the pooled liver S9 fraction, 12 to 15 individual livers are gathered together at an equal weight in a beaker.
3. Three times the weight (volume) of a cold homogenizing solution (0.25 *M* sucrose, 0.1 m*M* EDTA, and 3 m*M* Tris-HCl, pH 7.4) is added to the beakers containing the liver samples.
4. A liver sample is transferred to a Potter-Elvehjam apparatus with a polytron homogenizer and homogenized on ice.
5. The homogenate is transferred to a centrifuging tube and centrifuged for 20 min at 9000*g* at 4°C.
6. Fat (*see* **Note 10**) that appeared was carefully and completely removed (often as much as approx 2/5 vol of the supernatant after the centrifugation, depending on the fat content present in the liver used) using a spatula or aspirator (*see* **Note 11**).
7. The crude S9 fraction thus obtained is transferred to a new centrifuging tube and centrifuged for 20 min at 9000*g* at 4°C, and any remaining fat that appeared was scrupulously removed using an aspirator.
8. The purified S9 fraction thus obtained is transferred to a beaker on ice.
9. After adjustment of the protein concentration (20–21 mg/mL) with a cold homogenizing solution, the S9 fraction is dispensed to vials in 2-mL aliquots,

immediately frozen in liquid nitrogen, and stored at –80°C until use. At the same time, 0.05 mL of the S9 fraction is tested for sterility according to the procedure outlined in **Subheading 3.1.4.**, replacing the 0.5 mL of S9 mix with 0.05 mL of S9 fraction.

4. Notes

1. It is considered preferable for the Ames test to use an S9 fraction that has not been filtered through a membrane filter for sterilization because the possibility of losing some of the proteins concerned with metabolic activation/detoxication cannot be completely ignored, although there seems to be no practical difference in the *Salmonella* mutagenic activity of three mutagens (BP, IQ, and DMN) between S9 fractions obtained through a membrane filter and those prepared by the method in **Subheading 3.2.** (data not shown). However, in the event that the amount of human liver tissue that can be obtained is insufficient to prepare the S9 fraction according to the method in **Subheading 3.2.** (usually less than 1–2 g of tissue), bacterial contaminants may be removed by passage of the S9 mix through a 0.45-μm millipore filter for sterilization. Filtration of an S9 fraction before it is diluted into the S9 mix is difficult because it clogs the filter *(1)*.
2. Caution should be paid to biohazards. Human materials must be screened for specific kinds of known viruses that may cause serious diseases, such as hepatitis B, hepatitis C, and HIV, prior to S9 preparation, and the use of human samples suspected of being at risk should be avoided in the test. According to the Biosafety in Biomedical and Microbiological Laboratories (BMBL), human cells and tissues are recommended to be handled using Biosafety Level 2 practices and containment, and all work should be performed in a biosafety cabinet *(24)*. On the basis of this report, we recommend that any stages of the S9 preparation (particularly while homogenating tissue samples) with a risk of scattering should be conducted at Biosafety Level 2, and the Ames test using human S9 with a very low or low risk of scattering should be conducted as much as possible at Biosafety Level 2. Workers should protect themselves from hazards due to human materials, bacteria, and chemical exposure by wearing eyeglasses, disposable masks and gloves, and gowns. All experimental supplies polluted with human materials or bacteria should be autoclaved or discarded in biohazard bags for destruction by fire. Supplies or equipment that are not autoclavable should be decontaminated by using something such as cotton sheets dipped in 70% ethanol. Ethical considerations must also be taken into account when using human materials.
3. For preparation of the cell culture of TA100 and TA98, which carry the pKM101 plasmid, ampicillin might be added to NB to prevent its possible loss. However, its addition is not usually necessary because it seldom affects the test results (data not shown).
4. Because the experimental conditions (e.g., aeration and incubation period) of this stage for the preparation of the cell culture are known to affect the test results frequently and to a large extent, it is important to determine the best conditions matched to the equipment and supplies used in each laboratory in advance. Aerobic conditions are recommended, and over-long incubation should be avoided.

Table 1
Mutagenicity Data[a]

Chemical	Dose (μg/plate)	Bacterial strain	Revertants per plate[b]	
			Induced rat S9[c]	Human S9[d]
BP	0 (DMSO)	TA100	109	158
	27		874	280
IQ	0 (DMSO)	TA98	40	42
	0.005		1678	242
DMN	0 (DMSO)	YG7108	37	82
	50		435	3231

[a]The mutagenicity of positive compounds was determined by the Ames test with a modification of preincubation at 37°C for 20 min in the presence of S9 mix containing 1 mg S9 protein per plate.

[b]Mean of duplicate plates.

[c]Phenobarbital/5,6-benzoflavone-induced rat liver S9 fraction, which was purchased from Oriental Yeast Co., Ltd, Tokyo.

[d]Pooled human liver S9 fraction prepared from a mixture of an equal weight of 15 individual human livers at the HAB Biomedical Research Institute (Chiba, Japan) using frozen tissue.

Abbr: DMSO, dimethylsulfoxide; BP, benzo[*a*]pyrene; IQ, 2-amino-3-methylimidazo[4,5-*f*]quinoline; DMN, dimethylnitrosamine.

5. The flask containing the culture may be protected from direct fluorescent light by wrapping it in aluminum foil. This precautionary procedure is not required if the laboratories are equipped with yellow or red overhead lights *(2)*. We always use the cell culture on ice within 3 h after the end of the cultivation.
6. If test compounds are soluble in water, water will be used as the solvent. We usually use DMSO as the first choice of solvent because of its good ability to dissolve many kinds of organic compounds.
7. If the Ames test is performed by one person, then S9 mix (or phosphate buffer), chemical solutions, and bacterial culture will be added to each test tube set up in test tube stands and immersed in iced water to the flush level with the surface of the mixture in each test tube (**steps 1–3**). After incubation for 20 min (the preincubation procedure, **step 4**), the stands complete with the tubes will once again be dipped in iced water to stop the enzymatic reaction. After the water has been blotted off from the outside of the tubes with absorbent paper (e.g., Kimtowel, Kimberly-Clark Co.) or decontaminated with cotton sheets dipped in 70% ethanol, one by one, top agar will be added to each test tube and mixed, and the contents are immediately poured onto the surface of miminal-glucose agar medium (**step 5**). On the other hand, if the Ames test is performed by 2 to 4 persons, then the iced water will not be necessary to stop the reaction because of assembly line style of procedure.
8. Our data are shown in **Table 1** (mutagenicity results) and **Table 2** (analytical results of S9) for reference.

Table 2
Contents and Enzyme Activities of P450s in Human (21 mg protein/mL) and Induced Rat Liver (23 mg protein/mL) S9 Fractions Used in the Ames Test

		Enzyme activity[a] (pmol/min/mg protein)		
S9 Fraction	Total P450 content[b] (pmol/mg protein)	Ethoxyresorufin *o*-deethylation[c]	Chlorzoxazone 6-hydroxylation[d]	Testosterone 6β-hydroxylation[e]
Human S9	44	90	487	824
	(1.0)[f]	(1.0)	(1.0)	(1.0)
Induced rat S9	715	4670	1295	2733
	(16)	(52)	(2.7)	(3.3)

[a]Determined according to the method of Ikeda et al. ***(30)*** using high-performance liquid chromatography (HPLC) procedures.
[b]Measured by the method of Omura and Sato ***(29)***.
[c]Each value represents a specific activity for CYP1A1/2.
[d]Each value represents a specific activity for CYP2E1.
[e]Each value represents a specific activity for CYP3A.
[f]Figures in parentheses indicate the ratio relative to human S9.

9. Human liver samples used for the preparation of S9 at the Biomedical Research Institute (Chiba, Japan) were obtained from nontransplantable liver donors that, because of certain medical reason(s) such as immunological incongruence, could not be used. Liver samples were legally procured from the NDRI (National Disease Research Interchange) in Philadelphia, with permission for their use for research purposes only, based on the international partnership between the NDRI and the Human and Animal Bridge Research Organization (HAB) in Japan.
10. In general, human liver samples (particularly lipid) contain a large amount of fat, depending on the age, lifestyles, and dietary styles of organ donors. This is in contrast to the small amount of fat present in the livers of young experimental rats, which are kept in strictly controlled housing conditions and have often undergone fasting to reduce liver fat before sacrifice. Hence, crude human S9 fractions prepared according to conventional procedures ***(1)*** may have the potential risk of foreign bacterial contamination, leading to an increase in the number of colonies on negative (solvent) control plates. This is possibly attributable to the trapping of foreign bacteria by a large amount of fat through the S9 preparation process, starting with tissue removal from donors. Possible endogenous or exogenous mutagens present in human liver samples (particularly lipid) might also increase the number of colonies ***(25–28)***. Because a much higher increase in the number of colonies with a tester strain of YG7108 ***(23)*** was more frequently observed as compared with tester strains of TA100 and TA98, some alkylating mutagens, particularly methylating mutagens, might exist in human liver tissue (data not shown).
11. Fat layers may be carefully removed with a spatula at first, and then the floating fat that remains can be assiduously aspirated.

Acknowledgments

We are grateful to Dr. B. N. Ames of University of California, Berkeley, for his gift of the *Salmonella* tester strains TA100 and TA98. We also thank Drs. T. Nohmi and M. Yamada for their gift of the *Salmonella* tester strain YG7108.

References

1. Maron, D. M. and Ames, B. N. (1983) Revised methods for the *Salmonella* mutagenicity test. *Mutat. Res.* **113,** 173–215.
2. Mortelmans, K. and Zeiger, E. (2000) The Ames *Salmonella*/microsome mutagenicity test. *Mutat. Res.* **455,** 29–60.
3. Ames, B. N., Durston, W. E., Yamasaki, E., and Lee, F. D. (1973) Carcinogens are mutagens: a simple test system combining liver homogenates for activation and bacteria for detection. *Proc. Natl. Acad. Sci. USA* **70,** 2281–2285.
4. Tang, T. and Friedman, M. A. (1977) Carcinogen activation by human liver enzymes in the Ames mutagenicity test. *Mutat. Res.* **46,** 387–394.
5. Dybing, E., Bahr, C. V., Aune, T., Glaumann, H., Levitt, D. S., and Thorgeirsson, S. S. (1979) In vitro metabolism and activation of carcinogenic aromatic amines by subcellular fractions of human liver. *Cancer Res.* **39,** 4206–4211.

6. Bartsch, H., Malaveille, C., Barbin, A., and Planche, G. (1979) Mutagenic and alkylating metabolites of halo-ethylenes, chlorobutadienes and dichlorobutenes produced by rodent or human liver tissues: evidence for oxirane formation by P450-linked microsomal mono-oxygenases. *Arch. Toxicol.* **41,** 249–277.
7. Sabadie, N., Malaveille, C., Camus, A.-M., and Bartsch, H. (1980) Comparison of the hydroxylation of benzo(a)pyrene with the metabolism of vinyl chloride, *N*-nitrosomorpholine, and *N*-nitroso-*N*'-meth1ylpiperazine to mutagens by human and rat liver microsomal fractions. *Cancer Res.* **40,** 119–126.
8. Phillipson, C. E. and Ioannides, C. (1983) Activation of aromatic amines to mutagens by various animal species including man. *Mutat. Res.* **124,** 325–336.
9. Phillipson, C. E. and Ioannides, C. (1984) A comparative study of the bioactivation of nitrosamines to mutagens by various animal species including man. *Carcinogenesis* **5,** 1091–1094.
10. Beaune, P., Lemestré-Cornet, R., Kremers, P., Albert, A., and Gielen, J. (1985) The *Salmonella*/mammalian microsome mutagenicity test: comparison of human and rat livers as activating systems. *Mutat. Res.* **156,** 139–146.
11. Le, J., Jung, R., and Kramer, M. (1985) Dedicated to Prof. Med. Helmut Kewitz in honor of his 65th birthday: effects of using liver fractions from different mammals, including man, on results of mutagenicity assays in *Salmonella typhimurium. FdÅ@Chem. Toxic.* **23,** 695–700.
12. Neis, J. M., Yap, S. H., van Gemert, P. J. L., Roelofs, H. M. J., Bos, R. P., and Henderson, P. T. (1986) Activation of mutagens by hepatocytes and liver 9000 × *g* supernatant from human origin in the *Salmonella typhimurium* mutagenicity assay: comparison with rat liver preparations. *Mutat. Res.* **164,** 41–51.
13. Raineri, R., Andrews, A. W., and Poiley, J. A. (1986) Effect of donor age on the levels of activity of rat, hamster and human liver S9 preparations in the *Salmonella* mutagenicity assay. *J. Appl. Toxicol.* **6,** 101–108.
14. Yamazaki, H., Mori, Y., Toyoshi, K., Nagai, H., Koda, A., and Konishi, Y. (1986) A comparative study of the mutagenic activation of N-nitrosopropylamines by various animal species and man: evidence for a cytochrome P-450 dependent reaction. *Jpn. J. Cancer Res. (Gann)* **77,** 107–117.
15. Jongeneelen, F. J., Akker, W. v. d., Bos, R. P., Anzion, R. B. M., Theuws, J. L. G., Roelofs, H. M. J., et al. (1988) 1-Hydroxypyrene as an indicator of the mutagenicity of coal tar after activation with human liver preparations. *Mutat. Res.* **204,** 195–201.
16. Smith, A. J. and Chipman, J. K. (1988) Inter-individual variation in the mutagenic activation of 2-acetylaminofluorene by human liver in relation to animal metabolic models. *Mutagenesis* **3,** 323 328.
17. Phillipson, C. E. and Ioannides, C. (1989) Metabolic activation of polycyclic aromatic hydrocarbons to mutagens in the Ames test by various animal species including man. *Mutat. Res.* **211,** 147–151.
18. Johnson, T. E., Umbenhauer, D. R., and Galloway, S. M. (1996) Human liver S-9 metabolic activation: proficiency in cytogenetic assays and comparison with phenobarbital/β-naphthoflavone or aroclor 1254 induced rat S-9. *Environ. Mol. Mutagen.* **28,** 51–59.

19. Hakura, A., Suzuki, S., and Satoh, T. (1999) Advantage of the use of human liver S9 in the Ames test. *Mutat. Res.* **438,** 29–36.
20. Hakura, A., Suzuki, S., Sawada, S., Motooka, S., and Satoh, T. (2002) An improvement of the Ames test using a modified human liver S9 preparation. *J. Pharmacol. Toxicol. Methods.* **46,** 169–172.
21. Hakura, A., Suzuki, S., Sawada, S., Sugihara, T., Hori, Y., Uchida, K., et al. (2003) Use of human liver S9 in the Ames test: assay of 3 procarcinogens using human S9 derived from multiple donors. *Regul. Toxicol. Pharmacol.* **37,** 20–27.
22. Hakura, A., Shimada, H., Nakajima, M., Sui, H., Kitamoto, S., Suzuki, S., et al. (2001) The *Salmonella*/human S9 mutagenicity test: assay of 58 chemicals (collaborative study by JEMS/BMS). *Mutat. Res.* **483,** Suppl. 1, S151.
23. Yamada, M., Matsui, K., Sofuni, T., and Nohmi, T. (1997) New tester strains of *Salmonella typhimurium* lacking O^6-methylguanine DNA methyltransferases and highly sensitive to mutagenic alkylating agents. *Mutat. Res.* **381,** 15–24.
24. http://bmbl.od.nih.gov/appendh.htm
25. Obana, H., Hori, S., Kashimoto, T., and Kunita, N. (1981) Polycyclic aromatic hydrocarbons in human fat and liver. *Bull. Environm. Contam. Toxicol.* **27,** 23–27.
26. Martin, F. L., Carmichael, P. L., Crofton-Sleigh, C., Venitt, S., Phillips, D. H., and Grover, P. L. (1996) Genotoxicity of human mammary lipid. *Cancer Res.* **56,** 5342–5346.
27. Thompson, P. A., DeMarini, D. M., Kadlubar, F. F., McClure, G. Y., Brooks, L. R., Green, B. L., et al. (2002) Evidence for the presence of mutagenic arylamines in human breast milk and DNA adducts in exfoliated breast ductal epithelial cells. *Environ. Mol. Mutagen.* **39,** 134–142.
28. Philips, D. H., Martin, F. L., Williams, J. A., Wheat, L. M. C., Nolan, L., Cole, K. J., et al. (2002) Mutagens in human breast lipid and milk: the search for environmental agents that initiate breast cancer. *Environ. Mol. Mutagen.* **39,** 143–149.
29. Omura, T. and Sato, R. (1964) The carbon monooxide-binding pigment of liver microsomes: I. Evidence for its hemoprotein nature. *J. Biol. Chem.* **239,** 2370–2378.
30. Ikeda, T., Nishimura, K., Taniguchi, T., Yoshimura, T., Hata, T., Kashiyama, E., et al. (2001) In vitro evaluation of drug interaction caused by enzyme inhibition—HAB protocol. *Xenobio. Metabol. Dispos.* **16,** 115–126.

22

Screening for Chemical Mutagens Using the Mouse Lymphoma Assay

Tao Chen and Martha M. Moore

Summary

The mouse lymphoma assay (MLA) using the thymidine kinase (*Tk1*) gene is widely used to detect the potential genotoxicity of a wide variety of chemical agents. The assay is recommended as a part of the core battery of genetic toxicology tests. Although the assay was developed more than 30 yr ago, there have been some technical modifications and also an evolution of the guidelines for the proper conduct and interpretation of data from the assay. In this chapter, the authors provide the details for the conduct of both the agar and microwell versions of the assay. They include their strategy for test chemical concentration selection and also provide a summary of the recommendations of an expert MLA Workgroup of the International Workshop for Genotoxicity Testing (IWGT). This group has been working over the past few years to discuss and reach consensus on a number of important aspects of the assay. Issues addressed include the appropriate measure for cytotoxicity, 24-h treatment, acceptance criteria for valid assays, and a new strategy for interpreting data.

Key Words: Mouse lymphoma assay; thymidine kinase; mutagens; genotoxicity test; loss of heterozygosity, point mutations; large-colony mutants; small-colony mutants.

1. Introduction

The mouse lymphoma assay (MLA) using the thymidine kinase (*Tk1*) gene detects a broad spectrum of genetic damage, including both point and chromosomal mutations *(1–9)*. This assay is the most widely used mammalian cell gene mutation assay for regulatory purposes and is included in the core battery of genotoxicity tests for the registration of pharmaceuticals, pesticides, and other regulatory decision making *(10–12)*. Current specific guidance for the

From: *Methods in Pharmacology and Toxicology*
Optimization in Drug Discovery: In Vitro Methods
Edited by: Z. Yan and G. W. Caldwell © Humana Press Inc., Totowa, NJ

conduct of the MLA can be found in the *Red Book* located on the Web site of US Food and Drug Administration, Center for Food Safety and Applied Nutrition ***(13)***.

The MLA is conducted using the L5178Y/$Tk^{+/-}$-3.7.2C mouse lymphoma cell line, and it detects mutations that inactivate the gene product of the wild-type *Tk* allele (*Tk*1b) located on mouse chromosome 11. In this assay, *Tk*-deficient ($Tk^{-/-}$ or $Tk^{0/-}$) mutants are selected with the pyrimidine analog trifluorothymindine (TFT) because TFT inhibits division of normal cells ($Tk^{+/+}$ or $Tk^{+/-}$) but not the mutant cells. Because the mutant cells have a non-functional pyrimidine salvage pathway, they can grow in the TFT selective growth medium and develop into colonies.

A striking feature of *Tk* mutant colonies recovered in the MLA is the bimodal frequency distribution of colony sizes, with the large colonies growing at a normal growth rate and the small colonies at a slower rate. The relative frequency of the two colony classes is mutagen dependent ***(2)***. Chemicals whose major mechanism of action is to break chromosomes (clastogens) primarily induce small-colony mutants, whereas chemicals whose major mechanism of action is to induce point mutations tend to induce primarily large-colony mutants ***(1,2)***. *Tk* mutants can be characterized using a combination of molecular and cytogenetic analysis to determine the types of mutations induced by specific mutagenic agents, thus revealing their mechanisms of action ***(6–8,14,15)***.

The MLA was originally developed by Don Clive and his coworkers more than 30 yr ago, and many protocol improvements have been made since then ***(16–32)***. There are currently two equally acceptable methodologies for conducting the MLA. The assay was originally developed using cloning of cells immobilized in soft agar to enumerate mutants ***(16,22)***. In 1983, Jane Cole and her coworkers published a method using liquid medium and 96-well microwell plates for mutant frequency determination ***(21)***.

In this chapter, we describe the procedure for performing this assay and also our strategy for obtaining and interpreting MLA data. We are including summaries of the international consensus that is being formulated by MLA experts as a part of the International Workshop for Genotoxicity Testing (IWGT) ***(29,30,33)***. For information concerning the molecular characterization and other aspects of the MLA, the readers are referred to the reference list.

2. Materials

1. BBL agar (Baltimore Biological Laboratories, Baltimore, MD).
2. Benzo(a)pyrene (BP) (Sigma, St. Louis, MO).
3. Cyclophosphamide (CP) (Sigma).
4. Dimethylsulfoxide (DMSO) (Sigma).
5. Glucose-6-phosphate (Sigma).

6. Glycine (Sigma).
7. Horse serum (Invitrogen, Carlsbad, CA).
8. Hypoxanthine (Sigma).
9. Fischer's medium for leukemic cells of mice with glutamine (Quality Biologicals, Inc., Gaithersburg, MD).
10. Methotrexate (Sigma).
11. Methymethanesulfonate (MMS) (Sigma).
12. Nicotinamide adenine dinucleotide phosphate (NADP) (Sigma).
13. 4-Nitroquinoline-1-oxide (NQO) (Sigma).
14. Penicillin-streptomycin (Invitrogen).
15. Pluronic F68 (Invitrogen).
16. Thymidine (Sigma).
17. TFT (Sigma).
18. S9 (In Vitro Technologies, Baltimore, MD).
19. Sodium pyruvate (Sigma).

3. Methods

3.1. Culture Media and Solutions

Fischer's medium for leukemic cells of mice supplemented with horse serum is used for this assay (*see* **Note 1**). Freshly thawed horse serum should be heat inactivated at 56°C for 30 min before using. All media should be properly filter sterilized.

Basic medium (F_{0P}). Basic medium consists of Fischer's medium supplemented with 200 µg/mL sodium pyruvate, 100 U/mL penicillin, and 100 µg/mL streptomycin, 0.05% (v/v) pluronic F68 (*see* **Note 2**).

Growth medium (F_{10P}). F_{10P} is made by adding 10% (v/v) heat-inactivated horse serum into F_{0P}. F_{0P} and F_{10P} are stored in a light-tight refrigerator at 4°C.

Cloning medium F_{20P} can be prepared either by adding 10% (v/v) heat-inactivated horse serum to F_{10P} or by adding 20% (v/v) serum to F_{0P}. Media and heat-inactivated horse serum should be warmed to room temperature before use. F_{20P} is used as the cloning medium for the microwell method. For the agar method, prewarmed F_{20P} is measured into an Erlenmeyer flask, and autoclaved agar (at 95°C) is added with thorough mixing. We use BBL agar ***(34)*** at a final concentration of 0.22%, and the soft agar cloning medium should be made immediately prior to use and kept at 37°C.

Freezing medium. Cells can be frozen for storage in liquid N_2 using F_{20P} containing 5% DMSO. Freezing medium can be made and stored at –20°C for later use. It should be thawed just prior to use.

THMG and THG stock media. A 100X THMG stock medium is made with F_{0P} containing 300 µg/mL thymidine, 500 µg/mL hypoxanthine, 10 µg/mL methotrexate, and 750 µg/mL glycine. A 100X THG stock medium contains the same components as the THMG stock medium but without methotrexate. These stock media can be made and stored at –20°C for future use.

TFT stock solution. In a foil-wrapped bottle, mix 10 mg TFT with 100 mL physiological saline. Sterilize by filter and dispense 15-mL aliquots into sterile tubes. Label and store the solution at –20°C for up to 3 mo.

3.2. Cells

The L5178Y/$Tk^{+/-}$-3.7.2C mouse lymphoma cell line is used for this assay. The available sources include Dr. Don Clive's stock (now stored in our laboratory at the National Center for Toxicological Research/FDA, Jefferson, AR), Dr. Jane Cole's stock in the UK (Medical Research Council, Cell Mutation Unit, University of Sussex, Falmer, Brighton, United Kingdom), and the Japanese stock (contact Dr. Masamitsu Honma, National Institute of Health Sciences, Division of Genetics & Mutagenesis, Tokyo, Japan).

3.3. Cell Maintenance

The cultures are periodically replenished from frozen stocks of cells whose origin is as close as possible to the original source. Working stocks should not be carried longer than 3 mo. F_{10P} is used for cell maintenance and growth. The cultures are grown in glass mutagenicity flasks or polypropylene tissue culture flasks that are gassed with 5% CO_2-in-air and placed on a shaker incubator at 37°C with constant mixing. Stationary cultures incubated at 37°C in a humidified incubator gassed with 5% CO_2-in-air are also acceptable. The cells should be maintained in log phase, with a doubling time of 9 to 10 h. Cell density is determined by using a hemacytometer or a Coulter counter, and the cultures are routinely diluted with fresh F_{10P} medium each day to 2×10^5 cells/mL. Each Friday, the cells are diluted to 7×10^3 cells/mL to give a well-grown culture (1.5×10^6 cells/mL) on the following Monday. Doubling times should be carefully monitored, and cultures showing doubling times in excess of 10 h should not be used. The cells are periodically checked for mycoplasma contamination. Cells with normal karyotype and population doubling times that are free of mycoplasma contamination can be cryopreserved as master stocks for future experiments.

3.4. Cleansing Cultures of Preexisting Tk Mutants

Within the week preceding each assay, the stock cultures of cells are treated with THMG and THG to cleanse the culture of spontaneous *Tk* mutants. The cleansing procedure is performed as follows: (1) add 0.5 mL of THMG stock to 50 mL of the stock culture at 2×10^5 cells/mL F_{10P}, (2) mix and gas the culture with 5% CO_2-in-air and then place it in an incubator at 37°C for 24 h,

(3) perform a cell count (the cell count should not be less than 1.0×10^6 cells/mL), (4) centrifuge the cells at 200*g* for 10 min and resuspend the cell pellet at a concentration of 2×10^5 cells/mL in THG medium (F_{10P} medium containing 1% THG stock), and (5) gas the culture with 5% CO_2-in-air and place it in an incubator at 37°C for 2 d. The cells can be expected to grow at longer doubling times during cleansing than they do normally. Normal growth should resume after the first 24 h in THG medium. The cells should not be exposed to test chemicals until they have completely recovered from cleansing. Excessive or prolonged growth inhibition during or after cleansing can be indicative of mycoplasma contamination. Although we have successfully carried a stock culture and cleansed it every week, one can also carry an uncleansed culture and then subject a portion of the stock culture to THMG cleansing prior to its use in a mutagenicity experiment. Cleansed cells may be grown and cryopreserved at a density of 5×10^6 cells/mL/tube in freezing medium. New cultures for assays may be started directly from the cryopreserved cleansed stocks.

3.5. S9 Mix

A chemical must be adequately tested in the presence and absence of metabolic activation before declaring it to be negative in the MLA. Aroclor-induced rat liver S9 is routinely used for this purpose. S9 is available from commercial sources or made according to the published methods ***(21,22)***. For use in an assay, the standard S9 mix for each culture contains 3 mL of cofactor mix (F_{0P} supplemented with NADP [8 mg/mL] and sodium isocitrate [15 mg/mL], neutralized to an orange-red color with 1 *N* NaOH and filter sterilized) and 1 mL of S9 (equivalent of 25 mg of protein per milliliter). It should be prepared just before use and kept on ice prior to use.

3.6. Test Compound Stock Solutions and Exposure Concentrations

Test chemicals should be dissolved to make a 100X stock in a suitable solvent such as saline, DMSO, or F_{0P}. Serial dilutions with the sterile solvent are made as required to produce appropriate concentrations of the stock solutions. Treatment is initiated by adding these stock solutions into treatment medium containing cells in suspension. When DMSO or other nonaqueous solvents are used, the final volume should not exceed 1%.

The exposure concentrations of a test chemical are selected to give toxicity spanning from approx 100% to 10%–20% relative total growth (RTG, *see* **Subheading 3.12.** for calculation). Different laboratories use various strategies to identify the appropriate concentrations to be used. Generally, we use a strategy of performing the first assay using half-log concentrations (between 5000 and 0.1 µg/mL) of the chemical. If, based on the toxicity during the expression period, it appears that several of these concentrations are appropriate for the assay, we will continue with the experiment and evaluate the mutant frequency of those cultures. Generally, a second (and perhaps more) experiment is required to fine-tune the dose range and to obtain a sufficient number of cultures to adequately cover the dose range. It is important to have more than one data point that can be used to establish whether the chemical is positive or negative. For chemicals that induce high mutant frequencies, it may not be necessary to obtain doses covering the entire 100% to 10% RTG range. For chemicals that are negative or weakly positive, more concentrations are generally necessary. The current Organisation for Economic Co-operation and Department (OECD) and *Red Book* guidelines specify that at least four analyzable concentrations are required with duplicate test cultures and that eight analyzable concentrations are required for single cultures. At its meeting in New Orleans in 2000, the IWGT MLA Workgroup reached consensus on a number of details for concentration selection ***(30)***. Although we feel that the use of single cultures increases the probability that appropriate concentrations will be selected, the use of duplicate (or triplicate) cultures is acceptable. Duplicate (or triplicate) cultures should always be used for the negative/solvent control. For chemicals deemed to be noncytotoxic or weakly cytotoxic, the maximum concentration is 5 mg/mL, 5 μL/mL, or 0.01 *M*, whichever is the lowest. Compounds that have limited solubility should be tested at a concentration up to or beyond their limit of solubility under culture conditions. Evidence of insolubility should be present at the highest dose level. Compounds that are not soluble in any acceptable solvent cannot be appropriately evaluated for their mutagenicity in the MLA.

3.7. Positive and Negative Controls

Positive and negative controls are included with each experiment. The positive control chemicals commonly used include MMS (10–20 μg/mL) (*see* **Note 3**) and NQO (0.05–0.1 μg/mL) in the absence of S9, as well as BP (2–3 μg/mL) and CP (3–5 μg/mL) for testing with S9. MMS and CP 100X stocks should be freshly prepared with physiological saline, whereas NQO and BP can be prepared with DMSO as 100-fold concentrated stock solutions and stored as frozen aliquots at –80°C in the dark ***(30)***. If a solvent other than saline or F_{0P} is used, the solvent control should receive a dose of the solvent equivalent to the highest amount used for a treated culture, but should not exceed a final volume of 1%.

3.8. Treatment of Cell Cultures

Assays can be performed with and without activation conditions, or individual assays can be conducted for the two metabolic conditions. **Table 1** provides an example of an experiment including both metabolic conditions.

Table 1

Sample Data for Demonstrating the Treatment Condition, Main Parameters, and Calculation of Cell Cytoxicity and Mutant Frequency in the Mouse Lymphoma Assay

Culture no.	Concentration (μg/mL)	S9	SG_1	SG_2	RSG (%)	PE_v	RPE_v (%)	RTG (%)	PE_M ($\times10^{-6}$)	MF ($\times10^{-6}$)	%SC
Sol. Con.-100	0	–	4.60	6.02	100	0.92	103	103	40	44	49
Sol. Con.-101	0	–	4.64	5.98	100	0.87	97	97	44	51	47
Dose 1-102	10	–	4.61	6.03	100	0.94	105	105	45	48	48
Dose 2-103	20	–	4.49	5.82	94	0.80	89	84	50	62	52
Dose 3-104	40	–	4.22	5.83	89	0.78	87	77	120	154	60
Dose 4-105	80	–	3.88	5.74	80	0.74	83	66	164	222	62
Dose 5-106	160	–	3.53	5.62	72	0.68	76	55	271	399	68
Dose 6-107	320	–	2.92	5.02	53	0.60	67	36	419	698	71
Dose 7-108	640	–	2.31	4.77	40	0.51	57	23	441	865	79
Dose 8-109	1280	–	1.82	3.89	26	0.46	51	13	412	896	81
Pos. Con. 1-150	20	–	2.24	4.11	33	0.47	53	18	636	1353	51
Sol. Con.-200	0	+	4.51	5.83	96	0.94	103	99	51	54	51
Sol. Con.-201	0	+	4.72	6.01	104	0.89	97	101	54	61	53
Dose 1-202	10	+	3.89	5.88	84	0.90	98	82	65	72	50
Dose 2-203	20	+	3.63	5.62	75	0.78	85	64	180	231	62
Dose 3-204	40	+	3.46	5.71	72	0.73	80	58	290	397	70
Dose 4-205	80	+	3.15	5.79	67	0.70	77	52	340	486	67
Dose 5-206	160	+	2.77	5.19	52	0.65	71	37	440	677	76
Dose 6-207	320	+	2.04	4.52	34	0.55	60	20	520	946	74
Dose 7-208	640	+	1.10	4.29	19	0.53	58	11	602	1136	85
Dose 8-209	1280	+	0.20	Discard culture							
Pos. Con. 2-250	10	+	1.81	4.86	32	0.45	49	16	550	1222	66

SG_1, suspension growth rate between d 0 and d 1 of the expression time; *SG_2*, suspension growth rate between d 1 and d 2 of the expression time; *RSG*, relative suspension growth; *PE_v*, plating efficiency for viability; *RPE_v*, relative plating efficiency for viability; *RTG*, relative total growth; *PE_M*, plating efficiency for mutants; *MF*, mutant frequency; *SC*, small colony.

Within a few days of cleansing with THMG, the logarithmically growing mouse lymphoma cells can be used for treatment. The serum level in the cultures used for treatment should be reduced to 5% (v/v) with F_{0P}. This can be done by centrifuging cells and resuspending them in fresh medium containing 5% serum. Generally, for the individual test cultures, we use 50-mL sterile disposable centrifuge tubes containing 6×10^6 cells in 6 mL of F_{5P} (half-conditioned F_{10P} and half-fresh F_{0P}). To each tube, we add either 4 mL of F_{0P} (for without metabolic activation) or 4 mL of S9 mix (for with metabolic activation). The test chemical is added to each tube with gentle mixing. After the addition of the test chemical, all cultures are gassed with 5% CO_2-in-air (or placed in a CO_2 incubator for stationary cultures) and incubated in a roller drum at 37°C for 4 h (*see* **Note 4**). After the incubation period, the cells are centrifuged at 200*g* for 10 min, and the supernatant is discarded. Each culture is then washed with F_{0P} twice by resuspension and centrifugation, and the cell pellet is resuspended in 20 mL of fresh F_{10P}.

The cultures are either gassed with 5% CO_2-in-air or placed in a 5% CO_2 incubator. Most laboratories that conduct the microwell version of the assay have followed the practice of adjusting the density of the cell cultures and plating a portion of the cells immediately after treatment to obtain the relative survival (RS). They have used RS as their measure of cytotoxicity for concentration selection. Following extensive debate, the IWGT MLA workgroup reached consensus that RTG should be used as the cytotoxicity measure and that those laboratories that adjust cell density following treatment must adjust their RTG to take into account the cytotoxicity that occurs during treatment (*see* **refs. *31*,*32*** for a complete discussion and the proper procedure to adjust the RTG).

3.9. Expression Time

Cultures are incubated as noted above for an expression period of 2 d. Cell densities are determined approx 24 h following treatment and adjusted to approx 2×10^5 cells/mL with fresh F_{10P}. On completion of the 2-d expression period, cell densities are determined. The cell densities from d 1 and d 2 are used for calculating the relative suspension growth (RSG) (*see* **Subheading 3.12.**). Cultures with cell densities less than 2×10^5/mL will not be considered for cloning.

3.10. Cloning

Centrifuge and dilute each culture with F_{20P} to 3×10^5 cells/mL for the soft agar version of the assay and to 2×10^5 cells/mL for the microwell version of the assay. Mix and incubate the cultures for at least 30 min to minimize trauma and adapt to the medium. The cells then are diluted to the appropriate densities to plate for TFT resistance or cell viability.

Cloning for mutant selection. For both methods, it is imperative that a single cell suspension be used for cloning. For the soft agar version of the assay, 3×10^6 cells from each sample are centrifuged and the cell pellet is resuspended in 100 mL soft agar cloning medium with 1 mg/mL TFT and mixed thoroughly. Prior to the addition of the TFT, a 0.5-mL sample is taken and placed into a flask containing 50 mL of soft agar cloning medium. After thorough mixing, a 2-mL sample is taken and placed into a flask containing 98 mL of cloning medium, thus giving the 600 cells needed for determining cloning efficiency in the absence of TFT (*see* below). The cells in 100 mL of TFT-containing cloning medium are distributed into three 100-mm tissue culture dishes. The plates are chilled at –20°C for 12 min to solidify the agar. Stack the plates in an incubator after chilling them. For the microwell version of the assay, the cells are agitated to form a single cell suspension, and the cell concentrations are adjusted to 1×10^4/mL F_{20P}. TFT (3 mg/mL) is added following sampling for the dilution required for the cloning efficiency plates (*see* below). Using a multichannel pipette, place 200 µL of each TFT containing suspension into each well of four flat-bottom 96-well plates.

Cloning for Plating Efficiency. For the soft agar version of the assay, 600 cells in 100 mL soft agar cloning medium are used for each sample (*see* above). Following a 15-min mix in the 37°C shaker incubator, this medium is distributed into three 100-mm tissue culture dishes, and the plates are chilled at –20°C for 12 min. For the microwell version of the assay, cultures are adjusted to 10^4 cells/mL with F_{20P} (*see* above). Samples from these are diluted to 8 cells/mL with two-step dilution. Using a multichannel pipet, dispense 200 µL of the culture from each sample into each well of two flat-bottom 96-well microwell plates.

3.11. Incubation, Colony Counting, and Sizing

The plates with seeded cells are incubated at 37°C in a humidified incubator gassed with 5% CO_2-in-air for 11 to 14 d. For the soft agar version of the assay, colony counting and sizing from selection and viability plates is performed using an automatic colony counter fitted with the capability to evaluate the size of the colonies. Mutant colonies approx < 0.6 mm in diameter are considered to be small-colony mutants, and those that are larger are considered large-colony mutants. For the microwell version of the assay, colonies are identified by low-power microscope or eye; small colonies are defined as less than a quarter of the diameter of the well, whereas large colonies are more than a quarter of the diameter of the well. The morphology is generally compact for small colonies and may be diffuse for large colonies.

3.12. Calculations

Mutant frequency. The mutant frequency (MF) is determined by the plating efficiencies of mutant colonies (PE_M) and adjusted with plating efficiencies of viable cells (PE_v) from the same culture. The calculation is

$$MF = PE_M/PE_v$$

Table 1 shows a set of sample data for calculations of MF and RTG. For culture 100 in **Table 1**, the PE_M and PE_v are 40×10^{-6} and 0.92, respectively. Therefore, this spontaneous mutant frequency is $PE_M/PE_v = 40 \times 10^{-6}/0.92 = 44 \times 10^{-6}$. For the positive control 1, culture 150, the MF is $636 \times 10^{-6}/0.47 = 1353 \times 10^{-6}$.

PE_M and PE_v are calculated by using the number of colonies and the total number of cells used for the cloning:

$$PE_M = C_M/T_M$$

$$PE_v = C_v/T_v$$

where C_M is the number of colonies on the selective plates, T_M is the total number of cells used for selection, C_v is the number of colonies on the viability plates, and T_v is the total number of cells used for viability.

In soft agar version of the assay, C_M and C_v are obtained by directly counting the clones. When 600 cells are plated for cloning efficiency and 3×10^6 cells are used for mutant selection,

$$PE_M = C_M/(3 \times 10^6) = (C_M/3) \times 10^{-6}$$

$$PE_v = C_v/600$$

For example, if we count 150 mutants from TFT selection plates and 480 colonies from nonselection plates,

$$PE_M = (150/3) \times 10^{-6} = 50 \times 10^{-6}$$

$$PE_v = 480/600 = 0.80$$

$$MF = PE_M/PE_v = (50 \times 10^{-6})/0.80 = 62.5 \times 10^{-6}$$

In the microwell version of the assay, however, C_M and C_v are determined as the product of the total number of microwells (TW) and the probable number of colonies per well (P) on microwell plates.

$$C_M = P_M \times TW_M$$

$$C_v = P_v \times TW_v$$

From the zero term of the Poisson distribution, the P is given by

$$P = -\ln(EW/TW)$$

where EW is empty wells and TW is total wells ***(35)***. Therefore,

$$PE_M = C_M / T_M = (P_M \times TW_M)/T_M$$

$$PE_v = C_v / T_v = (P_v \times TW_v)/T_v$$

With the knowledge that 768,000 cells are plated in four 96-well plates (2×10^3 cells/well) for mutant selection and 307 cells are plated in two 96-well plates (1.6 cells/well) for viability,

$$PE_M = (P_M \times 384)/768{,}000 = P_M/(2 \times 10^3)$$

$$PE_v = (P_v \times 192)/307 = P_v/1.6$$

If we find 284 empty wells from 384 total wells in the four TFT selection plates and 50 empty wells from 192 total wells in the two viability plates,

$$PE_M = -\ln(284/384)/(2 \times 10^3) = 150 \times 10^{-6}$$

$$PE_v = -\ln(50/192)/1.6 = 0.84$$

$$MF = (150 \times 10^{-6})/0.84 = 179 \times 10^{-6}$$

Relative Total Growth. RTG is the measure for cytotoxicity of the test chemical. It is calculated as

$$RTG = RSG \times RPE_v$$

where RSG is the relative suspension growth and RPE_v is the relative plating efficiency for viability.

$$RSG = [SG_{1(\text{test})} \times SG_{2(\text{test})}]/[SG_{1(\text{control})} \times SG_{2(\text{control})}]$$

$$RPE_v = PE_{v(\text{test})}/PE_{v(\text{control})}$$

SG_1 is the growth rate between d 0 and d 1 (cell concentration at d 1/cell concentration at d 0), and SG_2 is the growth rate between d 1 and d 2 (cell concentration at d 2/cell concentration at d 1).

Here is an example for calculating the RTG of culture 107 in **Table 1**. First, we determine the means of $SG_1 \times SG_2$ and PE_v from the duplicate solvent controls:

$$SG_{1(\text{control})} \times SG_{2(\text{control})} = (4.60 \times 6.02 + 4.64 \times 5.98)/2 = 27.7$$

$$PE_{v(\text{control})} = (0.92 + 0.87)/2 = 0.90$$

Then, we calculate the *RSG* and RPE_v of culture 107:

$$RSG = (2.92 \times 5.02)/27.7 = 0.53$$

$$RPE_v = 0.60/0.90 = 0.67$$

Finally, we get the *RTG* as

$$RTG = 0.53 \times 0.67 = 0.36 = 36\%$$

Percentage of small-colony mutants. Percentage of small colony mutants is simply calculated as follows:

$$\%SC = [(\text{small colony } MF)/(\text{total } MF)] \times 100$$

3.13. Data Interpretation

The IWGT MLA Workgroup met in Plymouth, England, in the summer of 2002. This meeting was devoted to discussing the criteria for defining an acceptable assay and for appropriately evaluating the MLA data ***(33)***. A summary of the newly defined criteria is presented below. The reader is encouraged to refer to the Plymouth meeting summary for an extensive discussion for the proper steps to evaluate and interpret MLA data and for a discussion of the current workgroup activities toward developing a new method for data analysis.

Assay acceptability. An assay is considered acceptable and valid only if the negative/solvent control meets the following criteria.

Soft agar method:

Mutant frequency: $35–140 \times 10^{-6}$
Cloning efficiency: 65–120%
Suspension growth: 8- to 32-fold

Microwell method:

Mutant frequency: $50–200 \times 10^{-6}$
Cloning efficiency: 65–120%
Suspension growth (corrected for cytotoxicity during treatment and during expression): 8- to 32-fold

The positive control must also adequately demonstrate that the assay was properly conducted and that small-colony mutants were optimally detected. The IWGT Workgroup plans to provide more specific guidance once it completes its current evaluations.

Criteria for positive response. For acceptable assays, the test chemical can be classified as positive or negative. Historically, the twofold rule has been generally used with the soft agar method for deciding whether an agent is positive or negative ***(22)***. More recently, the Environmental Protection Agency's Gene-Tox Committee devised a method based on a somewhat arbitrary increase in mutant frequency (the delta 100 method) ***(36)***. For the microwell version of the assay, the United Kingdom Environmental Mutagen Society (UKEMS) developed a statistical method that uses heterogeneity factors, and this method has been generally used in Europe ***(35)***. More recently, Omori et al. ***(37)*** published a statistical method for evaluation of the data from the microwell version of the assay.

The IWGT MLA Workgroup members agree that none of these previously used methods is entirely satisfactory, and they are currently discussing the development of a new approach that would require that the induced mutant frequency exceed a certain value (a global evaluation factor) and that the data demonstrate a concentration-related increase. The proposal is outlined in the meeting report from the Plymouth meeting, and the group plans to finalize its recommendations during the 2003 meeting in Aberdeen ***(33)***.

Criteria for negative results. A compound is negative if it does not meet the criteria for a positive response. Before a negative response can be concluded, however, the treatment concentrations must exhibit sufficient cytotoxicity (10% to 20% RTG).

4. Notes

1. RPMI 1640 medium is also used for the assay and may provide better growth conditions for the cells. However, proper heat inactivation of the horse serum is required with RPMI 1640 ***(19,38)***. In addition, a threefold higher concentration of TFT (3 µg/mL) is required when using RPMI 1640. It should be noted that every laboratory must verify the stringency of its mutant selection conditions by confirming that mutants retain their TFT resistance upon isolation and reculture ***(1,18)***.
2. Pluronic F68 is used to prevent mechanical disruption of cells during shaking, and it is not necessary for stationary cultures.
3. Although MMS is widely used as a positive control chemical, there are some reservations over its use because it is volatile and hydrolytic. In addition, some commercial supplies of MMS are not as mutagenic as others.
4. Although we have generally used a 4-h treatment period, others, particularly those conducting the microwell version of the assay, normally use 3 h. In addition, according to the International Conference on Harmonization (ICH) guidelines ***(11,12)***, a 24-h treatment trial must be conducted in the absence of the S9 mix ***(29)*** if a test chemical yields negative responses in the 3- or 4-h treatment assay with and without the S9 mix. For the 24-h treatment incubations, cultures of 50 mL at 2×10^5 cells/mL culture medium are treated in flasks with a series of diluted test chemicals for 24 h in a 37°C, 5% CO_2 humidified incubator. The cells are then centrifuged and washed twice. They are transferred to new flasks and adjusted to 50 mL at 2×10^5 cells/mL with fresh medium for growth through the 2-d expression period. For the 24-h treatment, the RSG and the RTG should include the cytotoxicity that occurs during the 24-h treatment.

References

1. Moore, M. M., Clive, D., Hozier, J. C., Howard, B. E., Batson, A. G., Turner, N. T., et al. (1985) Analysis of trifluorothymidine-resistant (TFTr) mutants of L5178Y/$TK^{+/-}$ mouse lymphoma cells. *Mutat. Res.* **151,** 161–174.
2. Moore, M. M., Clive, D., Howard, B. E., Batson, A. G., and Turner, N. T. (1985) In situ analysis of trifluorothymidine-resistant (TFTr) mutants of L5178Y/$TK^{+/-}$ mouse lymphoma cells. *Mutat. Res.* **151,** 147–159.
3. Hozier, J., Sawyer, J., Clive, D., and Moore, M. M. (1985) Chromosome 11 aberrations in small colony L5178Y $TK^{+/-}$ mutants early in their clonal history. *Mutat. Res.* **147,** 237–242.
4. Blazak, W. F., Stewart, B. E., Galperin, I., Allen, K. L., Rudd, C. J., Mitchell, A. D., et al. (1986) Chromosome analysis of trifluorothymidine-resistant L5178Y mouse lymphoma cell colonies. *Environ. Mutagen.* **8,** 229–240.
5. Applegate, M. L., Moore, M. M., Broder, C. B., Burrell, A., Juhn, G., Kasweck, K. L., et al. (1990) Molecular dissection of mutations at the heterozygous *thymidine kinase* locus in mouse lymphoma cells. *Proc. Natl. Acad. Sci. USA* **87,** 51–55.
6. Liechty, M. C., Scalzi, J. M., Sims, K. R., Crosby, H., Jr., Spencer, D. L., Davis, L. M., et al. (1998) Analysis of large and small colony L5178Y $tk^{+/-}$ mouse lymphoma mutants by loss of heterozygosity (LOH) and by whole chromosome 11 painting: detection of recombination. *Mutagenesis* **13,** 461–474.
7. Chen, T., Harrington-Brock, K., and Moore, M. M. (2002) Mutant frequency and mutational spectra in the *Tk* and *Hprt* genes of *N*-ethyl-*N*-nitrosourea-treated mouse lymphoma cells. *Environ. Mol. Mutagen.* **39,** 296–305.
8. Chen, T., Harrington-Brock, K., and Moore, M. M. (2002) Mutant frequencies and loss of heterozygosity induced by *N*-ethyl-*N*-nitrosourea (ENU) in the *thymidine kinase* (*TK*) gene of L5178Y/$Tk^{+/-}$-3.7.2C mouse. *Mutagenesis* **17,** 105–109.
9. Blazak, W. F., Los, F. J., Rudd, C. J., and Caspary, W. J. (1989) Chromosome analysis of small and large L5178Y mouse lymphoma cell colonies: comparison of trifluorothymidine-resistant and unselected cell colonies from mutagen-treated and control cultures. *Mutat. Res.* **224,** 197–208.
10. Dearfield, K. L., Auletta, A. E., Cimino, M. C., and Moore, M. M. (1991) Considerations in the U.S. Environmental Protection Agency's testing approach for mutagenicity. *Mutat. Res.* **258,** 259–283.
11. ICH (1995) *Topic S2A Genotoxicity: Guidance on Specific Aspects of Regulatory Genotoxicity Tests for Pharmaceuticals*, International Conference on Harmonisation of Technical Requirements for Registration of Pharmaceuticals for Human Use, Harmonised Tripartite Guideline CPMP/ICH/141/95. Approved September 1995. Available: http://www.ifpma.org/ich1.html.
12. Department of Health and Human Services (1997) *Genotoxicity: A Standard Battery for Genotoxicity Testing of Pharmaceuticals*, International Conference on Harmonization of Technical Requirements for Registration of Pharmaceuticals for Human Use, Food and Drug Administration, Rockville, MD.
13. US Food and Drug Administration (2001) *Red Book 2000, Toxicological Principles for the Safety of Food Ingredients: IV.C.1.c. Mouse Lymphoma Thymidine*

Kinase Gene Mutation Assay. Available: www.cfsan.fda.gov/~redbook/redivc1c.html

14. Liechty, M. C., Rauchfuss, H. S., Lugo, M. H., and Hozier, J. C. (1993) Sequence analysis of *tka*$^{(-)}$-1 and *tk*b$^{(+)}$-1 alleles in L5178Y *tk*$^{+/-}$ mouse-lymphoma cells and spontaneous *tk*$^{-/-}$ mutants. *Mutat. Res.* **286,** 299–307.
15. Liechty, M. C., Hassanpour, Z., Hozier, J. C., and Clive, D. (1994) Use of microsatellite DNA polymorphisms on mouse chromosome 11 for in vitro analysis of *thymidine kinase* gene mutations. *Mutagenesis* **9,** 423–427.
16. Clive, D., Flamm, W. G., Machesko, M. R., and Bernheim, N. J. (1972) A mutational assay system using the *thymidine kinase* locus in mouse lymphoma cells. *Mutat. Res.* **16,** 77–87.
17. Clive, D. (1973) Recent developments with the L5178Y *TK* heterozygote mutagen assay system. *Environ. Health Perspect.* **6,** 119–125.
18. Clive, D. and Spector, J. F. (1975) Laboratory procedure for assessing specific locus mutations at the *TK* locus in cultured L5178Y mouse lymphoma cells. *Mutat. Res.* **31,** 17–29.
19. Moore-Brown, M. M., Clive, D., Howard, B. E., Batson, A. G., and Johnson, K. O. (1981) The utilization of trifluorothymidine (TFT) to select for *thymidine kinase*-deficient (*TK*$^{-/-}$) mutants from L5178Y/*TK*$^{+/-}$ mouse lymphoma cells. *Mutat. Res.* **85,** 363–378.
20. Moore, M. M. and Clive, D. (1982) The quantitation of *TK*$^{-/-}$ and *HGPRT*$^{-}$ mutants of L5178Y/*TK*$^{+/-}$ mouse lymphoma cells at varying times post-treatment. *Environ. Mutagen.* **4,** 499–519.
21. Cole, J., Arlett, C. F., Green, M. H., Lowe, J., and Muriel, W. (1983) A comparison of the agar cloning and microtitration techniques for assaying cell survival and mutation frequency in L5178Y mouse lymphoma cells. *Mutat. Res.* **111,** 371–386.
22. Turner, N. T., Batson, A. G., and Clive, D. (1984) Procedures for the L5178/*Tk*$^{+/-}$-*Tk*$^{-/-}$ mouse lymphoma assay, in *Handbook of Mutagenecity Test Procedures* (Kilbey, B., Legator, M., and Ramel, C., eds.), Amsterdam, Elsevier, pp. 239–268.
23. Majeska, J. B. and Matheson, D. W. (1990) Development of an optimal S9 activation mixture for the L5178Y *TK*$^{+/-}$ mouse lymphoma mutation assay. *Environ. Mol. Mutagen.* **16,** 311–319.
24. Clive, D., Bolcsfoldi, G., Clements, J., Cole, J., Homna, M., Majeska, J., et al. (1995) Consensus agreement regarding protocol issues discussed during the mouse lymphoma workshop: Portland, Oregon, May 7, 1994. *Environ. Mol. Mutagen.* **25,** 165–168.
25. Garriott, M. L., Casciano, D. A., Schechtman, L. M., and Probst, G. S. (1995) International workshop on mouse lymphoma assay testing practices and data interpretations: Portland, Oregon, May 7, 1994. *Environ. Mol. Mutagen.* **25,** 162–164.
26. Sofuni, T., Honma, M., Hayashi, M., Shimada, H., Tanaka, N., Wakuri, S., et al. (1996) Detection of in vitro clastogens and spindle poisons by the mouse lymphoma assay using the microwell method: interim report of an international collaborative study. *Mutagenesis* **11,** 349–355.

27. Sofuni, T., Wilcox, P., Shimada, H., Clements, J., Honma, M., Clive, D., et al. (1997) Mouse lymphoma workshop: Victoria, British Columbia, Canada, March 27, 1996 protocol issues regarding the use of the microwell method of the mouse lymphoma assay. *Environ. Mol. Mutagen.* **29,** 434–438.
28. Honma, M., Hayashi, M., Shimada, H., Tanaka, N., Wakuri, S., Awogi, T., et al. (1999) Evaluation of the mouse lymphoma *tk* assay (microwell method) as an alternative to the in vitro chromosomal aberration test. *Mutagenesis* **14,** 5–22.
29. Honma, M., Zhang, L. Z., Sakamoto, H., Ozaki, M., Takeshita, K., Momose, M., et al. (1999) The need for long-term treatment in the mouse lymphoma assay. *Mutagenesis* **14,** 23–29.
30. Clements, J. (2000) The mouse lymphoma assay. *Mutat. Res.* **455,** 97–110.
31. Moore, M. M., Honma, M., Clements, J., Awogi, T., Bolcsfoldi, G., Cole, J., et al. (2000) Mouse lymphoma *thymidine kinase* locus gene mutation assay: International Workshop on Genotoxicity Test Procedures Workgroup Report. *Environ. Mol. Mutagen.* **35,** 185–190.
32. Moore, M. M., Honma, M., Clements, J., Harrington-Brock, K., Awogi, T., Bolcsfoldi, G., et al. (2002) Mouse lymphoma *thymidine kinase* gene mutation assay: follow-up International Workshop on Genotoxicity Test Procedures, New Orleans, Louisiana, April 2000. *Environ. Mol. Mutagen.* **40,** 292–299.
33. Moore, M. M., Honma, M., Clements, J., Bolcsfoldi, G., Cifone, M., Delongchamp, R., et al. (2003) Mouse lymphoma *thymidine kinase* gene mutation assay: International Workshop on Genotoxicity Tests Workgroup Report—Plymouth, UK 2002. *Mutat. Res.*; in press.
34. Meyer, M., Brock, K., Lawrence, K., Casto, B., and Moore, M. M. (1986) Evaluation of the effect of agar on the results obtained in the L5178Y mouse lymphoma assay. *Environ. Mutagen.* **8,** 727–740.
35. Furth, E. E., Thilly, W. G., Penman, B. W., Liber, H. L., and Rand, W. M. (1981) Quantitative assay for mutation in diploid human lymphoblasts using microtiter plates. *Anal. Biochem.* **110,** 1–8.
36. Mitchell, A. D., Auletta, A. E., Clive, D., Kirby, P. E., Moore, M. M., and Myhr, B. C. (1997) The L5178Y/$tk^{+/-}$ mouse lymphoma specific gene and chromosomal mutation assay a phase III report of the U.S. Environmental Protection Agency Gene-Tox Program. *Mutat. Res.* **394,** 177–303.
37. Omori, T., Honma, M., Hayashi, M., Honda, Y., and Yoshimura, I. (2002) A new statistical method for evaluation of L5178Y$tk^{(+/-)}$ mammalian cell mutation data using microwell method. *Mutat. Res.* **517,** 199–208.
38. Moore, M. M. and Howard, B. E. (1982) Quantitation of small colony trifluorothymidine-resistant mutants of L5178Y/$TK^{+/-}$ mouse lymphoma cells in RPMI-1640 medium. *Mutat. Res.* **104,** 287–294.

23

A High-Throughput Binding Assay for HERG

Keith Finlayson and John Sharkey

Summary

The human homologue of the *ether-a-go-go*-related-gene (HERG) has been implicated in the "iatrogenic" long QT syndrome, with several products withdrawn from the market because of their interaction with this K^+ channel. The resultant impact on the pharmaceutical industry has been profound, with the need to assess whether compounds interact with HERG now at a much earlier stage in the drug development process. Electrophysiological assays for HERG have been used to evaluate drug candidates. However, these are time-consuming and expensive, and so a simple assay, suitable for general laboratory use, would be beneficial. The authors have established a radioligand binding assay that utilizes [^{3}H]dofetilide and membranes prepared from HEK293 cells stably expressing HERG. In assays performed at 25°C, [^{3}H]dofetilide (10 n*M*) binding equilibrium was achieved by 30 min and was stable for at least 120 min. The affinity (K_d) of [^{3}H]dofetilide for HERG was 22.3 ± 2.53 n*M* ($n = 11$; $nH = 0.93 \pm 0.06$) with a binding site density (B_{max}) of 8.92 ± 0.94 pmol/mg protein. A range of class III antiarrhythmics was shown to inhibit [^{3}H]dofetilide binding to HERG-transfected membranes in a concentration-dependent manner. Moreover, non-cardiac compounds associated with QT prolongation, such as pimozide, terfenadine, and haloperidol, also inhibit [^{3}H]dofetilide binding. This assay may therefore provide a simple method at an early stage in drug development to detect compounds that interact with HERG, potentially preventing QT prolongation in man.

Key Words: HERG; long QT syndrome; potassium channels; [^{3}H]dofetilide; radioligand assay; drug evaluation; preclinical.

From: *Methods in Pharmacology and Toxicology*
Optimization in Drug Discovery: In Vitro Methods
Edited by: Z. Yan and G. W. Caldwell © Humana Press Inc., Totowa, NJ

1. Introduction

The publication in 1997 by the European Agency for Evaluation of Medicinal Products, highlighting the association between various medicinal products and potentially fatal cardiac arrhythmias *(1)*, propelled the K^+ channel HERG (the human homologue of the *Drosophila ether-a-go-go* related gene) *(2)* to its current position as one of the most high-profile safety issues in preclinical research *(3,4)*. The safety issues surrounding HERG have been emphasised in the recent publication of draft guidelines outlining what pharmacological studies are desirable for assessing the potential for delayed ventricular repolarization (QT interval prolongation) by human pharmaceuticals (ICH S7B; *see* **Note 1**). HERG encodes for an inwardly rectifying potassium channel (I_{Kr}), which is essential for normal cardiac function *(5,6)*. Mutations in this K^+ channel are thought to be responsible for chromosome seven-linked congenital long QT syndrome, a potentially life-threatening disorder (LQTS) *(7)*. LQTS is associated with a form of polymorphic ventricular tachycardia called Torsades de Pointes, which can spontaneously resolve or degenerate into ventricular fibrillation and sudden death *(3)*. It is now clear that an interaction with HERG underlies the "iatrogenic" long QT syndrome seen with various drug classes *(3,8)*, and so the need for a simple, cost-effective, high-throughput screen is apparent. Class III methanesulfonanilide antiarrhythmic drugs, epitomized by dofetilide, are known to interact with this channel in cardiac tissue and so provide a pharmacological means with which to investigate HERG. Membranes were prepared from a HEK293 cell line stably expressing HERG *(9)* and a radioligand binding assay established using [^{3}H]dofetilide *(10,11)*. The establishment of this assay will be described and the pharmacological characteristics of [^{3}H]dofetilide binding sites in HERG-transfected membranes presented.

2. Materials

1. Cell culture incubator with CO_2 (5%), temperature (37°C), and humidity control (99%) and appropriate class II cell culture facilities.
2. HEK293 cells; American Type Culture Collection (ATCC; CRL-1573).
3. Minimum essential medium, fetal bovine serum (10%), nonessential amino acids (1%), L-glutamine (2 m*M*), trypsin-ethylenediaminetetraacetic acid (EDTA) (0.25%), and plasticware (Sigma, Poole, UK).
4. HERG channel complementary deoxyribonucleic acid (cDNA) *(12,13)*. Search engine terms such as KCNH2 or unigene cluster Hs.188021 reveal that a number of HERG channel clones may be available for purchase from various commercial sources (http://www.openbiosystems.com; http://www.origene.com; http://www.stratagene.com; http://clones.invitrogen.com; http://www.hgmp.mrc.ac.uk/geneservice/reagents/tools/MGC_Finder.shtml). As an alternative, Professor C. T. January, in association with the University of Wisconsin, will consider all requests for the provision of the cell line described herein, circumventing **items 2–7**.

5. pcDNA3 or an equivalent expression vector (Invitrogen, Paisley, UK; now replaced by pcDNA3.1), restriction enzymes, deoxyribonucleic acid (DNA) ligase, and agarose gel equipment.
6. Appropriate competent *Escherichia coli* strains such as TOP10 or DH5α (Invitrogen, Paisley, UK), LB agar and medium, and antibiotics (Sigma, Poole, UK).
7. Plasmid preparation kits, Lipofectamine or a comparable transfection reagent, G418 (Invitrogen, Paisley, UK), and cloning cylinders (Sigma, Poole, UK).
8. Cell lysis buffer; 5 m*M* Tris-HCl (pH 7.4) stored at 4°C. Hanks's balanced salt solution (HBSS; Invitrogen, Paisley, UK).
9. Assay buffer: 10 m*M* HEPES, 130 m*M* NaCl, 5 m*M* KCl, 0.8 m*M* $MgCl_2$, 1 m*M* NaEGTA, and 10 m*M* glucose, adjusted to pH 7.4 with 5 *M* NaOH and stored at 4°C.
10. Tris-wash buffer: 25 m*M* Tris-HCl, 130 m*M* NaCl, 5.5 m*M* KCl, 0.8 m*M* $MgCl_2$, 5 m*M* glucose, and 50 μ*M* $CaCl_2$, adjusted to pH 7.4 with 5 *M* NaOH and stored at 4°C.
11. [^{3}H]Dofetilide ([^{3}H]UK-68,798; 78–80 Ci/mmol prepared by APB, Little Chalfont, UK) and dofetilide (UK-68,798; *N*-[4-(2-{2-[4-(methanesulphonamido)phenoxy]-*N*-methylethylamino}ethyl)phenyl]methanesulphonamide) were kindly provided by Pfizer Central Research (Sandwich, UK). Storage, handling, use, and disposal of radioactive compounds should only be performed by registered users and adhere strictly to the appropriate institutional guidelines. [^{3}H]dofetilide was supplied as an ethanol solution and stored at –20°C in the absence of moisture, light, and air. Working aliquots (5 μ*M*) were prepared by dilution in milli-Q H_2O and stored under liquid N_2 or at –20°C for up to 3 mo. Dofetilide is a class III antidysrhythmic agent with teratogenic potential and should be handled with extreme care. In powder form, it is stable at room temperature, with (10^{-2}*M*) stock solutions routinely dissolved in Me_2SO and stored at –20°C in brown glass vials. No loss in binding affinity for dofetilide has been observed over periods of up to 3 mo.
12. E-4031 was kindly provided by Eisai Pharmaceutical (Tsukuba, Japan). Clofilium tosylate, haloperidol, and terfenadine were purchased from SigmaRBI (Poole, UK), and pimozide was purchased from Tocris (Avonmouth, UK).
13. Sterlin RT-30 tubes, Whatman GF/C filters (VWR International, Lutterworth, UK), and polyethylenimine (Sigma, Poole, UK).
14. Brandel 24-well (Brandel, Gaithersburg, MD) or appropriate harvester.
15. Emulsifier safe scintillation fluid, 6 mL polyethylene scintillation vials, and a Canberra Packard TRI-CARB 2500TR or equivalent scintillation counter (Perkin-Elmer, Groningen, The Netherlands).

3. Methods

3.1. Cell Culture and Membrane Preparation

HEK293 cells stably expressing HERG (HERG-HEK293) were kindly provided by Professor C. T. January of the Department of Medicine, University of Wisconsin *(9)*. This cell line had been generated by transfecting HEK293 cells

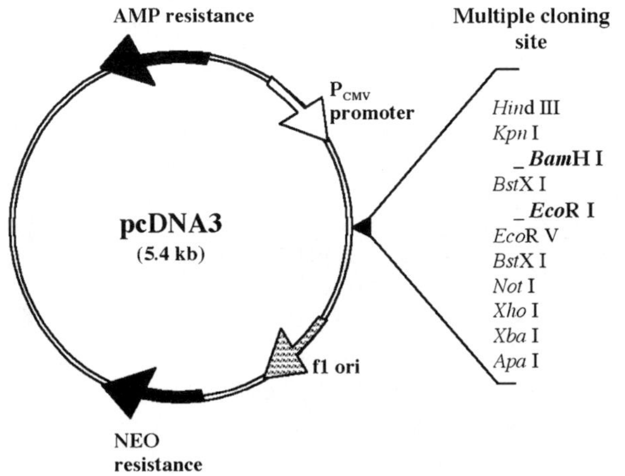

Fig. 1. Schematic representation of pcDNA3 expression vector modified from Invitrogen (Invitrogen, Paisley, UK; http://www.invitrogen.com/content/sfs/vectors/pcdna3.pdf). HERG cDNA was inserted at BamH1/EcoR1 sites, as described by Zhou et al. ***(9)***.

with a HERG cDNA subcloned into the BamH1/EcoR1 sites of pCDNA3 (**Fig. 1**), with individual colonies isolated and expanded by standard procedures. HERG-HEK293 cells were maintained in culture in supplemented minimal essential medium containing 400 µg/mL of G418 (passages 50–75; *see* **Note 2**). To prepare membranes from the stable cell line, flasks (175 cm²) of confluent cells were rinsed twice with 15 mL of prewarmed (37°C) HBSS, 15 mL of ice-cold 5 m*M* Tris-HCl, pH 7.4, was added, and the cells were dislodged by agitation/scraping. The suspension was decanted, homogenized using a glass/Teflon homogenizer, and then left on ice to lyse for a minimum of 120 min. Finally, the suspension was centrifuged at 50,000*g* for 20 min (4°C), resuspended in 1-mL/flask of assay buffer, rehomogenized, and stored at –20°C. On the day of use, membranes were thawed, homogenized, centrifuged as above, and resuspended in the appropriate volume of assay buffer. A 1-mL aliquot would routinely suffice for a 24-tube/well assay at 25°C, with no obvious reduction in specific binding being observed in more than 40 passages since use of the cell line was initiated (*see* **Note 3**).

3.2. [^{3}H]Dofetilide Binding Assay

[^{3}H]Dofetilide binding to HERG transfected membranes was assessed as described previously ***(10,11)***, with some modifications: HEPES assay buffer (10 µL; for total binding, use 30 µL) or test drug (20 µL) was incubated with 20 µL of [^{3}H]dofetilide (78–80 Ci/mmol, final concentration 10 n*M*) and 150 µL of membranes at 25°C for 60 min; protein content was determined subsequently, as described previously (***14***; *see* **Note 4**). Nonspecific binding was determined in the presence of 100 μ*M* E-4031. Stock solutions of compounds under investigation were prepared in either milli-Q H_2O (clofilium and E-4031) or Me_2SO (dofetilide, haloperidol, pimozide, and terfenadine; *see* **Note 5**), and drugs were serially diluted in the assay buffer, with the exception of pimozide, which was diluted in 10% Me_2SO. The final concentration of solvent did not exceed 0.1%, which had no effect on [^{3}H]dofetilide binding (data not shown; *see* **Note 6**). The binding assay was terminated by filtration onto glass filters (GF/C presoaked in 0.3% polyethylenimine) by use of a Brandel Cell Harvester, followed by three rapid washes (1 mL) with ice-cold Tris-HCl wash buffer (pH 7.4; *see* **Note 7**). Filter disks were transferred to scintillation vials and allowed to dry, scintillant was added (4 mL of Emulsifier Safe), and tubes were left overnight prior to radioactive determination in a Packard 2500TR liquid scintillation analyzer with automatic quench correction (*see* **Note 8**).

3.3. Data Analysis

For [^{3}H]dofetilide binding studies, data were analyzed using an iterative, nonlinear least squares curve-fitting program (SigmaPlot, Jandel; *see* **Note 9**) to a one-site logistic model: $Y = M \cdot IC_{50}{}^{P}/(I^P + IC_{50}{}^{P}) + B$, where P is the Hill coefficient and Y is bound ligand in the presence of an inhibitor concentration, I; M and B are specific binding in the absence of an inhibitor and nonspecific binding, respectively. Estimates of M and B were within 10% of experimentally determined values. If the inhibitor was the unlabeled form of dofetilide, the binding site affinity (K_d) and the binding site density (B_{max}) were calculated using the following equations: $K_d = IC_{50} - ([^3H]\text{dofetilide})$ and $B_{max} = (M \cdot IC_{50})/([^3H]\text{dofetilide})$. For other test compounds, K_i values were calculated using the following Cheng Prusoff approximation ***(15)***: $K_i = IC_{50}/(1 + [^3H]\text{dofetilide}/K_d)$.

3.4. Pharmacology of [^{3}H]Dofetilide-Binding Sites in HERG-Transfected Membranes

We have reported previously that the pharmacology of [^{3}H]dofetilide-binding sites could be characterized in a range of cell types, including whole HEK293 cells ***(10)***. However, when membranes prepared from these cells were used, very little specific [^{3}H]dofetilide binding was observed (**Fig. 2**; *see* **Note 2**). In contrast, membranes prepared from HEK293 cells overexpressing HERG exhibited specific, high-affinity, saturable [^{3}H]dofetilide binding (**Fig. 3**). Initial [^{3}H]dofetilide-binding studies using whole cells and membranes were conducted at 37°C to maintain cell integrity and for consistency with previous binding studies ***(10,11,16–23)***. However, to parallel most in vitro functional

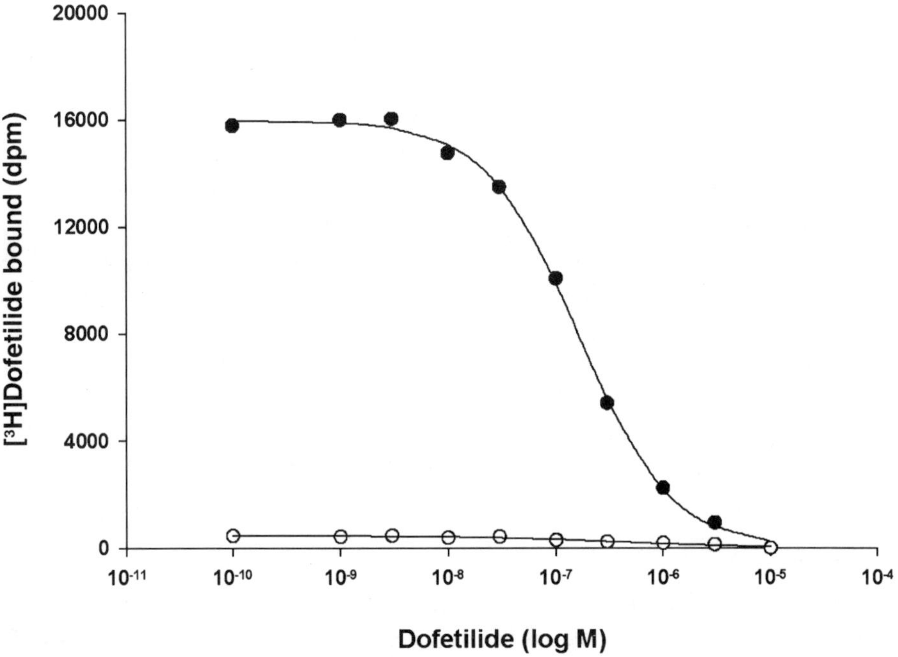

Fig. 2. Inhibition of [^{3}H]dofetilide binding to whole HEK293 cells (filled symbols) and to frozen HEK293 membranes (open symbols). Cells or membranes were incubated with [^{3}H]dofetilide (10 n*M*) in a 10-m*M* HEPES assay buffer containing increasing concentrations of unlabeled dofetilide. Binding was terminated after 60 min by rapid filtration using a Brandel Cell Harvester. Data shown are representative inhibition curves from an individual experiment.

studies on HERG and to make the assay more amenable for high-throughput screening, the assay was performed at 25°C. An initial time-course of [^{3}H]dofetilide (10 n*M*) binding to HERG-transfected membranes confirmed that at 25°C, equilibrium was attained between 30 and 45 min and was stable up to at least 2 h (**Fig. 4**). In contrast, when the incubation temperature was held at 4°C or 37°C, equilibrium was attained by approx 1 h or 10 min, respectively (data not shown; *see* **Note 10**). Therefore, subsequent studies were conducted at 25°C for 60 min (*see* **Note 11**). When inhibition studies were performed using increasing concentrations of unlabeled dofetilide, the affinity (K_d/K_i) of the compound was 22.3 ± 2.53 n*M* (**Fig. 5**; $n = 11$), with a binding-site density (B_{max}) of 8.92 ± 0.94 pmol/mg and a Hill slope near unity ($nH = 0.93 \pm 0.06$). No differences were observed in the affinity of dofetilide-binding sites between fresh and frozen membranes (*see* inset **Fig. 5**), although the level of specific binding was some fourfold lower when frozen membranes were

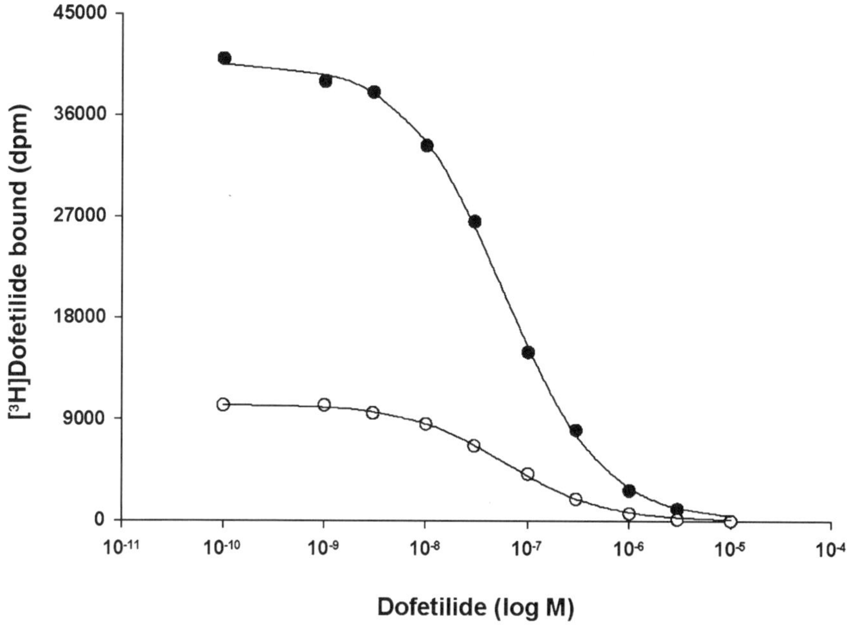

Fig. 3. Inhibition of [^{3}H]dofetilide binding to whole HEK293 cells, stably transfected with HERG (HERG-HEK293; filled symbols) and to frozen HERG-HEK293 membranes (open symbols). Cells or membranes were incubated with [^{3}H]dofetilide (10 n*M*) in a 10-m*M* HEPES assay buffer containing increasing concentrations of unlabeled dofetilide. Binding was terminated after 60 min by rapid filtration using a Brandel Cell Harvester. Data shown are representative inhibition curves from an individual experiment.

used. As a result of the limited availability of the radioligand, the concentration dependence of [^{3}H]dofetilide binding to HERG-transfected membranes was examined in one preliminary study. Although an asymptote was not reached, the K_d value of [^{3}H]dofetilide was approx 27.1 n*M* (**Fig. 6**), consistent with that seen in the inhibition studies above and similar to previously published data for dofetilide (*see* **Note 12**).

In addition to dofetilide, other class III antiarrhythmic drugs such as E-4031 and clofilium inhibited [^{3}H]dofetilide binding in a concentration-dependent manner. Furthermore, changes in assay temperature had no significant affect on the affinity of these agents for the [^{3}H]dofetilide-labeled HERG site (**Fig. 7**; *see* **Note 13**). Similarly, the antipsychotic drugs pimozide and haloperidol, as well as the antihistamine terfenadine—all of which cause QT prolongation in man—inhibited [^{3}H]dofetilide binding to HERG-transfected membranes (**Fig. 8**; *see* **Note 14**).

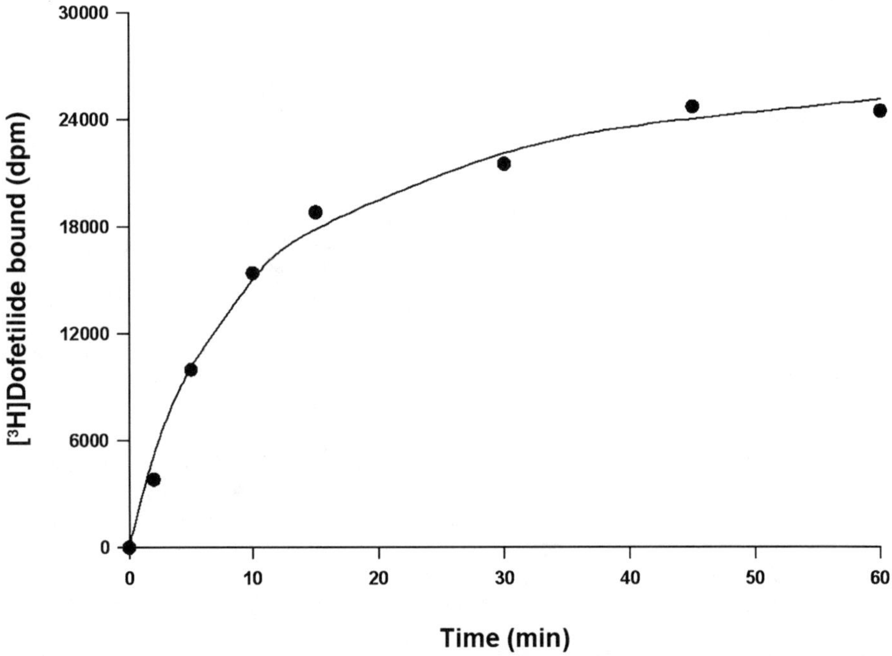

Fig. 4. Time-course of [^{3}H]dofetilide binding to frozen HERG-HEK293 membranes. Membranes were incubated with [^{3}H]dofetilide (10 n*M*) in a 10-m*M* HEPES assay buffer from 2 to 60 min at 25°C, with nonspecific binding determined by addition of E-4031 (100 μ*M*). Binding was terminated by rapid filtration using a Brandel Cell Harvester, with the data shown being a representative time-course from an individual experiment.

4. Notes

1. The International Conference on Harmonisation (www.ich.org) brings together international regulatory authorities to discuss scientific and technical aspects of product registration. ICH S7A and S7B discuss HERG and QT prolongation, with further coordination between preclinical (S7B) and clinical (E14) guidelines recently recommended (Chiba, February 2003).
2. As HEK293 cells contain endogenous voltage-gated K^+ currents that are apparently absent in Chinese hamster ovary (CHO) cells ***(24,25)***, the assay choice will dictate the most appropriate host cell line. We have shown previously that [^{3}H]dofetilide bound to both HEK293 and CHO-K1 cells, although dofetilide affinity was an order of magnitude lower in CHO-K1 cells ***(10)***. For both HEK293 (*see* **Fig. 2**) and CHO (data not shown) cell lines, the process of membrane preparation and subsequent storage at –20°C almost totally abolishes this endogenous binding. Loss of [^{3}H]dofetilide binding following membrane preparation has also been observed previously for guinea pig cardiac myocytes ***(16)***. Therefore, as

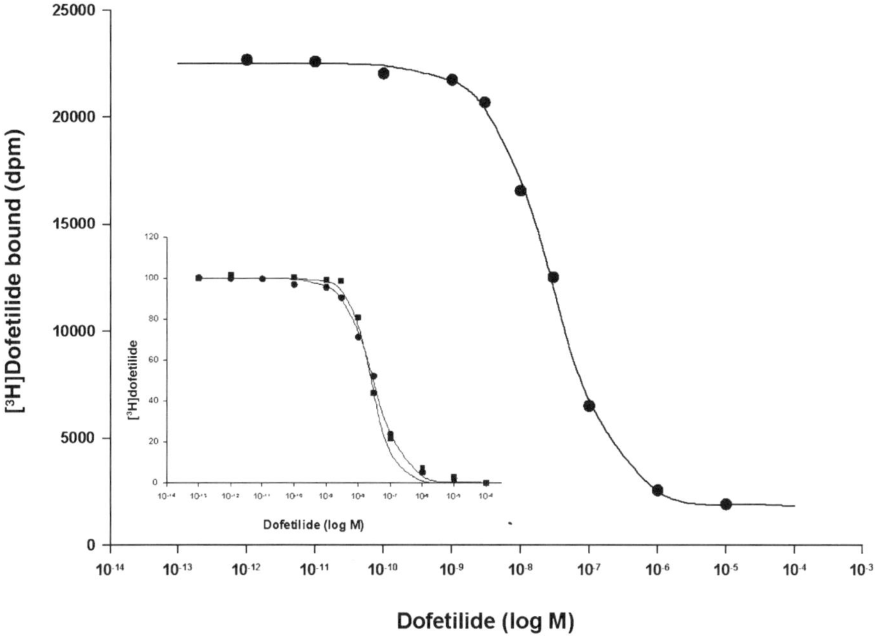

Fig. 5. Inhibition of [^{3}H]dofetilide binding to frozen and fresh (*see* insert) HERG-HEK293 membranes. Membranes were incubated with [^{3}H]dofetilide (10 n*M*) in a 10-m*M* HEPES assay buffer containing increasing concentrations of unlabeled dofetilide. Binding was terminated after 60 min at 25°C by rapid filtration using a Brandel Cell Harvester. Data shown are representative inhibition curves from an individual experiment; K_d/K_i values shown in text.

long as HERG channel expression is sufficient to render insignificant any endogenous binding, then either cell line can be used in the [^{3}H]dofetilide-binding assay. This also holds true for electrophysiological studies with the tail current amplitudes seen in the HERG-HEK293 cell line used here, totally overwhelming any endogenous voltage-gated K^+ currents ***(9)***. Preliminary studies using Molecular Device's FlexStation and membrane potential dye (FMP) indicate that CHO cells expressing HERG ***(26)*** are more suitable than HERG-HEK293 when KCl is used as the depolarizing stimulus because of the large endogenous response seen in the latter cell line (K. Finlayson, unpublished observations). In addition, when HERG channel blockers, including dofetilide, are added to cells preloaded with FMP dye, there is an immediate and gradual increase in fluorescence with drug alone, prior to KCl addition. Presumably, these effects occur as a result of the modification of the resting membrane potential, which is known to be hyperpolarized in cells expressing HERG ***(9,27)***. These observations suggest that thc use of membrane potential dyes for screening is complex, but further studies will be required to elucidate fully these preliminary findings. Whether

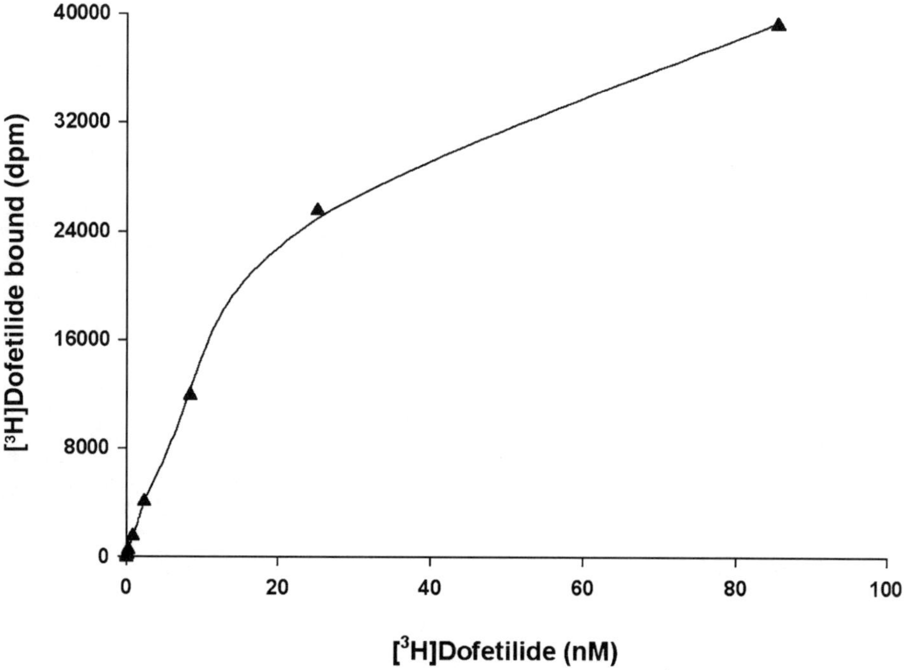

Fig. 6. Concentration dependence of [^{3}H]dofetilide binding to frozen HERG-HEK293 membranes. Membranes were incubated with increasing concentrations of [^{3}H]dofetilide in a 10-m*M* HEPES assay buffer; nonspecific binding was determined in the presence of E-4031 (100 μ*M*). Binding was terminated after 60 min at 25°C by rapid filtration using a Brandel Cell Harvester. Data shown are from an individual saturation experiment, with the calculated K_d value shown in the text.

these observations also hold true when radioactive rubidium (^{86}Rb) flux is used to examine HERG channel function remains to be determined *(27)*.

3. Thorough homogenization and resuspension of HERG-HEK293 membranes is required at all stages as occasional clumping can be observed. Membrane clumping is less apparent with CHO-HERG membranes. The electrophysiological characteristics of this cell line have now been evaluated over more than 100 passages, being routinely used up to passages 70–80 without any loss in functional response (C. T. January, 2003, personal communication).
4. As the total assay volume of 200 μL is small in the 5-mL Sterlin RT-30 tubes, following the final sample addition, tubes were vortexed, placed in centrifuge racks, and spun briefly up to 100*g* to ensure even mixing; this step would obviously not be required for a plate-based assay.
5. No loss in affinity has been observed for any of the drugs examined on reusing frozen stock solutions. In addition, both assay and wash buffers have been stored for reasonable periods of time (>2 mo) at 4°C.

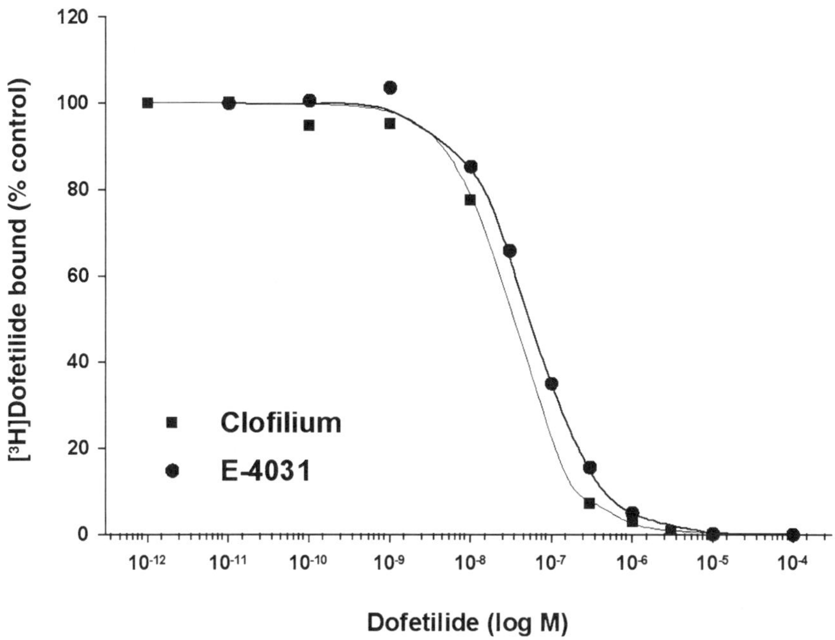

Fig. 7. Inhibition of [^{3}H]dofetilide binding to frozen HERG-HEK293 membranes by alternative class III antiarrhythmic drugs. Membranes were incubated with [^{3}H]dofetilide (10 n*M*) in a 10-m*M* HEPES assay buffer containing increasing concentrations of clofilium or E-4031. Binding was terminated after 60 min at 25°C by rapid filtration using a Brandel Cell Harvester, with data shown being representative inhibition curves.

6. Neither ethanol nor methanol has any effect on [^{3}H]dofetilide binding at concentrations up to 0.1%, the highest concentrations so far examined.
7. GF/C filters were soaked in polyethylenimine for a least 120 min prior to use. As the total volume in the assay tubes is only 200 µL, approx 500 µL of ice-cold Tris-HCl wash buffer was added to the samples at the onset of harvesting, ensuring efficient aspiration prior to the three rapid 1-mL washes. Total filtration time was less than 5 s, thereby minimizing any potential ligand dissociation.
8. Samples were vortexed thoroughly prior to scintillation counting. Leaving the samples overnight prior to counting resulted in a 10% increase in the level of specific binding when compared to immediate scintillation counting. The addition of formic acid to the scintillation tubes or extending the time prior to radioactive determination produced no further increase in specific binding.
9. Analysis of radioligand binding data can also be performed using simple less intuitive software such as GraphPad Prism (GraphPad.com).
10. The time-course of [^{3}H]dofetilide binding to HERG-transfected membranes at 37°C is similar to that reported for guinea pig ventricular myocytes and other cell

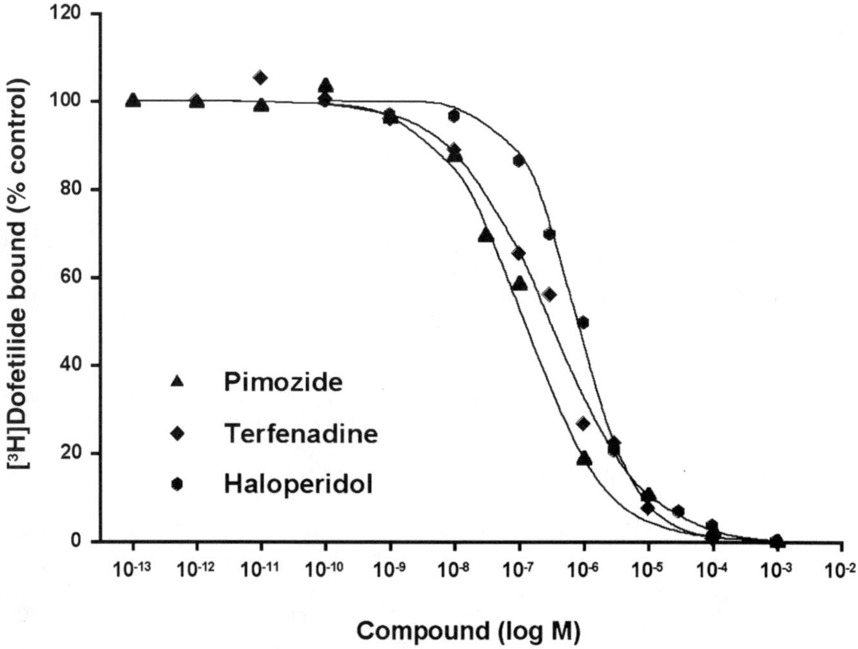

Fig. 8. Inhibition of [³H]dofetilide binding to frozen HERG-HEK293 membranes by structurally unrelated non-antiarrhythmic drugs. Membranes were incubated with [³H]dofetilide (10 n*M*) in a 10-m*M* HEPES assay buffer containing increasing concentrations of pimozide, terfenadine, and haloperidol. Binding was terminated after 60 min by rapid filtration using a Brandel Cell Harvester, with data shown being representative inhibition curves from individual experiments.

types ***(16–23)***. Although equilibrium was attained more slowly at 4°C and 25°C, as expected, at these temperatures, there was a substantial increase in the total amount of specific [³H]dofetilide bound (at 60 min, there is approx 2.5 and 5 times more specific binding, respectively). To date, no kinetic studies have been conducted to characterize fully the basis of this observation. At 25°C, the level of specific binding was greater than 90% and, during experiments, was kept to approx 15,000 dpm (approx 5% of total counts added), negating any residual endogenous binding (*see* **Note 2**). This observation is important as the presence of more than one site could lead to an underestimate in drug affinity ***(17)***.

11. Although some specific [³H]dofetilide binding has been observed in P2 rat hippocampal membranes ***(28)***, no further studies have been performed to characterize these observations.
12. To date, there are only a limited number of publications on [³H]dofetilide binding ***(16–23)***, with none previously examining the pharmacology of [³H]dofetilide binding sites in HERG-transfected membranes. Nevertheless, there is reasonable

agreement between our findings and the reported affinities for dofetilide in guinea pig ventricular myocytes: 19–100 n*M* for K_d/K_i (for the high-affinity site data) ***(16–18,20)***; 20 n*M* in neonatal mouse ventricular homogenates ***(18,21)***; 26 and 33 n*M* in human mononuclear cells and neutrophils, respectively ***(23)***; and 140 ± 60 n*M* in HL-1 mouse atrial myocytes ***(22)***.

13. It has been suggested by Finlayson et al. ***(11)*** that clofilium or its tertiary analog, LY97241, ***(29)*** may be useful ligands with which to study HERG. This observation is supported by Gessner and Heinemann ***(30)***, who reported low nanomolar affinity for clofilium and LY97241 in an electrophysiological study. Indeed, despite questions being raised about the utility of a nonfunctional binding assay to detect drugs that potentially interact with HERG ***(31)***, to date, we have not found any known HERG blockers that do not inhibit [^{3}H]dofetilide binding. The considerable heterogeneity in the methodology used to examine the effect of drugs on HERG precludes at this stage any meaningful attempt to draw any correlation between radioligand binding and functional data. Furthermore, major pharmaceutical companies such as Pfizer are using this assay ***(32)***, and Merck has subsequently used a radiolabeled version of its own class III methanesulfonanilide drug, MK-499, to characterize a second HERG binding assay ***(33)***. As both drugs (dofetilide and MK-499) act intracellularly, they may not detect compounds that act at an extracellular site or on the closed state of the channel, so perhaps a high-affinity blocker of closed channels such as ergtoxin could be used as a supplementary assay (***34,35***; H. J. Witchel, 2003, personal communication).
14. The affinity of the three nonantiarrhythmic drugs—pimozide, terfenadine, and haloperidol—in the [^{3}H]dofetilide-binding assay ***(11)*** is consistent with previous electrophysiological data ***(36–40)***.

Acknowledgments

We would like to thank Pfizer for kindly providing [^{3}H]dofetilide and unlabeled dofetilide and Eisai for E-4031. In addition, we would like to thank Professor C. T. January and Dr. H. J. Witchel for their helpful comments and for the HEK293 and CHO cell lines stably expressing HERG. Finally, we would like to thank Professor J. S. Kelly for all help given and Dr. B. R. Russell, J. McLuckie, and L. Turnbull for their technical assistance.

References

1. The European Agency for the Evaluation of Medicinal Products (EMEA): Committee for Proprietary Medicinal Products (CPMP), points to consider: the assessment of the potential for QT interval prolongation by non-cardiovascular medicinal products. Available: http://www.emea.eu.int/pdfs/human/swp/098696en.pdf
2. Warmke, J. W. and Ganetzky, B. (1994) A family of potassium channel genes related to EAG in *Drosophila* and mammals. *Proc. Natl. Acad. Sci. USA* **91,** 3438–3442.

3. De Ponti, F., Poluzzi, E., Cavalli, A., Recanatini, M., and Montanaro, N. (2002) Safety of non-antiarrhythmic drugs that prolong the QT interval or induce torsade de pointes. *Drug Saf.* **25,** 263–286.
4. Wakefield, I. D., Pollard, C., Redfern, W. S., Hammond, T. G., and Valentin, J.-P. (2002) The application of in vitro methods to safety pharmacology. *Fundam. Clin. Pharmacol.* **16,** 209–218.
5. Witchel, H. J. and Hancox, J. C. (2000) Familial and acquired long QT syndrome and the cardiac rapid delayed rectifier potassium current. *Clin. Exp. Pharmacol. Physiol.* **27,** 753–766.
6. Pond, A. L. and Nerbonne, J. M. (2001) ERG proteins and functional cardiac I_{Kr} channels in rat, mouse, and human heart. *Trends Cardiovasc. Med.* **11,** 286–294.
7. January, C. T., Gong, Q., and Zhou, Z. (2000) Long QT syndrome: cellular basis and arrhythmia mechanism in LQT2. *J. Cardiovasc. Electrophysiol.* **11,** 1413–1418.
8. Kiehn, J., Wible, B., Taglialatela, M., and Brown, A. M. (1995) Cloned human inward rectifier K^+ channel as a target for class III methanesulfonanilides. *Circ. Res.* **77,** 1151–1155.
9. Zhou, Z., Gong, Q., Ye, B., Fan, Z., Makielski, J. C., Robertson, G. A., et al. (1998) Properties of HERG channels stably expressed in HEK 293 cells studied at physiological temperature. *Biophys. J.* **74,** 230–241.
10. Finlayson, K., Pennington, A. J., and Kelly, J. S. (2001) [^{3}H]Dofetilide binding in SHSY5Y and HEK293 cells expressing a HERG-like K^+ channel? *Eur. J. Pharmacol.* **412,** 203–212.
11. Finlayson, K., Turnbull, L., January, C. T., Sharkey, J., and Kelly, J. S. (2001) [^{3}H]Dofetilide binding to HERG transfected membranes: a potential high throughput preclinical screen. *Eur. J. Pharmacol.* **430,** 147–148.
12. Trudeau, M. C., Warmke, J. W., Ganetzky, B., and Robertson, G. A. (1995) HERG, a human inward rectifier in the voltage-gated potassium channel family. *Science* **269,** 92–95.
13. Trudeau, M. C., Warmke, J. W., Ganetzky, B., and Robertson, G. A. (1996) HERG sequence correction [letter]. *Science* **272,** 1087.
14. Finlayson, K., Butcher, S. P., Sharkey, J., and Olverman, H. J. (1997) Detection of adenosine receptor antagonists in rat brain using a modified radioreceptor assay. *J. Neurosci. Meth.* **77,** 135–142.
15. Cheng, Y. C. and Prusoff, W. H. (1973) The relationship between the inhibition constant (K_i) and the concentration of inhibitor which causes 50% inhibition (IC_{50}) of an enzymatic reaction. *Biochem. Pharmacol.* **22,** 3099–3108.
16. Chadwick, C. C., Ezrin, A. M., O'Connor, B., Volberg, W. A., Smith, D. I., Wedge, K. J., et al. (1993) Identification of a specific radioligand for the cardiac rapidly activating delayed rectifier K^+ channel. *Circ. Res.* **72,** 707–714.
17. Duff, H. J., Feng, Z.-P., and Sheldon, R. S. (1995) High- and low-affinity sites for [^{3}H]dofetilide binding to guinea pig myocytes. *Circ. Res.* **77,** 718–725.
18. Duff, H. J., Feng, Z.-P., Fiset, C., Wang, L., Less-Miller, J., and Sheldon, R. S. (1997) [^{3}H]Dofetilide binding to cardiac myocytes: modulation by extracellular potassium. *J. Mol. Cell Cardiol.* **29,** 183–191.

19. Duff, H. J., Feng, Z.-P., Wang, L., and Sheldon, R. S. (1997) Regulation of expression of the [^{3}H]-dofetilide binding site associated with the delayed rectifier K^+ channel by dexamethasone in neonatal mouse ventricle. *J. Mol. Cell Cardiol.* **29,** 1959–1965.
20. Lynch, J. J., Baskin, E. P., Nutt, E. M., Guinosso, P. J., Hamill, T., Salata, J. J., et al. (1995) Comparison of binding to rapidly activating delayed rectifier K^+ channel, I_{Kr}, and effects on myocardial refractoriness for class III antiarrhythmic agents. *J. Cardiovasc. Pharmacol.* **25,** 336–340.
21. Fiset, C., Feng, Z.-P., Wang, L., Sheldon, R. S., and Duff, H. J. (1996) [^{3}H]Dofetilide binding: biological models that manifest solely the high or the low affinity binding site. *J. Mol. Cell Cardiol.* **28,** 1085–1096.
22. Claycomb, W. C., Lanson, N. A., Stallworth, B. S., Egeland, D. B., Delcarpio, J. B., Bahinski, A., et al. (1998) HL-1 cells: a cardiac muscle cell line that contracts and retains phenotypic characteristics of the adult cardiomyocyte. *Proc. Natl. Acad. Sci. USA* **95,** 2979–2984.
23. Geonzon, R., Exner, D. V., Woodman, R. C., Wang, L., Feng, Z.-P., and Duff, H. J. (1998) A high affinity binding site for [^{3}H]-dofetilide on human leukocytes. *J. Mol. Cell Cardiol.* **30,** 1691–1701.
24. Robertson, B. and Owen, D. G. (1993) Pharmacology of a cloned potassium channel from mouse brain (MK-1) expressed in CHO cells: effects of blockers and an inactivation peptide. *Br. J. Pharmacol.* **109,** 725–735.
25. Yu, S. P. and Kerchner, G. A. (1998) Endogenous voltage-gated potassium channels in human embryonic kidney (HEK293) cells. *J. Neurosci. Res.* **52,** 612–617.
26. Teschemacher, A. G., Seward, E. P., Hancox, J. C., and Witchel, H. J. (1999) Inhibition of the current of heterologously expressed HERG potassium channels by imipramine and amitriptyline. *Br. J. Pharmacol.* **128,** 479–485.
27. Cheng, C. S., Alderman, D., Kwash, J., Dessaint, J., Patel, R., Lescoe, M. K., et al. (2002) A high-throughput HERG potassium channel function assay: an old assay with a new look. *Drug Dev. Indust. Pharm.* **28,** 177–191.
28. Finlayson, K., McLuckie, J., Hern, J., Aramori, I., Olverman, H. J., and Kelly, J. S. (2001) Characterisation of [^{125}I]-apamin binding sites in rat brain membranes and HEK293 cells transfected with SK channel subtypes. *Neuropharmacology* **41,** 341–350.
29. Suessbrich, H., Schönherr, R., Heinemann, S. H., Lang, F., and Busch, A. E. (1997) Specific block of cloned *Herg* channels by clofilium and its tertiary analog LY97241. *FEBS Lett.* **414,** 435–438.
30. Gessner, G. and Heinemann, S. H. (2003) Inhibition of hEAG1 and hERG1 potassium channels by clofilium and its tertiary analogue LY97241. *Br. J. Pharmacol.* **138,** 161–171.
31. Netzer, R., Ebneth, A., Bischoff, U., and Pongs, O. (2001) Screening lead compounds for QT interval prolongation. *Drug Disc. Today* **6,** 78–84.
32. Volberg, W. A., Koci, B. J., Su, W., Lin, J., and Zhou, J. (2002) Blockade of human cardiac potassium channel human *Ether-a-go-go*-related gene (HERG) by macrolide antibiotics. *J. Pharmacol. Exp. Ther.* **302,** 320–327.

33. Wang, J., Della-Penna, K., Wang, H., Karczewski, J., Connolly, T. M., Koblan, K. S., et al. (2003) Functional and pharmacological properties of canine ERG potassium channels. *Am. J. Physiol. Heart Circ. Physiol.* **284,** H256–H267.
34. Gurrola, G. B., Rosati, B., Rocchetti, M., Pimienta, G., Zaza, A., Arcangeli, A., et al. (1999) A toxin to nervous, cardiac, and endocrine ERG K^+ channels isolated from *Centruroides noxius* scorpion venom. *FASEB J.* **13,** 953–962.
35. Padro-Lopez, L., Zhang, M., Liu, J., Jiang, M., Possani, L. D., and Tseng, G. N. (2002) Mapping the binding site of a human *ether-a-go-go*-related gene-specific peptide toxin (ErgTx) to the channel's outer vestibule. *J. Biol. Chem.* **277,** 16,403–16,411.
36. Suessbrich, H., Waldegger, S., Lang, F., and Busch, A. E. (1996) Blockade of HERG channels expressed in *Xenopus* oocytes by the histamine receptor antagonists terfenadine and astemizole. *FEBS Lett.* **385,** 77–80.
37. Mitcheson, J. S., Chen, J., Lin, M., Culberson, C., and Sanguinetti, M. C. (2000) A structural basis for drug-induced long QT syndrome. *Proc. Natl. Acad. Sci. USA* **97,** 12329–12333.
38. Kang, J., Wang, L., Cai, F., and Rampe, D. (2000) High affinity blockade of the HERG cardiac K^+ channel by the neuroleptic pimozide. *Eur. J. Pharmacol.* **392,** 137–140.
39. Kongsamut, S., Kang, J., Chen, X.-L., Roehr, J., and Rampe, D. (2002) A comparison of the receptor binding and HERG channel affinities for a series of antipsychotic drugs. *Eur. J. Pharmacol.* **450,** 37–41.
40. Suessbrich, H., Schönherr, R., Heinemann, S. H., Attali, B., Lang, F., and Busch, A. E. (1997) The inhibitory effect of the antipsychotic drug haloperidol on HERG potassium channels expressed in *Xenopus* oocytes. *Br. J. Pharmacol.* **120,** 968–974.

24

In Vitro Drug Metabolism

Thiol Conjugation

Wei Tang and Randy R. Miller

Summary

From a pharmaceutical research point of view, it seems reasonable in the early phase of discovery to eliminate those drug candidates that are subject to bioactivation to electrophilic intermediates. Although rarely detectable per se, the structures of these intermediates often can be deduced by analysis of the corresponding glutathione or *N*-acetylcysteine conjugates. A practical approach in this regard, therefore, is to screen drug candidates in vitro for the formation of reactive metabolites via incubations with liver microsomes or hepatocytes prepared from preclinical species or humans. These incubations are normally carried out at 37°C for a period of time in the presence of glutathione or *N*-acetylcysteine, followed by solid-phase extraction of the reaction mixture. The resulting samples are subject to reversed-phase chromatography. Further on-line detection and identification of thiol conjugates by mass spectrometry are performed in a stepwise manner from neutral loss and/or parent ion scans to multiple-stage mass fragmentations. This would eventually lead to elucidating the structures of reactive intermediates, from which the thiol conjugates result. The experiments require minimal sample preparation and method development and often afford ample structural information on the analytes.

Key Words: Glutathione; *N*-acetylcysteine; thiol conjugation; drug metabolism; bioactivation; reactive metabolites; HPLC; mass spectrometry.

1. Introduction

1.1. Glutathione

Glutathione, a tripeptide consisting of L-γ-glutamyl-L-cysteinyl-glycine (**Fig. 1**), is widely distributed in nature and virtually in all aerobic species. It

From: *Methods in Pharmacology and Toxicology*
Optimization in Drug Discovery: In Vitro Methods
Edited by: Z. Yan and G. W. Caldwell © Humana Press Inc., Totowa, NJ

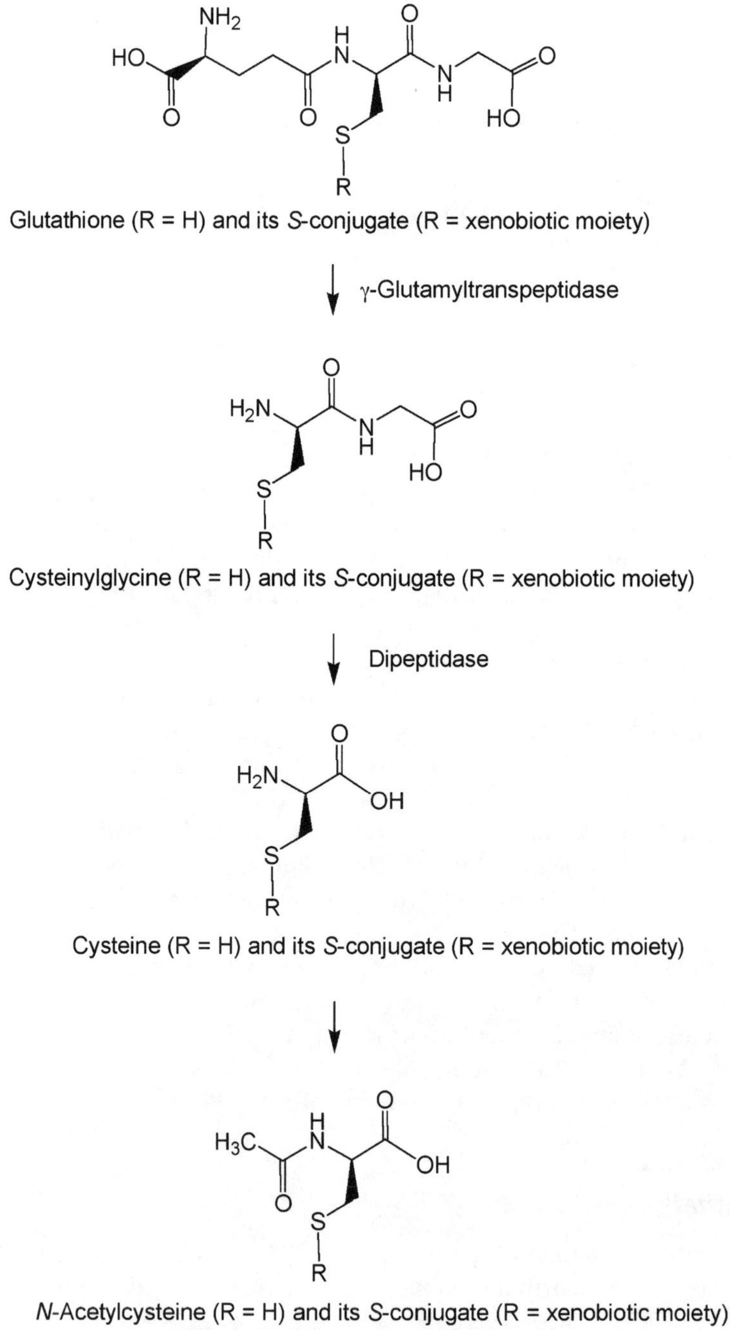

Fig. 1. Structures of glutathione and the metabolites formed via the mercapturic acid pathway.

represents the most important and abundant nonprotein thiol in mammalian cells; the concentrations of cellular glutathione normally range from 0.1 to 10 m*M*, nearly 90% of which is present in cytosol and 10% in mitochondria *(1,2)*. In hepatocytes, biosynthesis of glutathione occurs in the cytosolic compartment, wherein sequential coupling of L-glutamate with glycine and further with L-cysteine consumes two molecules of adenosine triphosphate (ATP) for every molecule of final product formed and is catalyzed by γ-glutamylcysteine synthetase and glutathione synthetase, respectively. Cytosolic glutathione is then subject to intracellular uptake transport by mitochondria and nuclei or export to extracellular biological fluids such as blood and bile *(1,3)*. The vital functions of glutathione in cells are to protect critical macromolecules from oxidative stress and to provide a storage and transport form of cysteine. Because of the free thiol-bearing structure, glutathione also serves as a scavenger in detoxifying reactive metabolites via conjugation reactions *(4,5)*. This, in fact, constitutes one of the primary cellular defense mechanisms against insult from xenobiotics and may be responsible for the drug resistance encountered during anticancer therapy, in which glutathione and glutathione-*S*-transferases, a group of enzymes catalyzing glutathione conjugation, sometimes are found to be overexpressed in tumor cells.

1.2. Metabolic Activation of Xenobiotics and Conjugation With Glutathione

Many xenobiotics pose no threat to human health until these compounds are biotransformed in the body to reactive metabolites. These metabolites often are electrophiles capable of covalent modification of proteins or nucleic acids and thereby have the potential to produce toxicity via disruption of critical cellular functions or elicitation of immunological responses *(6,7)*. Classic electrophiles include α,β-unsaturated carbonyls, epoxides, alkyl halides, isocyanates and isothiocyanates, nitrogen and sulfur mustards, quinones, quinone imines, and quinone methides. In addition to their ability to attack cellular macromolecules, electrophilic metabolites may form conjugates with glutathione via a thio linkage (**Fig. 2**). These conjugation reactions take place in cells either spontaneously, as a result of the highly reactive nature of the metabolites, or catalyzed by glutathione-*S*-transferases, a family of enzymes present predominantly in cytosol and, to a much lesser extent, in endoplasmic reticulum. Plausible mechanisms for catalysis by glutathione-*S*-transferase include (1) binding to an electrophile, in order for it to react preferentially with glutathione rather than other cellular nucleophiles, and (2) enhancing the nucleophilic potential of glutathione by promoting ionization of its sulfhydryl group *(8,9)*. Glutathione conjugates formed in hepatocytes are subject to active excretion into bile and/or blood and also undergo sequential hydrolysis cata-

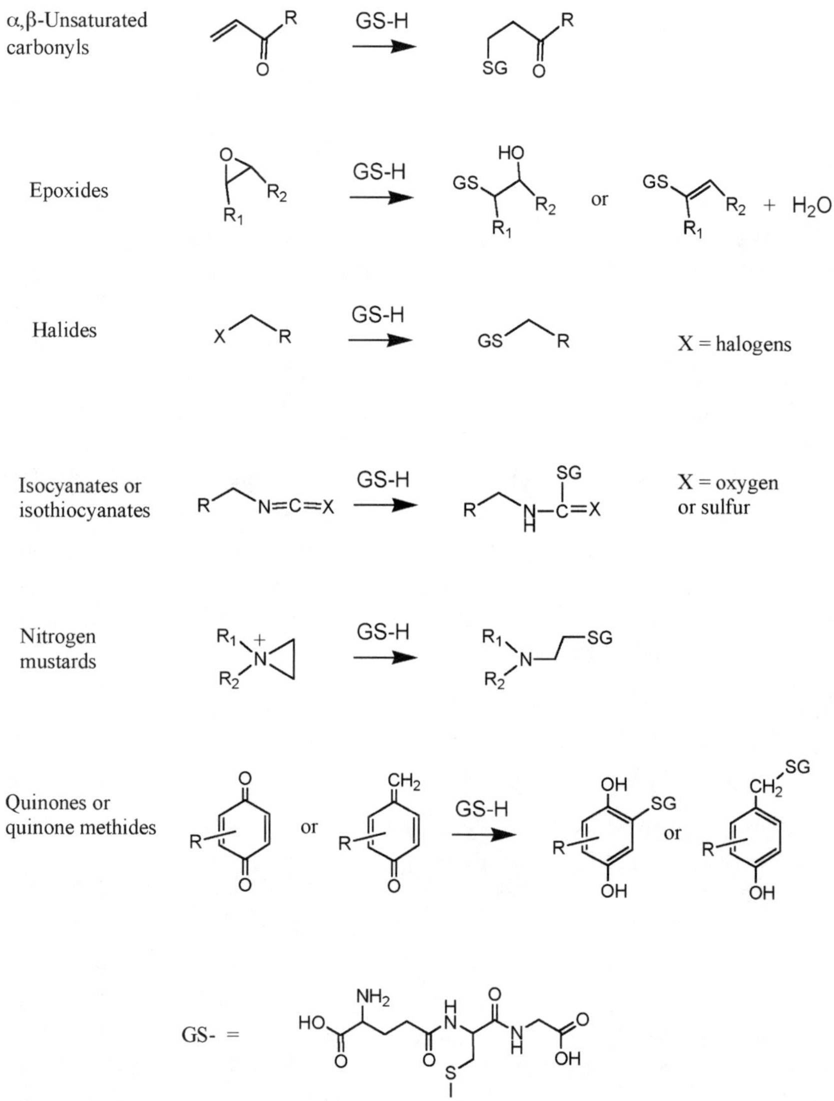

Fig. 2. Examples of electrophilic metabolites and their conjugation reactions with glutathione.

lyzed by γ-glutamyltranspeptidase and dipeptidase, leading to formation of the corresponding cysteinylglycine conjugates and further to the cysteine conjugates. *N*-Acetylation of the latter results in the formation of *N*-acetylcysteine conjugates, namely mercapturic acids (**Fig. 1**).

1.3. Identification of Thiol Conjugates by Mass Spectrometry

In numerous cases, the adverse effect of a drug may be attributed to its bioactivation to electrophilic metabolites. Classic examples include the severe hepatotoxicity caused by acetaminophen or tienilic acid, the metabolism of which leads to the formation of a quinone imine and an epoxide intermediate, respectively. As a result, toxicologic responses sometimes are characterized by the lack of a clear dose–response relationship with the parent drug and low incident rates even in patients with a prolonged exposure to the agent ***(10,11)***. To minimize the risk of idiosyncratic toxicity, it seems prudent to eliminate those molecules that are subject to bioactivation and limit the potential for covalent modification of cellular macromolecules in the early stage of drug discovery. In other words, a low propensity to form reactive metabolites may be included in the selection criteria for a drug candidate ***(12)***. A technical dilemma associated with this strategy, however, is that reactive metabolites often are short-lived in biological systems and rarely detectable per se even by the state-of-the-art modern instrumentation. This has been largely resolved via analysis of stable products resulting from the nucleophilic "trapping" of electrophilic metabolites. In this regard, screening for glutathione conjugates of compounds of interest by high-performance liquid chromatography (HPLC) coupled with mass spectrometry represents an experimental approach with the most practical utility ***(13,14)***. It has several advantages, including minimal sample preparation and method development, rapid detection with high sensitivity, and adequate structural information of the analytes.

2. Materials

2.1. Thiol Conjugation

1. Glutathione (reduced form) or *N*-acetylcysteine (Sigma Chemical Co., St. Louis, MO).
2. Glucose, glucose-6-phosphate, glucose-6-phosphate dehydrogenase, nicotinamide adenine dinucleotide phosphate (NADP), and the reduced form of nicotinamide adenine dinucleotide phosphate (NADPH) (Sigma Chemical Co., St. Louis, MO).
3. Potassium phosphate, ethylenediaminetetraacetic acid (EDTA), sodium chloride, magnesium sulfate, sodium bicarbonate, and calcium chloride (Sigma Chemical Co., St. Louis, MO).
4. Liver microsomes from preclinical species and humans. Human tissues are obtained from the Pennsylvania Regional Tissue Bank (Exton, PA) under the agreement for research use only.
5. Recombinant cytochrome P450 (CYP) enzymes (BD Biosciences/Gentest, Bedford, MA).

6. Hepatocytes, either freshly prepared or cryopreserved, from preclinical species or humans. Cryopreserved human hepatocytes are obtained from In Vitro Technologies (Baltimore, MD).

2.2. Sample Preparation

1. BondElut C_{18} solid-phase extraction cartridges (0.2 g; Varian Chromatography Systems, Walnut Creek, CA) or Oasis polymeric HLB extraction cartridges (Waters Corporation, Milford, MA) (*see* **Note 1**).

2.3. Identification of Thiol Conjugates

1. HPLC instrument.
2. Reversed-phase HPLC column (*see* **Note 1**).
3. HPLC mobile phase (*see* **Note 1**).
4. Mass spectrometry (*see* **Note 2**).

3. Methods

3.1. Thiol Conjugation

3.1.1. Incubations With Liver Microsomes or Recombinant CYP

Microsomes are isolated from livers of preclinical species or humans by differential centrifugation *(15)*. Incubation procedure:

1. 100 m*M* phosphate buffer, pH 7.4, containing 1 m*M* EDTA is prepared and stored at 4°C.
2. An aqueous solution of 50 m*M* glutathione or *N*-acetylcysteine is prepared daily, and the pH of the solution is adjusted to approx 7 with aqueous sodium hydroxide (*see* **Note 3**).
3. The compound of interest is dissolved in methanol at a concentration of 25 m*M*.
4. An NADPH-generating system is prepared by mixing 3.3 parts of 10 m*M* glucose-6-phosphate, 3.3 parts of 10 m*M* NADP, and 3.3 parts of 20 U/mL glucose-6-phosphate dehydrogenase, all dissolved in phosphate buffer.
5. 1 mg protein of liver microsomes from preclinical species or humans, or 0.1 nmol of recombinant CYP enzymes, is suspended in phosphate buffer in a round-bottom test tube (*see* **Notes 4** and **5**). The mixture is kept on ice.
6. 100 µL of the glutathione solution is added to the microsomal suspension. The mixture is kept on ice (*see* **Note 6**).
7. 2 µL of substrate (compound of interest) in methanol is added to the microsomal suspension. The mixture is incubated at 37°C for 5 min (*see* **Note 7**).
8. 100 µL of the NADPH-generating system is added to the incubation (*see* **Note 8**).
9. The final volume of incubations at this point is 1 mL, containing 1 mg/mL of liver microsomes or 0.1 nmol/mL of recombinant CYP. The concentration of glutathione or *N*-acetylcysteine is 5 m*M*, and the compound of interest is 50 µ*M*, whereas methanol is 0.2% (v/v). The pH is 7.4.
10. The reaction mixture is further incubated for 60 min at 37°C in a water bath with gentle rhythmic shaking, followed by solid-phase extraction.

3.1.2. Incubations With Hepatocytes

Hepatocytes are isolated according to a two-step perfusion procedure and are examined for viability by the trypan blue exclusion test ***(16)***. Incubation procedure:

1. Krebs-bicarbonate buffer, pH 7.4, is prepared daily, containing 125 m*M* sodium chloride, 5 m*M* potassium chloride, 1.25 m*M* monopotassium phosphate and magnesium sulfate, 25 m*M* sodium bicarbonate, 2.5 m*M* calcium chloride, and 15 m*M* glucose.
2. An aqueous solution of glutathione or *N*-acetylcysteine is prepared daily, and the pH of the solution is adjusted to approx 7 with aqueous sodium hydroxide. The concentration of glutathione is 50 m*M*.
3. The compound of interest is dissolved in dimethylsulfoxide at a concentration of 25 m*M*.
4. Hepatocytes are suspended in the Krebs-bicarbonate buffer at the density of approx 1 million cells/mL.
5. 100 μL of the glutathione solution is added to the cell suspension (*see* **Note 9**).
6. 2 μL of substrate (compound of interest) in dimethylsulfoxide is added to the cell suspension (*see* **Note 7**).
7. The final volume of hepatocyte suspensions is 1 mL. The concentration of glutathione or *N*-acetylcysteine is 5 m*M*, and the compound of interest is 50 μ*M*, whereas dimethylsulfoxide is 0.2% (v/v).
8. Incubations are performed, under the atmosphere consisting of 95% oxygen and 5% carbon dioxide, for 4 h at 37°C in a water bath with gentle rhythmic shaking. The mixture then is sonicated, followed by solid-phase extraction (*see* **Note 10**).

3.2. Sample Preparation

1. A BondElut C_{18} solid-phase extraction cartridge is conditioned with 1 mL of methanol, followed by equilibration with 1 mL of water.
2. 1 mL of reaction mixtures, from incubations with either liver microsomes or hepatocytes, is transferred to the extraction cartridge and loaded by applying vacuum suction until dryness (*see* **Note 11**).
3. The loaded cartridge then is washed with 1 mL of water, and the extracts are eluted with 2 mL of methanol into a clean test tube.
4. The methanol eluate is dried under a stream of nitrogen.
5. The residue is reconstituted in 200 μL of 40% aqueous acetonitrile containing 10% methanol and 0.05% trifluoroacetic acid (v/v), and the resulting sample is centrifuged to afford clean supernatant for further detection of thiol conjugates.

3.3. Identification of Thiol Conjugates

Aliquots of above samples (10 μL) are injected onto a DuPont Zorbax (Wilmington, DE) Rx-C8 column (4.6 × 250 mm, 5 μm) and delivered at a flow rate of 1 mL/min, with a 1:25 split to the ion source of a mass spectrometer. Chromatography is performed, with the mobile phase consisting of aqueous acetonitrile containing 10% methanol and 0.05% trifluoroacetic acid, and is programmed for a linear increase from 10% to 70% acetonitrile during a 30-min period (*see* **Note 1**). Mass spectrometry is performed either on a Perkin-Elmer Sciex API 3000 triple-quadrupole mass spectrometer (Toronto, Canada) or a Finnigan LCQ-DECA ion trap mass spectrometer (San Jose, CA). For the triple-quadrupole mass spectrometer, Turbo IonSpray® is interfaced to HPLC and is operated in the positive ionization mode. Generic calibration parameters include 150°C for the source temperature, 5 kV for the ionization voltage, and 50 V for the orifice potential. Nitrogen is used for tthe collision-induced dissociation of MH^+ ions with a collision energy at 35 eV. For the ion trap instrument, electrospray is the interface and is performed in the positive ionization mode. Generic calibration parameters are 4.1 kV for the spray voltage, 32 eV for the collision energy, and 200°C for the capillary temperature (*see* **Notes 12–17**).

4. Notes

1. The method for sample preparation, the HPLC column, and the mobile phase are normally selected based on physical-chemical properties of the analyte(s). However, certain generic approaches can meet with routine success. For example, solid-phase extraction of in vitro incubation mixtures is usually sufficient to partially purify and concentrate samples prior to liquid chromatography. A combination of a C_8 or C_{18} reversed-phase HPLC column, with a dimension of 4.6 × 250 mm and a particle size ranging from 3 to 5 µm, and a mobile phase consisting of aqueous acetonitrile buffered with ammonium acetate plus formic acid or trifluoroacetic acid generally serve well for the detection of glutathione or *N*-acetylcysteine conjugates. Phosphate buffer should be avoided in the HPLC mobile phase because it is incompatible with mass spectrometers operating in the online detection mode. If this is deemed essential, a postcolumn treatment is required to remove inorganic salts before introducing the analyte(s) into the ion source.
2. Current mass spectrometry in analytical laboratories includes triple-quadrupole and ion trap instruments, characteristics of which are easy to use and relatively inexpensive. Triple-quadrupole instruments may be used for product ion scan, parent ion scan and neutral loss scan, and are robust in either quantitative or qualitative studies, whereas ion trap instruments are designed to obtain sequential, multistage (MS^n) mass spectra and are preferable for qualitative analysis.
3. Commercial glutathione and *N*-acetylcysteine (Sigma) are in free acid forms and therefore need to be neutralized before adding into the incubation media.
4. Incubations should be performed in vessels that provide significant surface area at the liquid/air interface to avoid potential depletion of oxygen in the media. This is an important factor to consider when incubations are scaled up to larger volumes.

5. Liver microsomes, recombinant CYP, or hepatocytes are used as the source of enzymes for in vitro incubations, with the rationale being that clearance of xenobiotic compounds generally takes place in the liver, where oxidative metabolism and/or bioactivation are catalyzed primarily by CYP enzymes.
6. Addition of commercial glutathione-*S*-transferase (Sigma Chemical Co.) into liver microsomal incubations may enhance glutathione conjugation with an electrophilic metabolite. An aliquot (1/10 of total volume) of rat liver cytosolic fraction may serve the same purpose, except that it gives rise to the possibility of altering metabolism of the compound of interest. This becomes important if one's focus is on the mechanisms of bioactivation.
7. Optimal substrate concentrations are dependent on the rate of turnover in a particular in vitro system. In the absence of data from detailed kinetic studies, 50 μ*M* of the compound of interest may be used as an entry point for a preliminary experiment.
8. Alternatively, NADPH may be used at the final concentration of 1 mg/mL.
9. The intracellular concentrations of glutathione decrease rapidly during the isolation of hepatocytes. Thiol conjugates frequently are not detected unless glutathione is added to hepatocyte incubations.
10. Sonication is required to disrupt cell membranes and to ensure a good recovery of metabolites. This may be performed either in an ultrasonic tank or with a probe-type sonicator (Fisher Scientific) under relatively low temperature (<25°C).
11. Prior to extraction by a cartridge, the reaction mixtures (1 mL) may be acidified with 10% aqueous trifluoroacetic acid (50 μL) and centrifuged to remove precipitates. This would diminish the potential plugging of the cartridge as a result of the protein load. When the metabolite(s) is susceptible to an acidic environment, the reaction mixtures (1 mL) are diluted with 8 *M* aqueous urea (pH ~7.0, 1 mL), followed by extraction with a cartridge. Protein precipitation is an alternative approach, in which acetonitrile (3 mL) is added to the reaction mixtures (1 mL). Following centrifugation, the supernatant is transferred to a clean tube and dried under a stream of nitrogen. The residue is reconstituted in the HPLC mobile phase for further analysis of thiol conjugates.
12. Identification of intact glutathione or *N*-acetylcysteine conjugates by mass spectrometry often is carried out under the positive ion detection mode. Diagnostic mass fragmentations of MH^+ ions of the conjugates upon collision-induced dissociation include the following: (1) cleavage of an aromatic thioether bond with charge retention on the aromatic moiety; (2) neutral loss of glutathione or *N*-acetylcysteine from respective aliphatic thioether conjugates via a retro-Michael reaction; (3) neutral loss of 129 Da, corresponding to the loss of pyroglutamate from a glutathione conjugate or the loss of *N*-acetylaminoacrylic acid from an *N*-acetylcysteine conjugate; and (4) neutral loss of cysteine from a glutathione conjugate (**Fig. 3**).
13. With a triple-quadrupole instrument, a neutral loss scan of 129 Dalton may afford initial detection of glutathione conjugates derived from a diverse array of struc-

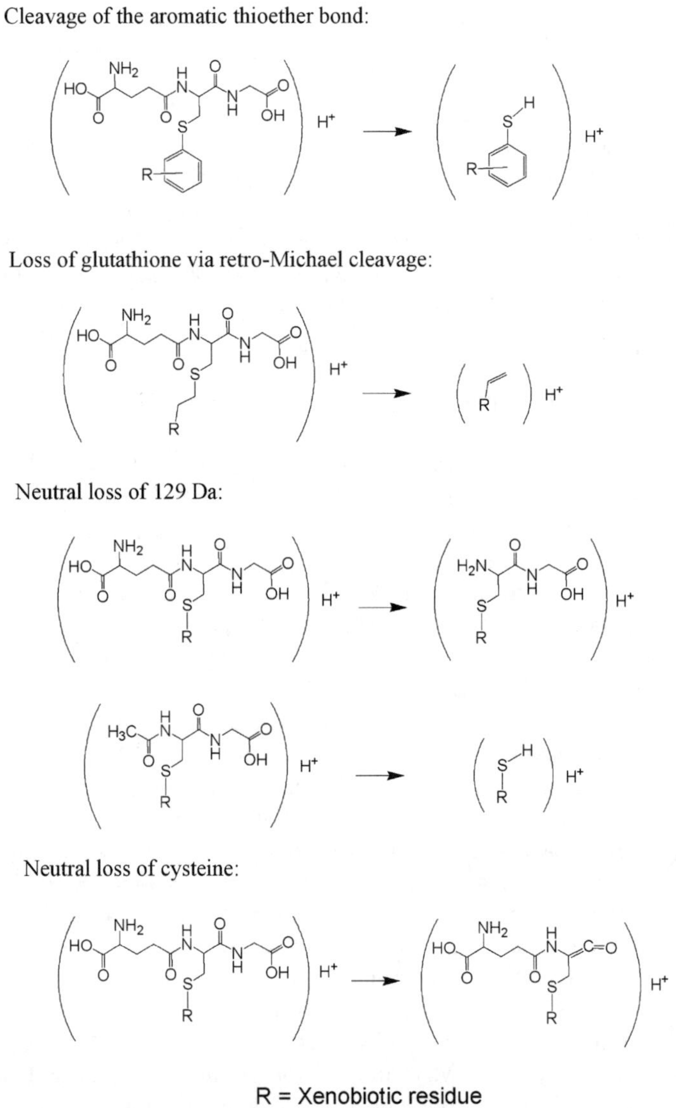

Fig. 3. Characteristic fragmentations of thiol conjugates following collision-induced dissociation of the corresponding MH^+ ions.

tural classes of electrophiles. It also is a common practice to extract from the Q1 scans for MH^+ ions that have the *m/z* ratio equal to the molecular weight of parent compound plus either 322 Dalton or 306 Dalton; the former corresponds to glutathione conjugation with a monohydroxylated metabolite, whereas the latter is indicative of a direct coupling between the thiol and unchanged parent molecule.

Further structural elucidation of a conjugate is based on collision-induced dissociation of the MH^+ ions. In this regard, data generated with sequential mass spectrometry (MS^n) can be very informative.

14. Some of the techniques described previously were used for identifying glutathione conjugates of raloxifene, a modulator of estrogen receptors ***(17)***. Briefly, three metabolites of raloxifene, with their MH^+ ion at *m/z* 779, were detected by mass spectrometry (triple-quadrupole) in samples from incubations of the drug with human liver microsomes in the presence of glutathione (**Fig. 4**). The mass of the MH^+ ions (i.e., a sum of the molecular weight of raloxifene plus 306 Dalton) was indicative of glutathione conjugation with the drug. Further structural evidence was obtained from collision-induced dissociation of the MH^+, which led to the formation of fragment ions at *m/z* 704 and 650, corresponding to losses of the elements of glycine and pyroglutamate, respectively. Additional informative fragment ions included those at *m/z* 112, which suggests the presence of an intact ethylpiperidine moiety in the conjugates, and *m/z* 506, which most likely results from cleavage of the thioether bond with charge retention on the raloxifene residue (**Fig. 4**). The three metabolites then were purified for nuclear magnetic resonance (NMR) analysis, and their structures were assigned as 7-glutathionyl-raloxifene, 5-glutathionyl-raloxifene, and 3'-glutathionyl-raloxifene, respectively ***(17)***.
15. Identification of thiol conjugates by mass spectrometry may be facilitated by the use of stable isotope-labeled tracers, an example of which was illustrated in the detection of a glutathione-glucuronic acid diconjugate of valproic acid, an anticonvulsant ***(18)***. Briefly, bile samples from the treatment of rats with either unlabeled or $^2H_7$-labeled valproic acid derivatives were subject to parent ion scans of the product ion at *m/z* 162, which often is diagnostic for glutathione conjugates. A pair of MH^+ ions with a difference of 7 Dalton was therefore registered at *m/z* 624 and 631, respectively (**Fig. 5**). The collision-induced dissociation of the MH^+ ions was characterized by losses of the elements corresponding to glucuronic acid, glutamate, and glycine moieties, resulting in the formation of two sets of fragment ions, among which the mass of paired ions was 7 Dalton apart (**Fig. 5**). The metabolite was eventually assigned as 5-glutathionyl-3-ene valproic acid-glucuronide, based on analysis of data generated by mass spectrometry and NMR ***(18)***.
16. In some cases, however, glutathione conjugates undergo further reactions, including degradation via the mercapturic acid pathway or cyclization between the amino group on the glutamate residue of glutathione and a reactive group on the xenobiotic moiety ***(19,20)***. As a result, the tactics described above are of no utility. In that instance, *N*-acetylcysteine may be a better trapping agent, in that mass spectra of the resulting conjugates are easier to interpret because of the lack of complications from further reactions.
17. Quantification of known thiol conjugates formed in incubations (or in biological matrices) is accomplished by HPLC separation in conjunction with detection by mass spectrometry. Three characteristic fragment ions are selected for multiple reaction monitoring, one of which usually corresponds to the transition from MH^+ to (MH^+ – 129).

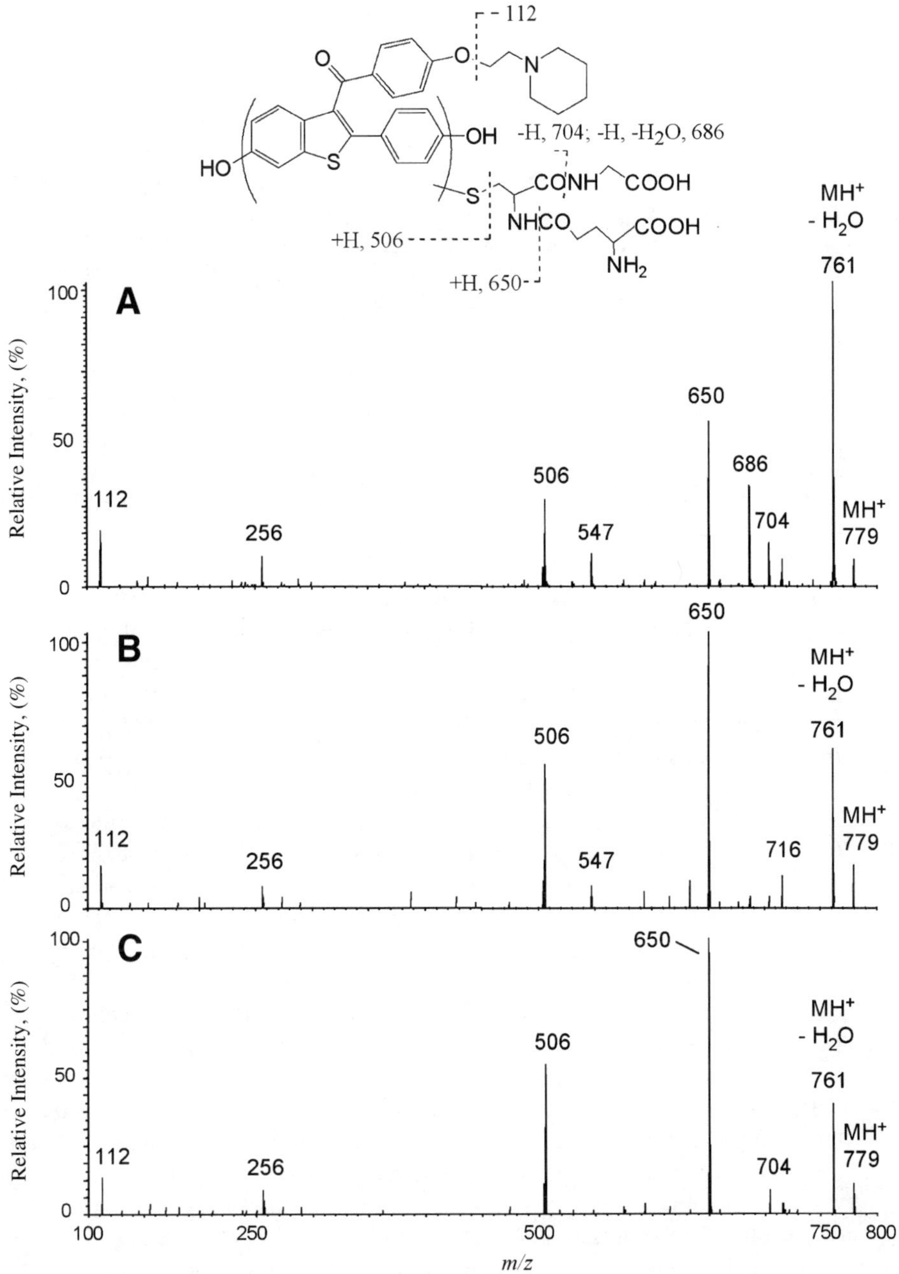

Fig. 4. Product ion mass spectra of **(A)** 7-glutathionyl-raloxifene, **(B)** 5-glutathionyl-raloxifene, and **(C)** 3'-glutathionyl-raloxifene derived from incubations of raloxifene with human liver microsomes ***(17)***. Fragmentation patterns are discussed in **Note 14**.

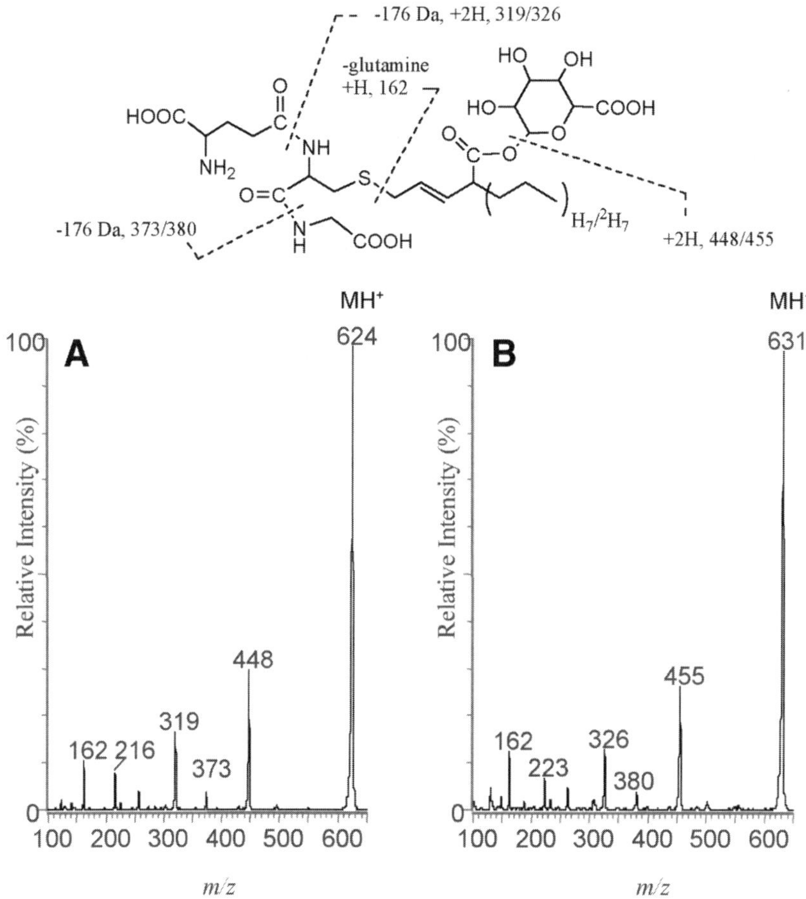

Fig. 5. Product ion mass spectra of **(A)** 5-glutathionyl-3-ene valproic acid-glucuronide and **(B)** 5-glutathionyl-3-ene [$^2H_7$]valproic acid-glucuronide in bile samples from rats treated with valproic acid derivatives ***(18)***. Fragmentation patterns are discussed in **Note 15**.

Acknowledgment

The authors would like to thank Dr. Ralph Stearns (Merck Research Laboratories) for valuable discussions.

References

1. DeLeve, L. D. and Kaplowitz, N. (1991) Glutathione metabolism and its role in hepatotoxicity. *Pharm. Ther.* **52,** 287–305.
2. Lu, S. C. (1999) Regulation of hepatic glutathione synthesis: current concepts and controversies. *FASEB J.* **13,** 1169–1183.

3. Smith, C. V., Jones, D. P., Guenthner, T. M., Lash, L. H., and Lauterburg, B. H. (1996) Compartmentation of glutathione: implications for the study of toxicity and disease. *Toxicol. Appl. Pharmacol.* **140,** 1–12.
4. Reed, D. J. (1986) Regulation of reductive processes by glutathione. *Biochem. Pharmacol.* **35,** 7–13.
5. Orrenius, S. and Moldeus, P. (1984) The multiple roles of glutathione in drug metabolism. *Trends Pharmacol. Sci.* **5,** 432–435.
6. Cohen, S. D., Pumford, N. R., Khairallah, E. A., Boekelheide, K., Pohl, L. R., Amouzadeh, H. R., et al. (1997) Selective protein covalent binding and target organ toxicity. *Toxicol. Appl. Pharmacol.* **143,** 1–12.
7. Uetrecht, J. P. (1999) New concept in immunology relevant to idiosyncratic drug reactions: the "danger hypothesis" and innate immune system. *Chem. Res. Toxicol.* **12,** 387–395.
8. Chasseaud, L. F. (1979) The role of glutathione and glutathione-S-transferases in the metabolism of chemical carcinogens and other electrophilic agents. *Adv. Cancer Res.* **29,** 175– 274.
9. Ketterer, B. and Mulder, G. (1990) Glutathione conjugation, in *Conjugation Reaction in Drug Metabolism* (Mulder, G. J., ed.), Taylor & Francis, New York, pp. 307–364.
10. Park, B. K., Pirmohamed, M., and Kitteringham, N. R. (1992) Idiosyncratic drug reactions: a mechanistic evaluation of risk factors. *Br. J. Clin. Pharmacol.* **34,** 377–395.
11. Park, B. K., Pirmohamed, M., and Kitteringham, N. R. (1998) Role of drug disposition in drug hypersensitivity: a chemical, molecular, and clinical perspective. *Chem. Res. Toxicol.* **11,** 969–988.
12. Baillie, T. A. and Kassahun, K. (2001) Biological reactive intermediates in drug discovery and development: a perspective from the pharmaceutical industry, in *Biological Reactive Intermediates VI: Chemical and Biological Mechanisms Insusceptibility to and Prevention of Environmental Diseases* (Dansette, P. M., Snyder, R., Delaforge, M., Gibson, G. G., Greim, H., Jollow, D. J., et al., eds.), Kluwer Academic/Plenum, New York, pp. 45–51.
13. Baillie, T. A. and Davis, M. R. (1993) Mass spectrometry in the analysis of glutathione conjugates. *Biol. Mass Spectrom.* **22,** 319–325.
14. Nikolic, D., Fan, P. W., Bolton, J. L., and van Breemen, R. B. (1999) Screening for xenobiotic electrophilic metabolites using pulsed ultrafiltration-mass spectrometry. *Combin. Chem. High Through. Screen.* **2,** 165–175.
15. Raucy, J. L. and Lasker, J. M. (1991) Isolation of P450 enzymes from human liver. *Meth. Enzymol.* **206,** 557–587.
16. Pang, J.-M., Zaleski, J., and Kauffman, F. C. (1997) Toxicity of allyl alcohol in primary cultures of freshly isolated and cryopreserved hepatocytes maintained on hydrated collagen gels. *Toxicol. Appl. Pharmacol.* **142,** 87–94.
17. Chen, Q., Ngui, J. S., Doss, G. A., Wang, R. W., Cai, X., DiNinno, F. P., et al. (2002) Cytochrome P450 3A4-mediated bioactivation of raloxifene: irreversible enzyme inhibition and thiol adduct formation. *Chem. Res. Toxicol.* **15,** 907–914.

18. Tang, W. and Abbott, F. S. (1996) Bioactivation of a toxic metabolite of valproic acid, (E)-2-propyl2,4-pentadienoic acid, via glucuronidation: LC/MS/MS characterization of the GSH-glucuronide diconjugates. *Chem. Res. Toxicol.* **9,** 517–526.
19. Samuel, K., Yin, W., Stearns, R. A., Tang, Y. S., Chaudhary, A. G., Jewell, J. P., et al. (2003) Addressing the metabolic activation potential of new leads in drug discovery: a case study using ion trap mass spectrometry and tritium labeling techniques. *J. Mass Spectrom.* **38,** 211–221.
20. Alt, C. and Eyer, P. (1998) Ring addition of the α-amino group of glutathione increases the reactivity of benzoquinone thioethers. *Chem. Res. Toxicol.* **11,** 1223–1233.

25

In Vitro Screening Assay of the Reactivity of Acyl Glucuronides

Sébastien Bolze

Summary

Acyl glucuronides are unstable at physiologic pH and thus can result in free aglycone by hydrolysis and lead to positional isomers by acyl migration. Acyl-migrated glucuronide isomers were shown to bind covalently to proteins in vitro and in vivo, causing potential toxicity, but the toxicological mechanisms are still unknown. Several molecules metabolized into acyl glucuronides were withdrawn from the market after adverse events of the immune allergic type were observed (zomepirac, tolmetin, benoxaprofen, ibufenac). The early identification of such reactivity for future development candidates would permit one to select equipotent products with less reactivity. The methodology to be followed in setting up an in vitro screening model of acyl glucuronide reactivity is presented. Molecules are screened according to their capacity to be metabolized into acyl glucuronides and their propensity to form covalent binding. This tool uses a linear relationship between the in vitro instability of acyl glucuronides (determined by the quantity of parent drug released) and the covalent binding levels reached with human albumin. A direct relationship between the covalent binding level obtained in this model and that observed in vivo in treated subjects also allows predicting the human in vivo level of covalent binding. Finally, these two relationships enable one to compare future development candidates to reference products that are known to be toxic (zomepirac, tolmetine) or not toxic (ibuprofen).

Key Words: Acyl glucuronides; covalent binding; reactivity; in vitro screening; in vitro/in vivo rclationship.

From: *Methods in Pharmacology and Toxicology*
Optimization in Drug Discovery: In Vitro Methods
Edited by: Z. Yan and G. W. Caldwell © Humana Press Inc., Totowa, NJ

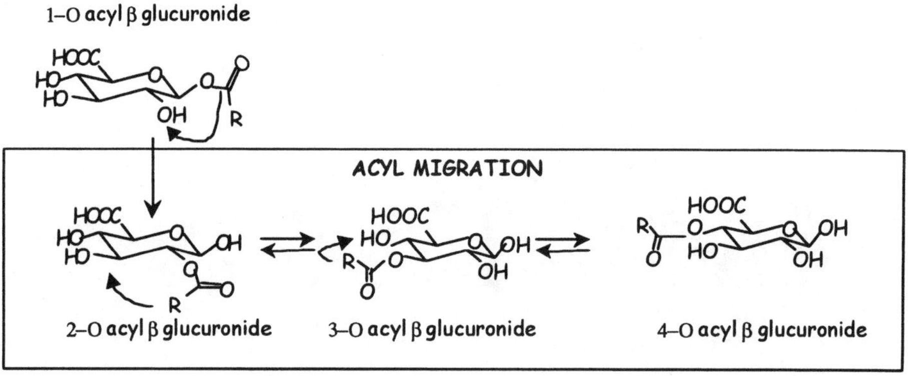

Fig. 1. Rearrangement of acyl glucuronides by intramolecular transesterification. After formation of the C-1-*O*-acyl glucuronide, the acyl residue can migrate within the glucuronic acid molecule, forming positional C-2, C-3, and C-4 isomers. The rearrangement between the last three isomers is reversible.

1. Introduction

Acyl glucuronides, resulting from the glucuroconjugation of free carboxylic acid compounds, are unstable at physiologic pH and thus can result in free aglycone by hydrolysis and lead to positional isomers by acyl migration. Acyl migration involves the transfer of the acyl group from the position 1β to the C-2, C-3, or C-4 position of the glucuronic acid ring, which results in the formation of isomeric acyl glucuronides (*see* **Fig. 1**) *(1,2)*. Acyl-migrated glucuronide isomers were shown to bind covalently to proteins in vitro and in vivo. According to the type of proteins involved, the formation of these adducts may lead to direct cytotoxicity or activate the immune system and result in autoimmune reactions against the organism. Some molecules generating this type of metabolites were withdrawn from the market after adverse events of the immune allergic type were observed (zomepirac, tolmetin, benoxaprofen, ibufenac). The early identification of such reactivity for future development candidates would permit one to select equipotent compounds that show less reactivity. The methodology to be followed in setting up an in vitro screening model of acyl glucuronide reactivity will be presented. Molecules are screened according to their capacity to be metabolized into acyl glucuronides and their propensity to form covalent binding *(3)*. The model was set up and validated with eight acidic drugs metabolized into acyl glucuronide: tolmetin, zomepirac, diclofenac, fenoprofen, ketoprofen, ibuprofen, suprofen, and furosemide. These drugs have been studied extensively and represent a large scale of reactive products *(4–13)*. The screening tool presented uses a linear in vitro relationship between the instability of acyl glucuronides (determined by the quantity of parent drug released) and the covalent binding levels reached with human albumin. A direct relationship between the covalent binding level obtained in this model and that observed in vivo in treated subjects also allows predicting the human in vivo level of covalent binding. These two relationships enable one to compare the expected in vivo reactivity in humans of future development candidates to reference products that are known to be toxic (zomepirac, tolmetin) or not toxic (ibuprofen). This chapter describes the methodology used to screen the in vitro reactivity of acyl glucuronide. The experimental protocol will be presented first, and then the interpretation of data generated will be discussed. Some modifications have been made recently to this assay method and will be presented in **Subheading 4.**

2. Materials

2.1. In Vitro Biosynthesis of Acyl Glucuronides

1. Pooled human hepatic microsomes from 29 donors (BIOPREDIC INTERNATIONAL, Rennes, France).
2. UDPAG (Sigma, U 4375).
3. UDPGA (Sigma, U 6751).
4. Potassium dihydrogen phosphate (Merck, 4873).
5. Sodium hydrogen phosphate (Merck, 6346).
6. $MgCl_2$ (Prolabo, 29 761.152).
7. TRIS (Sigma, G 2128).
8. H_2O (Carlo Erba, 307586).
9. Trifluoroacetic acid (TFA) (Aldrich, T6,220-0).
10. Dimethylsulfoxide (DMSO) (Merck, 1.02952.1000).

2.2. In Vitro Biosynthesis of Acyl Glucuronides

1. Human serum albumin (HSA) (Sigma, 040K7606) V fraction of human serum, 96% to 99% per agarose gel.
2. β-Glucuronidase (Sigma, G 0501).
3. β-Glucuronidase (Boehringer, 127051).
4. Phenolphtalein-1-*O*-glucuronic acid (Sigma, P0501).
5. 4-Nitrophenyl glucuronic acid (Sigma, N 1627).

2.3. Analytical Method

1. Acetonitrile (Merck, 1.14291.2500).
2. Methanol (Merck, 152506).
3. Ethyl acetate (Prolabo, 23 882.296).
4. Formica acid (Sigma, 503721).
5. Acetic acid (Carlo Erba, 401422).
6. Hydrochloric acid, 37% RPE (Sigma, G 3126).

7. Ammonium acetate (Sigma, A 7330).
8. High-performance liquid chromatography (HPLC) pumps (Perkin-Elmer series 200).
9. Autosampler (Perkin-Elmer, series 200).
10. Mass spectrometer (Applied Biosystems API 365 operating with a turbo ion spray).
11. Analytical column (Thermoquest Hypersil BDS 150 × 4.6 mm, 5 μ*M*).
12. SPE cartridges (Waters Oasis HLB).
13. Vortex.
14. Centrifuge (Heraeus Instrument Megafuge 1.0 R).
15. Analytical balance (Mettler, AE 240).

3. Methods

3.1. General Principle

The reactivity of acyl glucuronides is assessed by their instability (hydrolysis + isomerization) and by their propensity to form covalent binding to human serum albumin. The model developed allows in a single experiment the study of (1) the percentage of acyl glucuronide produced by human microsomal UGTs, (2) the determination of relevant hydrolysis and isomerization rates, and (3) the extent of covalent binding to human albumin.

The experiment is divided into two steps. The first phase (phase of enzymatiÄ∏synthesis) allows the synthesis of acyl glucuronides using human hepatic microsomes. The second phase (reactivity phase) is dedicated to determining the hydrolysis and isomerization rate constants of 1-*O*-acyl glucuronide and the extent of covalent binding.

3.2. In Vitro Biosynthesis of Acyl Glucuronides

Test compounds are incubated at 400 μ*M* in triplicate for 4 h at 37°C with human liver microsomes (3 mg/mL) in 100 m*M* Tris buffer, pH 7.4, containing 1% DMSO, 5 m*M* $MgCl_2$, 5 m*M* UDPGA, and 1 m*M* UDPAG (final volume: 4.8 mL) (*see* **Note 1**). Two 400-μL aliquots are withdrawn after 0 and 4 h incubation to know the exact concentration of aglycone incubated at the beginning and to determine the amount of 1-*O*-β acyl glucuronide and acyl glucuronide isomers formed, as well as the residual amount of aglycone in the medium. The reaction is stopped by protein precipitation with the addition of TFA (pH lowered to 3.0–4.0). After centrifugation at 2560*g* for 10 min, the supernatants are collected and frozen at –80°C until analysis to determine the amount of synthesized acyl glucuronides.

3.3. Acyl Glucuronide Reactivity

At the end of the 4-h incubation, the residual mixture is centrifuged at 640*g* for 20 min (withdrawal of microsomes). The supernatant (3 mL) is transferred into new capped tubes and incubated with 0.5 m*M* HSA. At the sampling times of 15 min, 30 min, 1 h, 2 h, 4 h, 6 h, and 24 h, a 300-µL aliquot is withdrawn and transferred into a tube containing 1 mL 4% TFA in acetonitrile, then centrifuged at 640*g* for 10 min. Supernatants are collected and frozen at –80°C. Protein pellets are washed with 1 mL 5% aqueous TFA (gentle shaking for 10 min, then centrifugation at 640*g* for 10 min), then three times successively with 1 mL methanol (*see* **Note 2**). Washed protein pellets, as well as dry residues from supernatants from the last washing step only, are frozen at –80°C. Controls are performed in parallel and treated identically, except that no glucuroconjugation cofactors are added during the incubation phase with microsomes. One 400-µL aliquot is withdrawn after 0 and 4 h incubation and treated like the aliquots from the biosynthesis phase. The residual mixture is centrifuged at 640*g* for 20 min, and the supernatant (1 mL) is transferred into a new capped tube and undergoes the reactivity phase of acyl glucuronides (i.e., incubation for various times with 0.5 m*M* HSA). After an incubation period of 6 h and 24 h, a 300-µL aliquot is withdrawn and treated like the other aliquots from the reactivity phase.

3.4. Analytical Method

The samples generated by the various incubations are analyzed by a generic liquid chromatography/tandem mass spectrometry (LC/MS-MS) method. This method was developed with the objective to separate the different acyl glucuronide isomers from their aglycone. This separation was achieved using a gradient elution mode. The same analytical column was used for all compounds, that is, the hypersylBDS column (150 × 4.6 mm id, 5 µ*M*, Thermoquest). The mobile phase is composed of solvent A and solvent B. Solvent A is a mixture of 10 m*M* acetonitrile-acetate ammonium buffer (70:30 [v/v]) + 0.5% acetic acid. Solvent B is a mixture of 10 m*M* acetonitrile-acetate ammonium buffer (4:96 [v/v]). Because the chemical structures of the studied compounds may differ from the others, it is necessary to adjust the gradient profile for each compound while keeping a flow rate of 1 mL/min and a runtime of approx 15 min.

A number of peaks higher than four acyl glucuronide isomers may be observed sometimes. This is because of the resolutive properties of the column compared to the anomeric and enantiomeric forms. Examples of separation

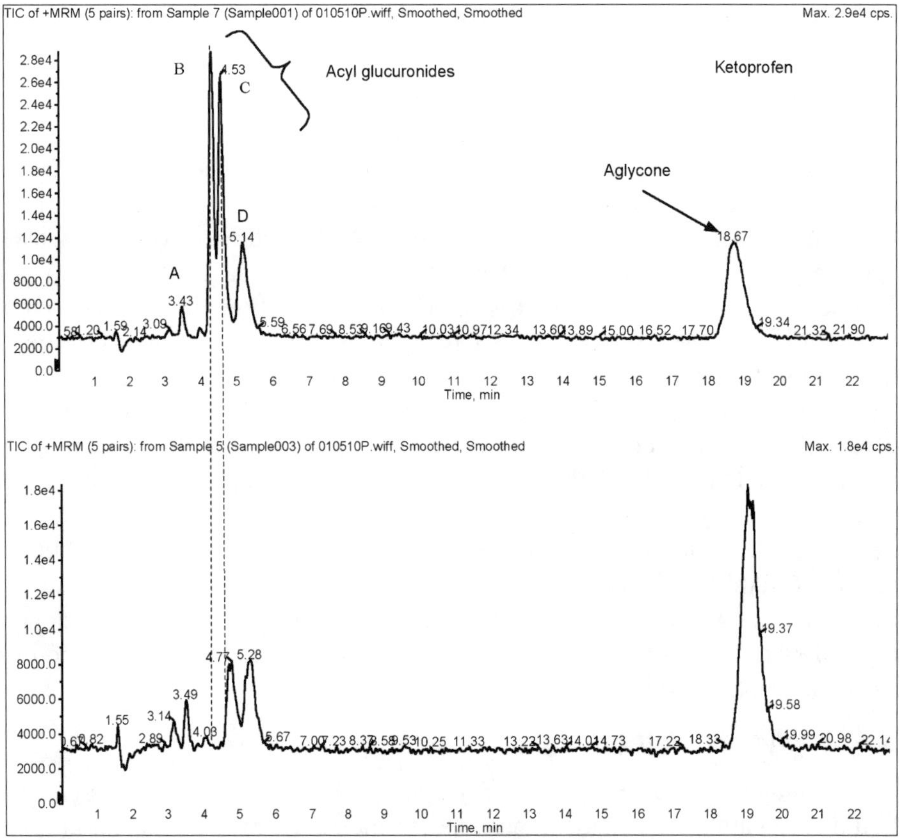

Fig. 2. Representative separation by LC/MS-MS of acyl glucuronides of a chiral compound ketoprofen (top) and identification of 1-*O*-β-acyl glucuronide after hydrolysis with β-glucuronidase (bottom).

obtained for chiral (ketoprofen) and achiral (zomepirac) compounds are presented in **Figs. 2** and **3** (*see* **Note 3**).

Detection and quantification are achieved by tandem mass spectrometry using an ionization source: *turbo ion spray* (API 365 Applied Biosystems, Toronto, Canada).

Concentrations of aglycone, 1-*O*-β-acyl glucuronide, and acyl glucuronide isomers are determined in the supernatants collected during the biosynthesis and reactivity phases of acyl glucuronides. The principle of the assay is summarized in **Fig. 4**. Each sample is divided into three aliquots. In the first aliquot, the aglycone concentration is determined. The second aliquot is incubated with 1000 U of bovine β-glucuronidase at 37°C for 2 h to hydrolyze $β_1$ conju-

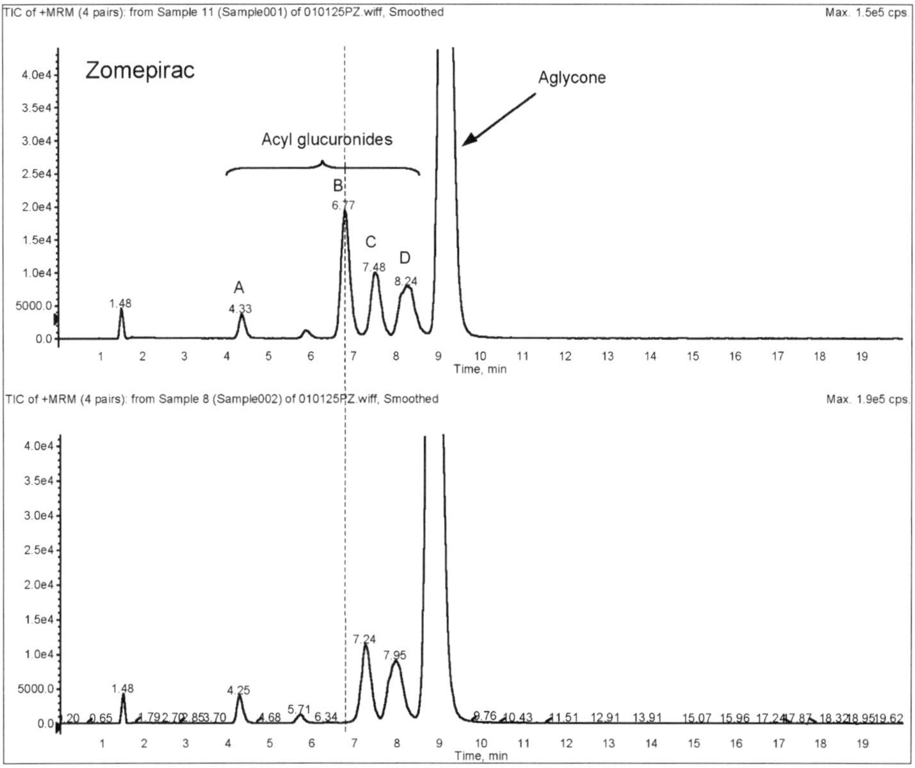

Fig. 3. Representative separation by LC/MS-MS of acyl glucuronides of an achiral compound zomepirac (top) and identification of 1-*O*-β-acyl glucuronide after hydrolysis by β-glucuronidase (bottom).

gates and release the corresponding aglycone part. A positive control (i.e., phenolphtalein-1-*O*-glucuronide) is examined to verify the β-glucuronidase enzyme activity. The aglycone concentration found after hydrolysis minus the aglycone concentration determined earlier will correspond to the 1-*O*-β-acyl glucuronide concentration. In the same way, the third aliquot will be submitted to alkaline hydrolysis (1 *N* KOH at 80°C for 3 h) to hydrolyze all acyl glucuronides into their corresponding aglycone. The concentration of acyl glucuronide isomers is estimated as the difference between total aglycone concentration and aglycone concentration resulting from β_1 conjugate cleavage.

The extent of covalent binding to human serum albumin is evaluated for each molecule. Protein pellets obtained during the reactivity phase after extensive washing are submitted to alkaline hydrolysis (1 *N* KOH at 80°C for 3 h). Moles of aglycone released by this procedure are considered as irreversibly

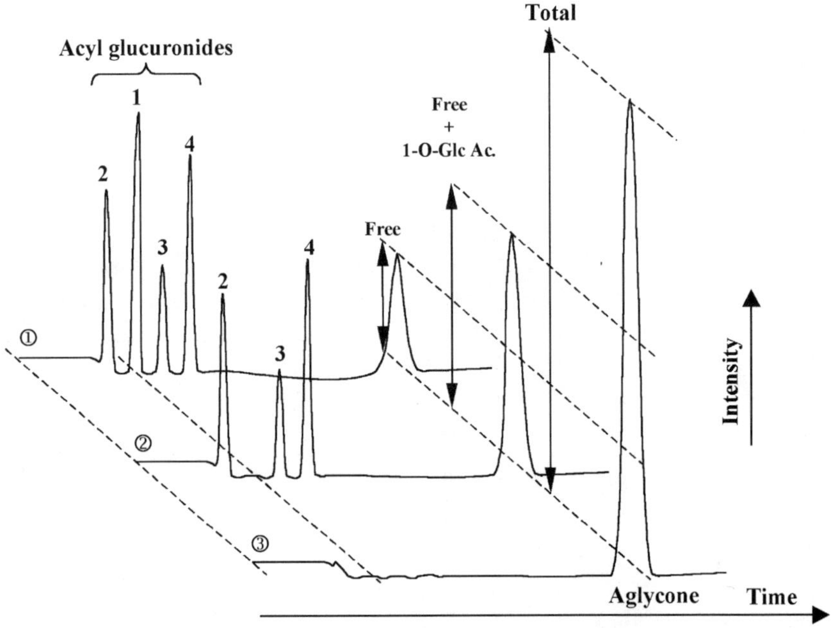

Fig. 4. Principle of the assay. (1) Theoretical chromatogram obtained after drug incubation with microsomes or HSA: 1-, 2-, 3-, and 4-*O*-acyl glucuronide are separated, and aglycone is assayed. (2) Samples are hydrolyzed with β-glucuronidase to determine the 1-*O*-acyl glucuronide concentration (difference [2] – [1]). (3) Concentration of acyl glucuronide isomers is obtained after alkaline hydrolysis ([3] –[1]).

bound to HSA. Protein pellets from control samples performed without cofactors are also submitted to alkaline hydrolysis. Although no aglycone release is expected, the detected levels are considered as background noise of the assay and are subtracted from the results obtained.

Samples for the determination of aglycone and 1-*O*-β-acyl glucuronide concentrations are diluted in the mobile phase 10-fold to 40-fold, depending on the sensitivity of the compound in MS/MS, before injection into the analytical system. Calibration curves are prepared by using the appropriate amount of blank matrix (microsomes or HSA). Samples for the determination of 1-*O*-β-acyl glucuronide concentration are incubated for 2 h at 37°C with β-glucuronidase. The calibration curves are prepared by using the appropriate amount of blank matrix (microsomes or HSA) as well as the appropriate amount of β-glucuronidase. Samples for the determination of the acyl glucuronide isomer and covalent binding concentrations are extracted by a solid/liquid extraction method (SPE) using Oasis HLB cartridges. Briefly, cartridges are conditioned by 1 mL of methanol followed by 1 mL of water. Then, samples are loaded onto the cartridges. The cartridges are washed with 1 mL of water. Elution is based on 1 mL of the acetonitrile/10 m*M* ammonium acetate buffer (75:25 [v/v]) + 0.05% acetic acid mixture. The collected phase is evaporated to dryness and then taken up with the mobile phase before injection into the analytical system.

Calibration ranges are prepared in the chromatographic mobile phase. Dry residues from the last washing fraction of protein pellets are dissolved in 1 mL of the chromatographic mobile phase and analyzed to ensure the exhaustiveness of the washing procedure previously developed. Only traces of free aglycone or free acyl glucuronide should still remain. The chromatographic peak area of each analyte calculated by the mass spectrometry software is used for quantification together with a calibration curve of 50 to 10,000 ng/mL. Quality control (QC) samples are prepared for each phase of the model at three concentrations (15, 150, and 300 μ*M*). Cofactors are added only at the end of the incubation period for QCs of the biosynthesis phase. QCs of the reactivity phase are incubated with HSA for a selected duration and then treated like the samples of the experiment. QCs are used to ensure accuracy and precision of the assay.

3.5. Data Analysis

Data generated during the incubation of diclofenac in the screening model conditions will be used to illustrate the data analysis procedure. Similarly, this procedure can be applied for new compounds tested in the model.

3.5.1. Determination of the Extent of Metabolization

The first step of the model consists of acyl glucuronide synthesis by human liver microsomes in straight conditions. The conditions chosen and fixed allow an estimation of the capability of each drug to be metabolized into acyl glucuronide. In those conditions, the metabolization of diclofenac is important and leads to 90% of acyl glucuronide.

3.5.2. Determination of the Degradation Rate Constant

The degradation rate is defined as the initial loss of the 1-*O*-β-acyl glucuronide component. Hydrolysis is defined as the initial formation of the aglycone, and acyl migration (isomerization) is defined as the formation of positional isomers. According to Sidelmann et al. ***(14)***, the hydrolysis rate is calculated as the degradation rate corrected for the formation of positional isomers, and the acyl migration rate is calculated as the degradation rate corrected for hydrolysis. Kinetic data of the degradation of acyl glucuronides are calculated by nonlinear regression analysis of the measured data using the equation for first-order reaction kinetics: $C = C(0)e^{-kt}$. In the same way, aglycone release

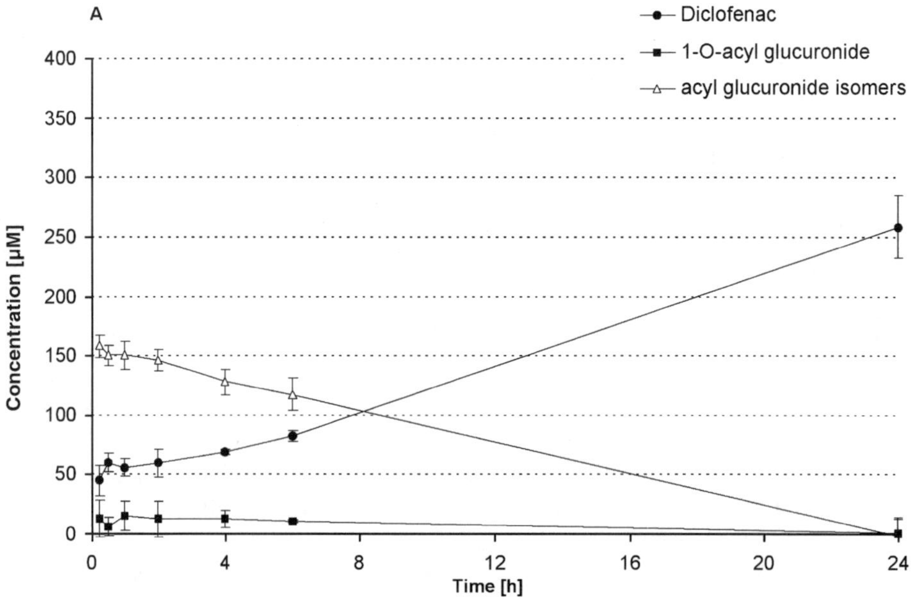

Fig. 5. Time-courses of rearrangement and hydrolysis of diclofenac acyl glucuronide in 0.15 m*M* phosphate buffer containing 0.5 m*M* of HSA, pH 7.4, at 37°C. (Each point and vertical bar represent the mean ± SD of three independent series.)

kinetic data are analyzed by nonlinear regression analysis using the equation for first-order reaction kinetics: $C = C(0)e^{kt}$.

During the second incubation step, supernatant from the first incubation is incubated with 0.15 m*M* phosphate buffer containing 0.5 m*M* HSA for 24 h. The disposition kinetics of 1-*O*-acyl glucuronide and its isomers and aglycone are monitored. An example of diclofenac acyl glucuronides behavior is shown in **Fig. 4**. Extensive acyl migration could occur during the process between the two steps. So, a majority of acyl glucuronide isomers could be detected from early kinetic points, as shown in **Fig. 5** (*see* **Note 3**). Therefore, the acyl glucuronide degradation rate calculated represents the degradation of acyl glucuronide isomers. Apparent first-order degradation of acyl glucuronide isomers and the aglycone appearance constant are determined by nonlinear regression analysis (*see* **Fig. 6**). The percentage of isomerization observed between the two incubation steps is calculated according to the following equation: [(acyl glucuronide isomers at the beginning of the second incubation – acyl glucuronide isomers at the end of the fist incubation)/(total acyl glucuronide) × 100]. The result is that 72% of diclofenac acyl glucuronide undergoes isomerization between the two steps.

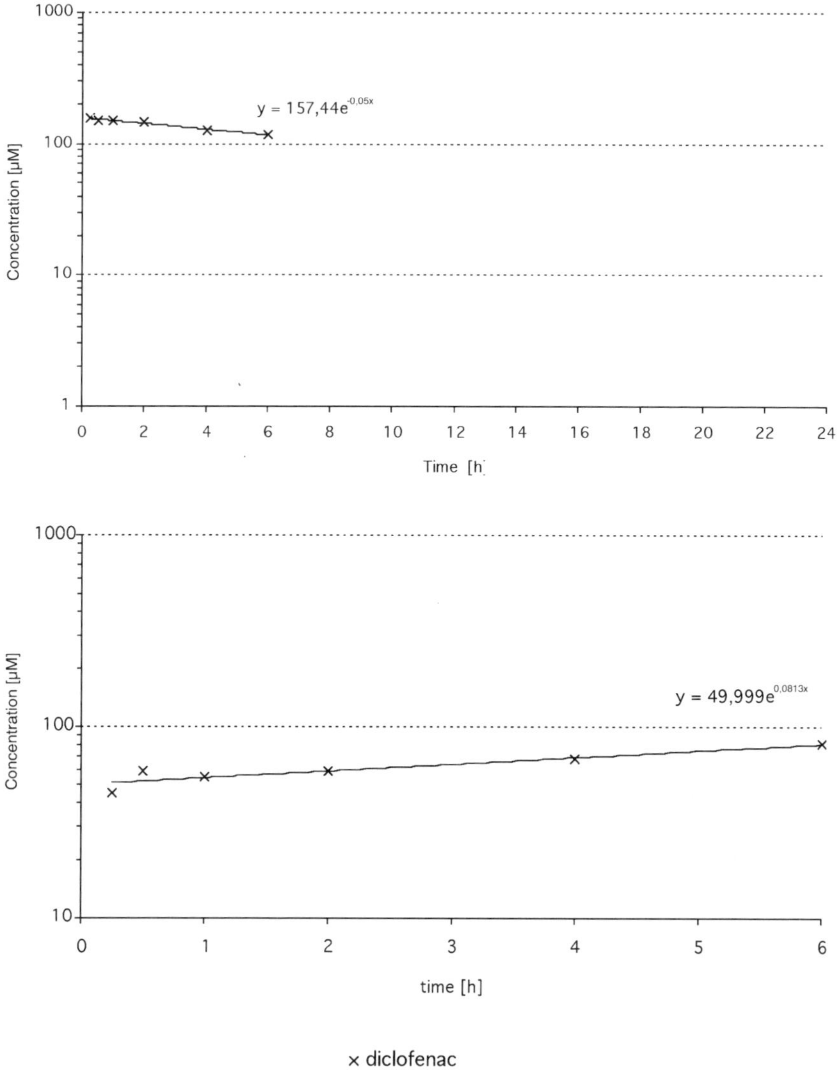

Fig. 6. Nonlinear regression analysis of the degradation of whole acyl glucuronide (top) and appearance of diclofenac (bottom) during incubation at 37°C, pH 7.4, with HSA.

3.5.3. Determination of Covalent Binding Levels

The time dependence for irreversible binding to HSA of each acyl glucuronide studied is also investigated during the second incubation step. The extent of covalent binding is expressed in mmoles of aglycone covalently bound

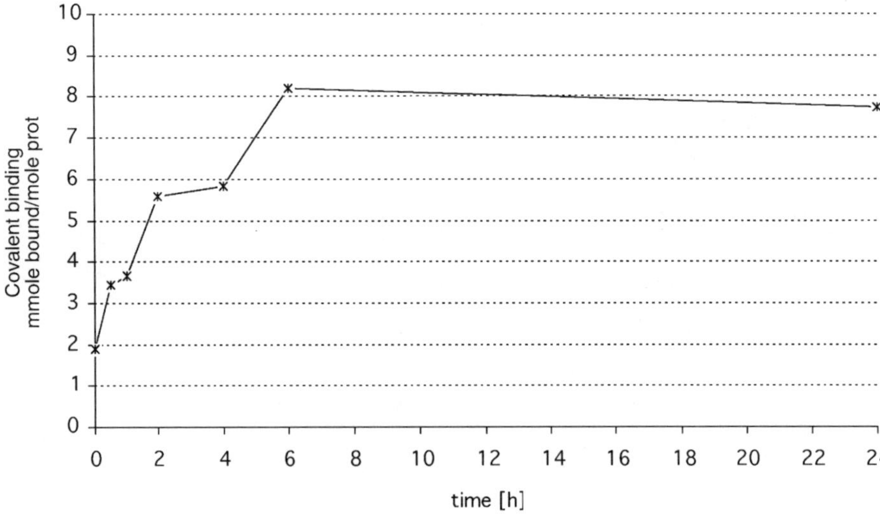

Fig. 7. Time-dependent irreversible binding of diclofenac after incubation of its acyl glucuronide (produced by HLM: incubation of 400 μ*M* aglycone) in 0.5 m*M*, pH 7.4, human serum albumin solution at 37°C. Data are the average of triplicate measurements.

per mole of protein. The time-course of covalent binding of diclofenac acyl glucuronide is shown in **Fig. 7**. The amount of drug irreversibly bound is obviously related to the amount of acyl glucuronide present at the beginning of the "reactivity phase." Thus, the extent of covalent binding is normalized to protein content and expressed as the percentage of total acyl glucuronide present at the beginning of the "reactivity phase." The maximum of the covalent binding reach with diclofenac acyl glucuronide is 8.2 mmol bound per mmol of protein incubated. When taking into account the amount of acyl glucuronide present at the beginning, the maximum of covalent binding observed represents 2.5% of the acyl glucuronide synthesized.

3.5.4. In Vitro Reactivity Scale

During the setup and validation of this in vitro screening method of the reactivity of acyl glucuronide ***(3)***, an excellent correlation was described between the maximal amount of drug bound, expressed as the percentage of acyl glucuronide present in the incubation medium, and the aglycone appearance rate constant weighted by the percentage of isomerization observed between the two incubation steps ($r^2 = 0.94$) (*see* **Fig. 8**). The extent of covalent binding could be predicted on the basis of the acyl glucuronide hydrolysis rate combined with the acyl migration propensity. The combination of these two

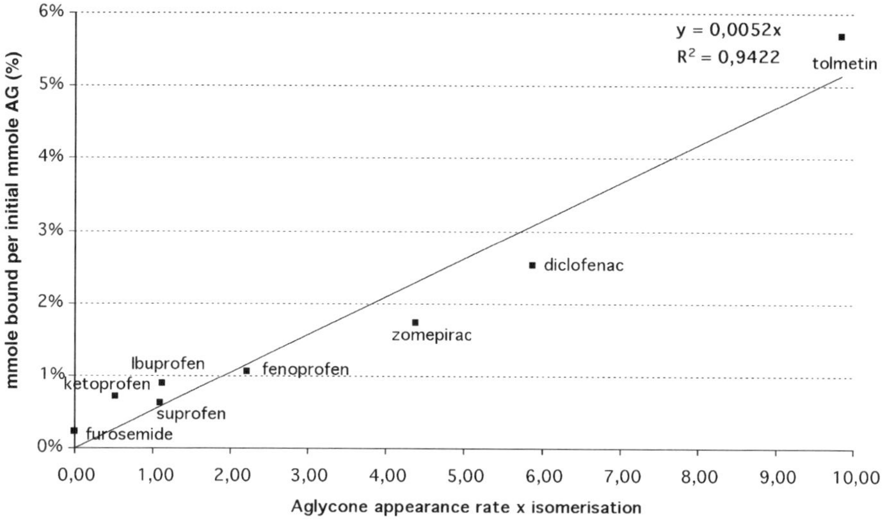

Fig. 8. Correlation between the extent of covalent binding (protein content normalized and expressed as a percentage of total acyl glucuronide present at the beginning of the reactivity phase) vs the aglycone appearance rate constant weighted by the percentage of isomerization (between the "biosynthesis" and "reactivity" phases) (h^{-1}) during in vitro incubation of various acyl glucuronides with HSA (0.5 m*M*).

parameters seems to be more accurate for the covalent binding prediction than the 1-*O*-acyl glucuronide degradation rate used by Benet et al. ***(15)***. An in vitro reactivity scale was thus established with eight reference compounds from the literature (tolmetin, zomepirac, fenoprofen, ketoprofen, ibuprofen, suprofen, diclofenac, and furosemide). This in vitro reactivity scale allows the ranking of new drugs screened on the model according to their covalent binding potential.

Diclofenac, as with any new drug tested, can be positioned on the scale because of its *x*-axis value, 5.87 (0.081 aglycone appearance rate × 72.2 isomerization %), and its *y*-axis value, 2.5% (amount of compound bound/initial amount of acyl glucuronides × 100).

The protocol recently has been optimized, and the modifications made are described in **Note 4**.

3.5.5. In Vitro/In Vivo Relationship

The different presented models allow for the assessment of the intrinsic instability of acyl glucuronides. We saw that the latter is directly related to the extent of covalent binding to albumin observed in vitro. The final objective is of course to predict the expected extent of covalent binding in vivo in humans. Even if the covalent binding limit that should not be exceeded is difficult to determine, this prediction would allow a comparison based on clinical criteria between the extents obtained with new compounds and those obtained with toxic reference compounds such as zomepirac and tolmetin.

In our in vitro model, the extent of covalent binding is expressed as the ratio (amount of bound compound/initial amount of acyl glucuronides). A literature data review showed that it was possible to obtain a similar criterion in vivo ***(15)***. In fact, Benet et al. ***(15)*** proposed normalizing the amount of covalent binding found in vivo by the area under the curve of acyl glucuronide plasma concentrations (AUC_{AG}). It would be ideal if a relation could be found between these two criteria so that in vitro data could be linked to the in vivo situation. Unfortunately, few published studies are giving results of covalent binding and AUC_{AG} in vivo. Benet et al. presented such results for five compounds (tolmetin, zomepirac, fenoprofen, carprofen, beclofibric acid). Castillo et al. ***(16)*** also published this type of data for ibuprofen. Furthermore, this type of data is also available for the two internal compounds: drug 1 and drug 2 (in-house data).

A relation could be established between the published values of the ratio (amount of covalent binding in vivo/AUC_{AG}) and the value of the ratio (amount of covalent binding in vitro/initial AG amount) experimentally found and is presented in **Fig. 8**. The correlation found between the ratios assessing in vivo and in vitro covalent binding was satisfactory for the six compounds (r^2 = 0.957). The extent of covalent binding in vivo could be predicted from values obtained in vitro with our model. As an example, the in vivo covalent binding levels are predicted for two compounds (ketoprofen, suprofen) tested in the in vitro screening model (open circles in **Fig. 9**).

In conclusion, we have described the methodology to be used for implementing a screening tool for the prediction of acyl glucuronide reactivity in early development phases.

This in vitro model allows the synthesis of acyl glucuronide metabolites from the test compound by human liver microsomes, as well as the assessment of their reactivity. A linear relation between in vitro acyl glucuronide instability (measured by the release of parent drug) and the extent of covalent binding to human albumin can be used for ranking new chemical entities. A direct relation between the extent of in vitro covalent binding in our model and that observed in vivo in treated subjects can also serve to predict in vivo covalent binding levels. Even if there is still no answer to one of the fundamental questions ("Is there a limit extent to trigger off toxic effects?"), these two relations enable one to compare future development candidates with a free carboxylic acid function to reference compounds known to be toxic (zomepirac, tolmetin) or not toxic (ibuprofen).

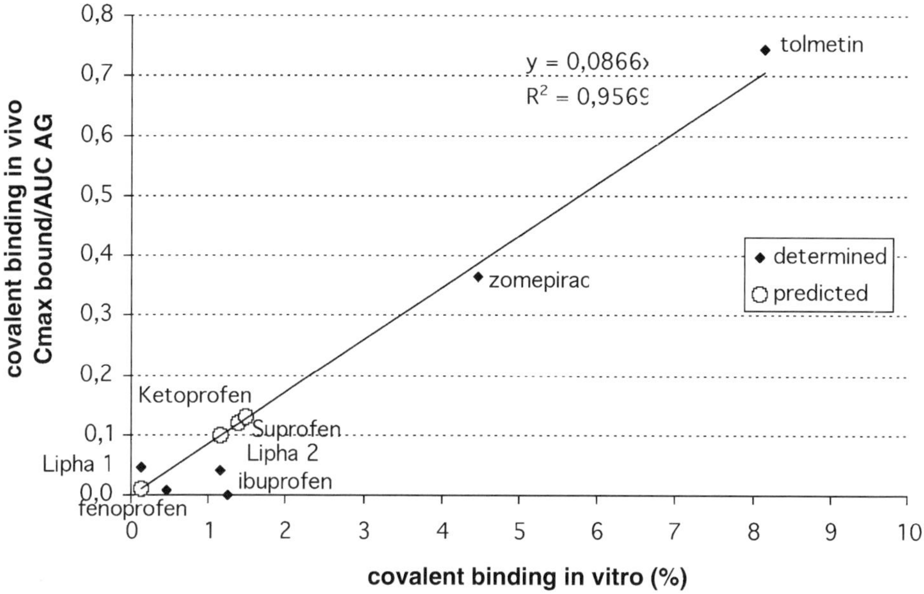

Fig. 9. In vitro/in vivo correlation of the extent of acyl glucuronide covalent binding to human albumin.

4. Notes

1. The first "biosynthesis" phase was designed with straightforward experimental conditions for standardization purposes. Human liver microsomes were used for the production of acyl glucuronides because they are easy to work on. High protein concentration (3 mg/mL), high drug concentration (400 μ*M*) of incubation, and long incubation duration (4 h) were chosen as standard conditions to maximize the biosynthesis of acyl glucuronide but were not specifically optimized for each case. They should allow for the comparison of the acyl glucuronidation potential between compounds from the same chemical family. In the same way, human serum albumin was chosen as a reference target protein to assess the extent of covalent binding during the "reactivity" phase. The extent of covalent binding was shown to vary greatly depending on the nature of the albumin preparation used ***(6,17)***. Thus, in vitro assays on covalent binding to proteins can be expected to be highly variable. Moreover, plasmatic proteins are not the only targets of covalent binding. Acyl glucuronides could irreversibly bind to several tissues or organ macromolecules. However, HSA remains the most extensively studied protein. It is largely distributed in the plasmatic compartment and easily related to the immune system. The knowledge accumulated about the covalent binding of acyl glucuronide and HSA allowed the comparison and validation of the results obtained with this model.

2. The washing procedure of the protein pellet used has been validated for eight reference compounds. The exhaustiveness of this washing procedure is very important. Indeed, the covalent binding level is determined by the amount of parent drug released after alkaline hydrolysis of the pellet, and any unspecific binding to the pellet of the parent drug or the acyl glucuronide may lead to over-estimation of the covalent binding level. The protein pellet is washed several times with solvants showing different polarities. The following protocol may be applied:

   First washing: 1 mL TFA 5%, moderate agitation 10 min.

   Second, third, and fourth washings: 1 mL methanol, moderate agitation 10 min.

   Fifth, sixth, and seventh washings: 1 mL ethyl acetate, moderate agitation 10 min.

   Each washing fraction is collected and analyzed by LC/MS-MS to determine the residual amount of parent drug or acyl glucuronide. The first washing fraction that does not have any trace of aglycone or acyl glucuronide is considered the last washing step to be performed. The washing by TFA and the third washing by methanol seem sufficient to withdraw all residual traces of the parent drug from the protein pellet for the eight drugs tested. This washing procedure has to be optimized before starting incubations for each new chemical series of drugs.
3. Extensive acyl migration could occur during the process between the two incubation steps. A majority of acyl glucuronide isomers can be detected from early kinetic points. The generic analytical method developed allows a good separation between 1-*O*-acyl glucuronide and its isomers but not always between the isomers themselves. This isomer resolution is time-consuming and not compatible with a screening purpose and thus is not always optimized. Therefore, high isomerization could not be seen because levels of isomers remain constant. Only the time-dependent degradation of acyl glucuronide isomers by hydrolysis can be followed.
4. When developing our screening model of acyl glucuronide reactivity, we were faced with several problems:

   Difficulties in separating acyl glucuronide isomers from each other.

   Heaviness of the assays with β-glucuronidase.

   Loss of compound between the two phases.

   Extensive isomerization between the two phases.

   Significant traces of residue in the last washing fraction for three compounds.

   To solve these problems, we decided to introduce radioactivity in our model. The use of the labeled glucuroconjugation cofactor allows the synthesis of ^{14}C-labeled acyl glucuronides. The radioactivity specificity could therefore allow a better follow-up of the evolution of synthesized acyl glucuronides. We also modified the end of the first phase in the protocol and replaced the centrifugation step to withdraw microsomes by a better performing and faster ultracentrifugation (15 min at 150,000*g* and at 4°C) to reduce the isomerization phenomenon and the loss of compound between the two phases. The general principal of the model is unchanged. The experiment is still divided into two phases: the first one (enzyme synthesis phase) allows the synthesis of acyl glucuronides by human liver microsomes, and the second one (reactivity phase) is

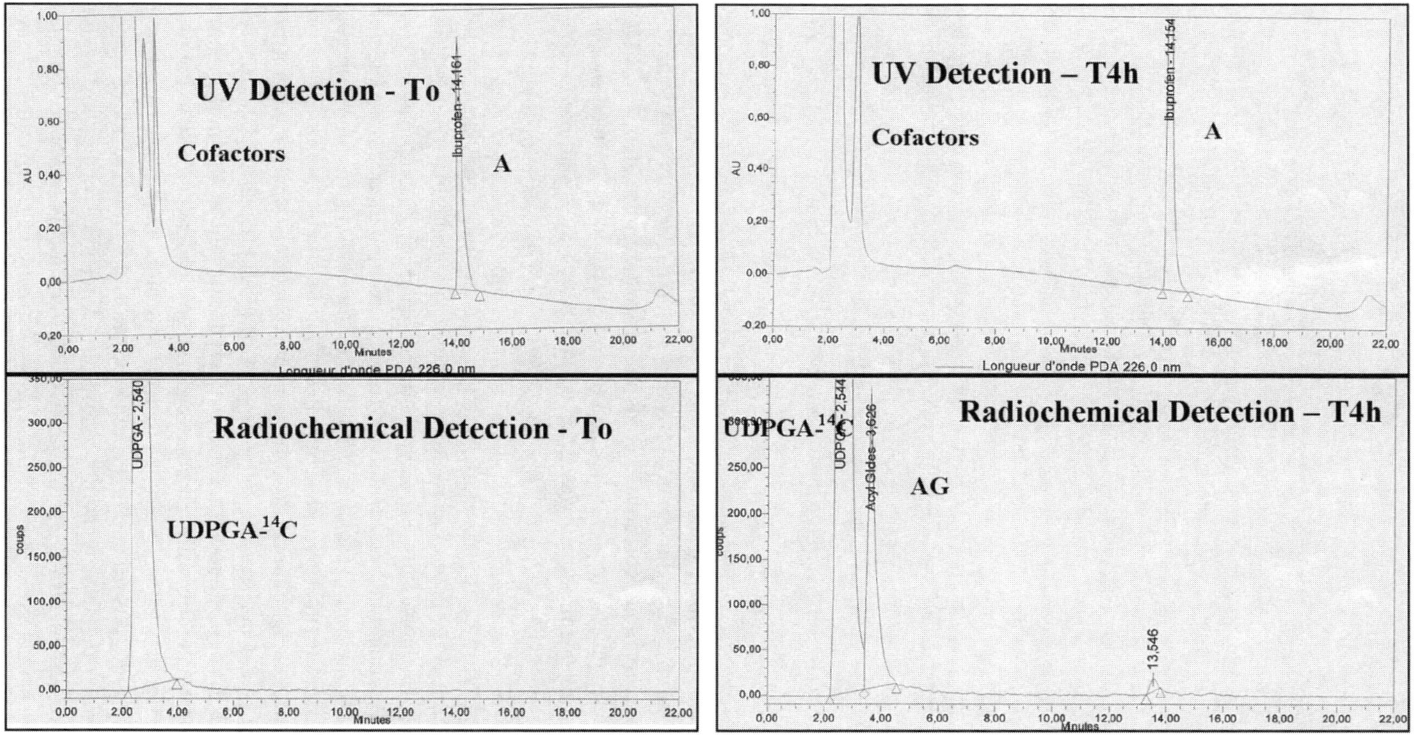

Fig. 10. Biosynthesis phase of acyl glucuronides. Example of chromatograms obtained by UV and radioactivity detection at T0 and T4 h. A, aglycone; AG, acyl glucuronides.

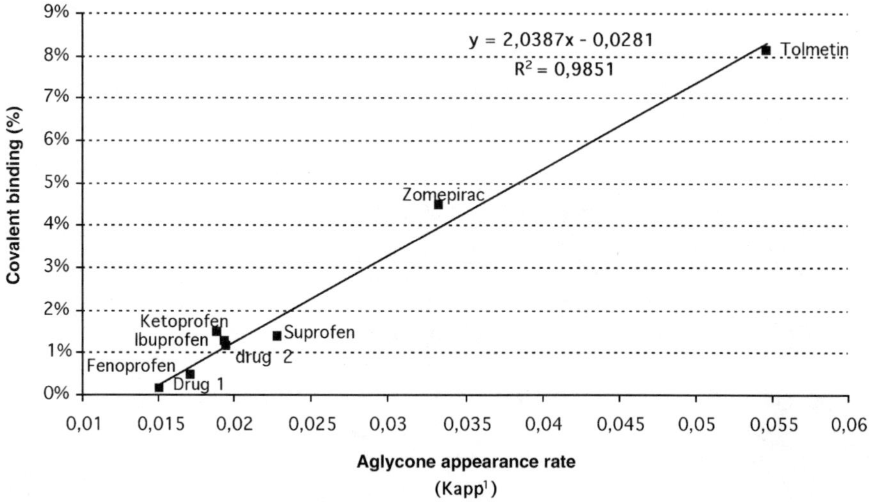

Fig. 11. Correlation between the extent of covalent binding (%) vs aglycone appearance constant.

dedicated to determining the hydrolysis and isomerization rate constants of 1-*O*-acyl glucuronides and the extent of covalent binding. The only modification made to the experimental protocol concerns the first incubation step. [^{14}C]-UDPGA was added to the medium to radiolabel the acyl glucuronides formed. The amount of radioactivity introduced was 222 kBecquerels (6 μCi), and the ratio of cold UDPGA to labeled UDPGA was approx 300. All other experimental conditions remained strictly equivalent.

The integration of the peaks detected by the radiodetector allowed a direct quantitation of the acyl glucuronide concentration. The intensity of the detected signal was proportional to the concentration of labeled compound. Aglycones were detected and quantitated by UV (at λ_{max}) using a diode array detector (*see* **Fig. 10**). A calibration range was determined for each matrix type (supernatants of the various incubations, protein pellets).

In the new selected conditions, the phenomenon of isomerization between the two phases did not seem to be as important as that observed previously. The phenomenon of isomerization obviously predominated earlier in the incubation with albumin and thus slowed down the aglycone release. The maximum covalent binding achieved for each compound was more important than that found when the model was set up. This could be explained by the absence of isomerization between the two incubation phases. In fact, covalent binding is directly related to isomerization. During the first hours of incubation with albumin, the neo-synthesized acyl glucuronides will, according to their own reactivity, undergo isomerization and thus covalently bind to albumin. The same reactivity scale as previously described was obtained, relating the maximum amount of compound (expressed as the percentage of the initial amount of acyl glucuronides) bound per mole of protein with the acyl glucuronide degradation rate expressed as the rate of aglycone appearance ($K_{app.\,A}{}^{-1}$) (*see* **Fig. 11**). The correlation does not need a weighting by isomerization because the phenomenon is taken directly into account in assessing the aglycone appearance rate in the medium. The modified protocol just described was tested on eight carboxylic drugs. Six were tested on the previous model—tolmetin, zomepirac, suprofen, ketoprofen, ibuprofen, and fenoprofen—and two internal compounds, drugs 1 and 2, were added.

References

1. Faed, E. M. (1984) Properties of acyl glucuronides: implications for studies of the pharmacokinetics and metabolism of acidic drugs. *Drug Metab. Disp.* **15,** 1213–1249.
2. Spahn-Langguth, H. and Benet, L. Z. (1992) Acyl glucuronides revisited: is the glucuronidation process a toxification as well as a detoxification mechanism? *Drug Metab. Rev.* **24,** 5–48.
3. Bolze, S., Bromet, N., Gay-Feutry, C., Massiere, F., Boulieu, R., and Hulot, T. (2002) Development of an in vitro screening model for the biosynthesis of acyl glucuronide metabolites and the assessment of their reactivity toward human serum albumin. *Drug Metab. Disp.* **30,** 404–413.
4. Hyneck, M. L., Smith, P. C., Mufano, A., McDonagh, F. A., and Benet, L. Z. (1988) Disposition and irreversible plasma protein binding of tolmetin in humans. *Clin. Pharmacol. Ther.* **44,** 107–114.
5. Smith, P. C., McDonagh, A. F., and Benet, L. Z. (1986) Irreversible binding of zomepirac to plasma protein in vitro and in vivo. *J. Clin. Invest.* **77,** 934–939.
6. Ebner, T., Heinzel, G., Prox, A., Beschke, K., and Wachsmuth, H. (1999) Disposition and chemical stability of telmisartan 1-0-acylglucuronide. *Drug Metab. Disp.* **27,** 1143–1149.
7. Volland, C., Sun, H., Dammeyer, J., and Benet, L. Z. (1991) Stereoselective degradation of the fenoprofen acyl glucuronide enantiomers and irreversible binding to plasma protein. *Drug Metab. Disp.* **19,** 1080–1086.
8. Dubois, N., Lapicque, F., Magdalou, J., Abiteboul, M., and Netter, P. (1994) Stereoselective binding of the glucuronide of ketoprofen enantiomers to human serum albumin. *Biochem. Pharmacol.* **48,** 1693–1699.
9. Dubois, N., Lapicque, F., Maurice, M. H., Pritchard, M., Fournel-Gigleux, S., Magdalou, J., et al. (1993) In vitro irreversible binding of ketoprofen glucuronide to plasma proteins. *Drug Metab. Disp.* **21,** 617–623.
10. Castillo, M. and Smith, P. C. (1991) Covalent binding of ibuprofen acyl glucuronide to human serum albumin in vitro. *Pharm. Res.* **10**(suppl.), S242.
11. Castillo, M., Lam, Y. W. M., Dooley, M. A., Stahl, E., and Smith, P. C. (1995) Disposition and covalent binding of ibuprofen and its acyl glucuronide in the elderly. *Clin. Pharmacol. Ther.* **57,** 636–644.

12. Smith, P. C. and Liu, J. H. (1993) Covalent binding of suprofen acyl glucuronide to albumin in vitro. *Xenobiotica* **23,** 337–348.
13. Mizuma, T., Benet, L. Z., and Lin, E. T. (1999) Interaction of human serum albumin with furosemide glucuronide: a role of albumin in isomerization, hydrolysis, reversible binding and irreversible binding of a 1-0-acyl glucuronide metabolite. *Biopharm. Drug Dispos.* **20,** 131–136.
14. Sidelmann, U., Hansen, S. H., Gvaghan, C., Nicholls, A. W., Carless, H. A. J., Lindon, J. C., et al. (1996) Development of simple liquid chromatographic method for the separation of mixtures of positional isomers and anomers of synthetic 2-, 3-, and 4-fluorobenoic acid glucuronides formed via acyl migration reactions. *J. Chromatogr.* **685,** 113–122.
15. Benet, L. Z., Spahn-Langguth, H., Iwakawa, S., Volland, C., Mizuma, T., Mayer, S., et al. (1993) Predictability of the covalent binding of acidic drugs in man. *Life Sci.* **53,** 141–146.
16. Castillo, M., Lam, Y. W. M., Dooley, M. A., Stahl, E., and Smith, P. C. (1995) Disposition and covalent binding of ibuprofen and its acyl glucuronide in the elderly. *Clin. Pharmacol. Ther.* **57,** 636–644.
17. Williams, A. M. and Dickinson, R. G. (1994) Studies on the reactivity of acyl glucuronides: IV. Modulations of reversible and covalent interaction of diflunisal acyl glucuronide and its isomers with human plasma protein in vitro. *Biochem. Pharmacol.* **47,** 457–467.

Index

A

Absorption and permeability, 21
Acetonitrile
  in CYP inhibition studies, 242
  in metabolic stability assays, 152
  and NCE solubility, 157, 160
Acetonitrile and plasma-protein binding assays, 120
Acyl glucuronides. *See also* Glucuronidation
  biosynthesis, in vitro, 387, 388, 401
  degradation, regression analysis, 395
  instability, assessing, 397–398
  isomeric, 386, 400, 402
  kinetic data, calculating, 393–394
  LC-MS/MS assay of, 389–393
  LC-MS/MS separation profile, 390, 391
  migration of, 400
  production of, 399
  quantitation of, 402
  reactivity
    described, 389
    scale, in vitro, 396–397
    in vitro screening model of, 385, 387–388, 392, 393–399, 400
  rearrangement of, 386
  washing procedures, importance of, 400
ADMET properties, evaluating, 2–3
AG337, permeability of, 21
α-glycoprotein (AGP) described, 128–129, 142
Alamethicin and glucuronidation assays, 192–193
Albumin. *See* Human serum albumin (HSA)
Alcohol and lipids in PAMPA, 44
Ames test
  CYP450 in human S9 fractions, 334
  described, 325–326
  materials, 326–328
  methods, 328–331, 332
Amlodipine, permeability of, 21
Amphotericin B in BMEC assays, 78, 79, 80
Association constant (K_a), 129–131
Atenolol, permeability of, 21
ATPase activity coupled enzyme assay, 90–98, 101

B

Bacteria in genotoxicity testing, 315
Barium chloride in ITC, 135–139
β-Galactosidase assay, 319–320, 322
Binding. *See also* Proteins, binding
  capacity number *(n)*, 127, 129–131
  curves, determining, 146
  thermodynamics of, 125–127
Binding in plasma-protein binding experiments, 113–114, 118
Biohazards in drug testing, 331
Biosensor methods for protein binding described, 113

Bjerrum plot, obtaining, 5
Black lipid membrane (BLM)
described, 39, 41
Blood, human, 112, 119, 127–129
Blood–brain barrier (BBB)
cell lines for, 77
and PAMPA, 49, 54
UWL in, 47
BMECs. *See* Bovine brain microvessel endothelial cells (BMECs)
Bovine brain microvessel endothelial cells (BMECs)
culture of, 77–78
materials, 78–82
methods, 82–86
Bovine pancreatic ribonuclease A (RNase A) in ITC, 139–141
Brain microvessels, isolation of, 82–85

C

Caco-2 cell cultures
applications, 20–21, 22
cells, freezing method, 32
CPY3A4 expression in, 22–23, 24
described, 19–20, 22, 41
materials, 23–25
methods, 25–27
model compounds, 21, 24
reproducibility of, 38
transepithelial electrical resistance in, 20
uniformity, maintaining, 32
validating, 21, 32
Calibration curves, preparing, 392, 393
Calorimetry methods of investigation described, 124, 135. *See also* Isothermal titration calorimetry (ITC)
Capacity factor *(k)*, calculating, 117
Cells
Ames test preparation, 331–332
Comet assay, 306–310
counting, 210
cultures
dishes, collagen-coated, 207
hepatocytes, 204, 207, 209, 210–211
inserts, preparing, 25–26
Tk mutant colonies, cleansing, 340–341
trypsin and, 32
yeasts, storage of, 319
hepatic S9
in Ames testing, 325–326, 331
and drug metabolite profiling, 165–166, 167–169
obtaining, 178, 326, 332
preparation of, 179, 330–331, 332–333
MLA, maintenance of, 340–341, 342, 344, 345
seeding onto transwells, 85–86
viability of, measuring, 159
Cephalexin, permeability of, 21
Chinese hamster ovary (CHO)
[^{3}H]Dofetilide binding in, 360–362
and epithelial transport experiments, 104
transfection of, 108–110
Chlophendianol
described, 3, 6
ionization percentage, calculating, 6
lipophilicity/pH profile of, 12
solubility/pH profile of, 8, 9
CHO. *See* Chinese hamster ovary (CHO)

Chromatographic hydrophobicity indices (CHI) and logP values, 10
Chromatographic methods for protein binding described, 113, 116, 117, 120
Chromatography solvents and phosphate content, 297
Cimetidine, metabolism of, 173
Ciprofloxacin, permeability of, 21
Clofilium
  [^{3}H]Dofetilide binding, inhibition of, 359, 365
Cloning in MLA, 344–345
  2'CMP in ITC, 139–141
Collagen/dispase in BMEC assays, 80
Comet assay
  applications, 302, 312
  described, 301–302
  materials, 303–305
  method, 301, 302–303, 305–310
  modifications of, 310–311, 312
  results analysis, 310, 311–312
Comparative enzyme kinetic analysis, 194–195
Concentration-dependent (K_i) inactivation constant, determining, 258
Covalent binding levels, determination of, 391–392, 395–399, 402–403
CPY3A4 expression in Caco-2 cells, 22–23, 24
  18-Crown-6 ether in ITC, 135–139
Cyclosporin A and P-gp activity, 100
Cytochrome P450 (CYP). *See also* Drug-DNA adduct formation
  activity, decreasing, 160
  Ames test in human S9 fractions, 334
  drug–drug interactions and, 231–233, 246
  enzymes
    classification of, 280
    in mammals, 280, 334
    metabolizing, location of, 152, 164
    specificity of, 242
    and toxicity, 280–281
  function of, 163, 164, 246
  human, in drug metabolism, 252
  induction
    by DMSO, 211
    mechanisms, monitoring, 205
    by NCEs, 203–204, 280
    species differences in, 204, 205
  inhibition
    assays, 249–256
    classification of, 238–239, 246
    curves, abnormal, 243
    and drug interaction studies, 231–233, 246
    free radical scavengers, effect of, 250, 258–259
    LC/MS/MS methods, 232–242, 254, 255–256
    and organic substances, 242–243, 253, 260
    screening, processes in, 251
    trapping agents, effect of, 250, 258–259
  inhibitors
    mechanism-based, 245–248
    preparation of, 237, 253–254
    screening of, 248
  kinetic parameters in, 234–235
  microsomal, measuring, 296
  N-oxide metabolites in, 182

probe substrates
Michaelis-Menten plot (K_m, V_{max}), 234, 241
in vitro, 232, 242, 251
recombinant and thiol conjugation, 374–375, 377
stability of, 192, 260
Cytotoxicity, measuring, 344, 347

D

Degradation rate constant, determining, 393–395
Deoxyribonucleic acid. *See* DNA
Desipramine, log permeability vs pH plots, 47, 48
Dexamethasone in hepatocyte culture, 204–205
Dialysis assay
in CYP inhibition, 250, 257, 260
96 well equilibrium dialysis methods described, 113, 114, 115, 117–119, 120
Diclofenac in acyl glucuronide evaluation, 393, 394, 395, 396, 397
Difference curve, obtaining, 5
Dimensionless numbers, creating, 126
Dimethylsulfoxide (DMSO)
in Ames testing, 332
and CYP induction, 211
in drug–transporter interaction assays, 110
and logD values, 12
in PAMPA, 50
solubility and, 13–14
Dispase in BMEC assays, 79, 80
Distribution coefficient *(D)*
defined, 8–9
logD values, 9, 12, 15
and pK_a, 11
Dithiothreitol (DTT) and ITC, 146–147
DMPK, 7, 259
DMSO. *See* Dimethylsulfoxide (DMSO)
DNA
adducts (*See also* Drug-DNA adduct formation)
covalent, formation of, 281
detection of, Comet assay, 302, 312
highest separation of, 276
labeling, 283–284, 294–295
levels, calculating, 292–293
phosphate buffer dosage for, 297
^{32}P labeled, measuring, 266–267, 271–276, 290, 296
TLC evaluation of, 269, 284, 292, 295
binding, radioactive detection of, 296
contamination, avoiding, 267, 268, 275, 297
damage
assessment of, 315–322
detecting, 301, 302, 308–309, 311
damage, detection of, 316–317
enzymatic digestion of, 265, 267–268
extraction efficiency, estimating, 273, 275
hydrolysis of, 282–283, 293–294
isolation of, 264, 267, 282, 287–289
migration, decreasing, 311
repair kinetics, studying, 312
spectrophotometric determination of, 289–290
storage of, 296, 297
[^{3}H]Dofetilide in HERG assays
binding
in CHO, 360–362
concentration dependence, 362

inhibition of, 358, 359, 360, 361, 363, 365
time-course dependence, 360, 363–364
described, 356–357
pharmacology of, 357–360, 364
Drug candidates. *See* New Chemical Entities (NCEs)
Drug-DNA adduct formation. *See also* Cytochrome P450 (CYP); DNA, adducts
assay for evaluating
defined, 281
detection procedures, 282–284, 289–296
DNA isolation, 282, 287–289
incubation procedures, 281–282, 285–287
modifications to, 293
sample preparation, 281, 284–285
Drug–drug interactions and CYP, 231–233, 246
Drug excretion, studying, 20
Drug metabolism and pharmacokinetics (DMPK) studies, 7, 259
Drug metabolite profiling, in vitro
chromatographic methods, 165, 167, 169, 171–172
hepatic cells in, 165–166, 167–169
metabolic pathways, proposed, 172–178
metabolite derivatization, 172
microsomes in, 152, 165–166, 167–169
overview, 163–165
sample preparation, 169, 181
Drug–protein complexes, formation of, 125
Drug–transporter interactions
materials, 104–105
methods, 105–110
overview, 103–104
Dulbecco's modified Eagle's medium recipe, 206–207

E

E-4031 and [^{3}H]Dofetilide inhibition, 359
Eadie-Hofstee plot, 194
EDTA in plasma-protein binding assays, 120
Enthalpy, observed (ΔH), 129–131
Entropy (ΔS) defined, 126, 127
Enzyme-activated irreversible inhibitors. *See* Mechanism-based inhibition
Enzymes
CYP, 152, 164, 242, 280–281, 334
and dialysis, 257
drug-metabolizing, phenotyping, 186
and free radical scavengers, 259
induction of, 203–204
solutions, storage of, 296
Epithelial transport experiments, 20, 104
96 well equilibrium dialysis methods for protein binding described, 113, 114, 115, 117–119, 120
Erythrocytes described, 127
Ethanol
in [^{3}H]Dofetilide assay, 363
in PAMPA, 50
Ethylenediaminetetraacetic acid (EDTA) in plasma-protein binding assays, 120

F

Fibronectin in BMEC assays, 81, 86
Filter properties, PAMPA, 42–44
96 well fluorescence method, 112, 113

Free energy (ΔG) defined, 125–126
Free fraction, calculating, 119
Free radical scavengers, effect of on CYP inhibition, 250, 258–259

G

Genistein, permeability of, 21
Genotoxicity
  and carcinogenesis, 280–281
  DNA damage in, 311
  evaluating, 301–302, 315–322, 337
Gentamycin in BMEC assays, 79, 80, 81
GLpKa described, 5, 11, 13
Glucuronidation. *See also* Acyl glucuronides
  activities, isoform-selective, 195, 196, 199
  assay
    development of, 190–193
    HPLC, 198. 200
    materials, 189
    optimization of, 192–193
  and β-glucuronidase, 200
  described, 185–186, 200
  linearity, ensuring, 200–201
  and the liver, 186
  λmax, determining, 200
Glutathione (GSH)
  classic fragmentations of, 378
  conjugation and raloxifene, 379
  described, 369–371
  electrophilic metabolites and, 372
  hepatocytes and, 371–372
  identification of, 377–379
  and mechanism based inactivation studies, 258–259
  and xenobiotics, 279, 371–372
Glycylsarcosine uptake, inhibition of, 107–108, 109
GSH. *See* Glutathione (GSH)
Guanabenz, permeability of, 21

H

Haloperidol and [^{3}H]Dofetilide inhibition, 359, 365
Heat capacity (ΔCp) defined, 126–127, 138
Heat effect and matrix dilutions, 146
Heat of binding (ΔH_{bind}) defined, 132, 133
HEK293 and epithelial transport experiments, 104
Hela and epithelial transport experiments, 104
Heparin, 81, 120
Hepatic S9 cells
  in Ames testing, 325–326, 331
  and drug metabolite profiling, 165–166, 167–169
  obtaining, 178, 326, 332
  preparation of, 179, 330–331, 332–333
Hepatocytes
  and compound stability, 153
  confluency in, 210–211
  cryopreserved, thawing, 158
  culture/treatment of, 204, 207, 209, 210–211
  and drug metabolite profiling, 165
  enzyme induction in, 203–204
  and glutathione, 371–372
  harvesting of, 208, 210
  isolation of, 206–207, 208–209, 375
  metabolic stability assessment, 155–156, 158–159
  microsomal CYP, measuring, 211–212
  obtaining, 152
  plated, 153–154
  in vitro incubation of, 377

HEPES in BMEC assays, 79, 80, 81, 86
HERG gene
binding
concentration dependence, 362
inhibition of, 358, 359, 360, 361, 365
time-course dependence of, 360, 363–364
and drug candidate evaluation, 353–354
high-throughput binding assay for, 354–356
High performance liquid chromatography (HPLC)
in drug metabolite profiling, 167, 170, 171
enhancements of, 199, 200, 201
glucuronides, assay methods, 198, 200
phosphate buffer in, 376
^{32}P labeled DNA adducts, measuring, 266–267, 272–273, 274, 276
^{32}P postlabeling/PAGE analysis described, 263, 264
reverse-phase HPLC and logP values, 10
thiol conjugates, detecting, 373, 376
Homogenization buffer, liver perfusion, 208
HPLC. *See* High performance liquid chromatography (HPLC)
HSA. *See* Human serum albumin (HSA)
Human serum albumin (HSA)
binding sites in, 128
covalent binding, evaluating, 391–392, 399
in ITC, 143–146
Hydrocarbons in PAMPA, 44–45
Hydrodynamic methods of investigation described, 124
Hydrolysis defined, 393

I

IC_{50} values
determining, 237–238, 240–242, 256, 260
and irreversible inhibitors, 239
Inactivation rate constants, determination of, 258
Indole binding site, 128, 143
Inhibitor molecule defined, 97, 100
International Conference on Harmonisation described, 360
Intestinal barrier-based metabolism, predicting, 38, 72–73
Intrinsic clearance values (V_{max}/K_m). *See* Michaelis-Menten plot (K_m, V_{max})
Intrinsic clearance values (V_{max}/K_m), calculating, 194
Ionization percentage, calculating, 6
Irreversible inhibition of CYPs described, 238–239
Isoforms, identification of, 194
Isomerization
in acyl glucuronides, 386, 400, 402
and covalent binding, 402–403
defined, 393, 394
Isothermal titration calorimetry (ITC)
2'CMP in, 139–141
18-Crown-6 ether in, 135–139
barium chloride in, 135–139
binding capacity number *(n)*, determining, 129–131
binding-site models in, 132–134
calculations, 129–131
described, 123–125, 132
dithiothreitol (DTT) and, 146–147

human serum albumin (HSA) in, 143–146
injection parameters in, 147
materials, 129–130, 134–135
and pH, 136
RNase A in, 139–141
warfarin and sample preparation, 144

K

Kinetic parameters, determining, 235–237
Kinetic solubility, measuring, 7

L

LC/MS assay
adducted molecular ions in, 181–182
in drug metabolite profiling, 167, 171–172
gradient issues, 14
ionization, enhancing, 181
lipophilicity, 3, 10–11, 14–15
in metabolic stability assays, 155
pK_a, 3–6
solubilizers and permeability, 3, 6–8, 53, 57
sonication in, 14
LC/MS/MS
and acyl glucuronide screening, 389–393
and compound stability, 242
in CYP inhibition studies, 232–242, 254, 255–256
in drug metabolite profiling, 167, 171–172
in metabolic stability assays, 154–155, 159–160
Li formate, preparation of, 297
Linopirdine, permeability of, 21
Lipophilicity
described, 1, 2, 8–9
LC/MS assay, 3, 10–11, 14–15
profile and pH, 9–10
Lipoproteins, binding in, 129
Liver perfusion
efficiency, increasing, 210
materials, 205–208
methods, 208–210
logD values, 9, 12, 15. *See also* Distribution coefficient *(D)*
logP values, 9, 10, 11, 15. *See also* Partition coefficient *(P)*
Long QT syndrome and HERG, 353, 354

M

Madin Darby canine kidney (MDCK) and epithelial transport experiments, 20, 104
Mammals, 280, 315, 334
Mannitol, permeability of, 21
Mass spectrography methods described, 376, 379
MDCK. *See* Madin Darby canine kidney (MDCK)
Mechanism-based inhibition
defined, 245, 246–248, 256
high-throughput screening for, 251–256
identifying, 255, 257
MEM in BMEC assays, 79, 80, 81
Metabolic stability, 151–154
Metabolism-based inhibition
defined, 245, 246, 256
identifying, 255, 257
Metabolites
efflux rate, calculating, 29, 38
identity, confirmation of, 192
multiple specific detecting, 239–240
Methanol
[^{3}H]Dofetilide assay for HERG binding, 363
in the Comet assay, 304

in CYP inhibition studies, 242, 253, 260
in metabolic stability assays, 152
and NCE solubility, 157, 160
Michaelis-Menten plot (K_m, V_{max})
CYP probe substrates, 234, 241
intrinsic clearance values (V_{max}/K_m), calculating, 194
non-Michaelis-Menten kinetics defined, 243
transport values, estimating, 66
validity of, 242
Microscale shake-flask method, 3, 10–11, 14
Microsomes
assay method, 156–158, 161
coincubation, 254–255
and drug metabolite profiling, 152, 165–166, 167–169
incubation, 155, 236–237, 238, 254, 374, 376
isolation of, 374
sources, 232
substrate mixtures, 238
MLA. *See* Mouse lymphoma assay (MLA)
Modified Chee's Medium (MCM), 207
Mouse lymphoma assay (MLA)
calculations, 346–348
cells, maintenance of, 340–341, 342, 344, 345
cloning, 344–345
controls in, 342
criteria for, 348–349
culture media for, 339–340, 344, 349
described, 337–338
materials, 338–339
mycoplasma contamination in, 341
S9 mix, 341
sample data for, 343
stock solutions/concentrations, 341–342
Mutagenicity testing, 328–330, 333
Mutant frequency (MF), calculating, 346, 347
Mycoplasma contamination in MLA, 341

N

Nadolol, permeability of, 21
NADPH
dependency, evaluating, 256–257
regenerating system in metabolic stability assessment, 157, 181, 236
Naproxen and transport, 51
n-Butanol enrichment procedure, 283, 284, 293, 294, 295
NCEs. *See* New Chemical Entities (NCEs)
New Chemical Entities (NCEs)
absorption characteristics, classifying, 19, 20, 65, 66
approval requirements for, 280
blood concentration, determining, 112, 119
CNS, screening, 77
cytochrome induction by, 203–204, 205, 280
and drug-drug interaction studies, 248–249
energetics, investigating, 123–125
free fraction, calculating, 119
genotoxicity screening of, 302, 315
and HERG interaction, evaluating, 353
intestinal metabolism, determining, 22
leaching of in assays, 106–107
low solubility, analyzing, 45
mutagenicity, evaluating, 325

permeability, calculating, 27
plasma-protein binding experiments, conduct of, 114–116
ranking, 7, 151
solubility limits in, 6–7, 45, 157, 160
stability, assessing, 33, 74–75, 120, 159, 160
stock solution preparation for metabolic stability assessment, 157, 161

Nicardipine and P-gp activity, 100
Non-Michaelis-Menten kinetics defined, 243
Nuclease P1 enrichment procedure, 283, 284, 293, 294, 295
Nucleotides
adducted, labeling, 266, 268
quantifying, 295–296

O

Octadiene in PAMPA, 50
Oligomer concentration, determining, 273

P

PAMPA. *See* Parallel artificial membrane permeability assay (PAMPA)
Parallel artificial membrane permeability assay (PAMPA)
assay variables, 42–46, 48–49
basis of, 39
BBB models in, 49, 54
BM-PAMPA, 49–51
buffer solutions, properties of, 45–46, 58–59
cosolvents in, 57
described, 37–39, 41, 42
detection methods in, 46
DS-PAMPA, 51–52, 53
filter properties, 42–44
in formulation research, 53
gradient pH methods, 56–57
history of, 39–42
hydrocarbons in, 44–45
impure compounds, 58
international symposium url, 41
iso-pH conditions in, 51, 56
lamella schematic, 44
lipid composition in, 44–45
low water solubility compounds, 57
materials, 50, 54–55
methods, 54, 55–59
pION system solution, 58–59
scavengers in, 51–52
and unstirred water layers (UWL), 46–48

Partition coefficient (P)
defined, 8–9
determining via PAMPA, 53
factors influencing, 247
logP values, 9, 10, 11, 15
and pK_a, 11

pcDNA3 expression vector schematic, 356
Penicillin G in BMEC assays, 78–79, 80, 81
PEPT1, 104–110
Percent recovery, calculating, 27–28, 30
Perfusion. *See* Liver perfusion; Rat *in situ* perfusion
Permeability
absorption and, 21
calculating, 27, 38, 43, 49, 52
coefficient expressed, 86
K_m values in transport, estimating, 66
and LC/MS assay solubilizers, 3, 6–8, 53, 57
pH and, 47–48, 50

rat *in situ* perfusion, 53, 71–73
of various compounds, 21
P-glycoprotein (P-gp)
ATPase activity
materials, 91
measuring, 90–91
methods, 91–98
troubleshooting, 98
binding sites on, 100
data analysis, 96–98
described, 89–90, 97, 98–99, 100
membrane preparation, 99
multispecific recognition property of, 101
plate properties, 92–93, 95–96
reagent distribution protocol, 94
and temperature regulation, 99
pH
chlophendianol, profile of, 8, 9, 12
and ITC, 136
lipophilicity profile, 9–10
and logP values, 11
and PAMPA, 46, 51, 56–57
permeability and, 47–48, 50
solubility and, 13
titration table for, 60
Phenylalanine, permeability of, 21
Phosphate buffer preparation, 156–157, 161, 200
Phosphatidylcholine in PAMPA, 44–45
Pimozide and [^{3}H]Dofetilide inhibition, 359, 365
pK_a
association constant (K_a), 125, 131
described, 1, 2, 4, 11
distribution coefficient *(D)* and, 11
LC/MS assay, 3–6
potentiometric titration method, 4–5
water-insoluble compounds, 5
Yasuda-Shedlovsky plot and, 5–6, 13
Plasma
harvesting, 120
obtaining, 127
to protein binding methods, 6, 111–116, 118, 120
proteins, properties of, 127–128
Plating efficiency (PE), calculating, 346, 347
Polymixin B in BMEC assays, 78, 79, 80
Porosity, apparent calculating, 43
^{32}P postlabeling analysis
described, 263–264, 265, 290–291
in DNA adduction formation analysis, 266–267, 271–276, 290, 296
materials, 264–267
^{32}P postlabeling/PAGE analysis, 263, 264, 266, 269–271
Progesterone and P-gp activity, 91, 97, 100
Propanolol
and AGP binding, 142–143
in PAMPA, 50
permeability of, 21
Proteins
binding
chromatographic methods for described, 113, 116, 117, 120
96 well equilibrium dialysis methods described, 113, 114, 115, 117–119, 120
minimizing, 242
sites in, 127
96 well ultrafiltration methods described, 113, 114, 116–119, 120
encoded, measuring, 103–104
plasma, properties of, 127–128
plasma-protein binding methods, 6, 111–116, 118, 120

recombinant, limitations of, 146
removal of, 287
starting concentration, estimating, 146

Q

Quinine in PAMPA, 50

R

RAL, calculating, 271–272, 273, 292–293
Raloxifene, 379, 380
Rat *in situ* perfusion
described, 65–67
materials, 67–68, 73–74
methods, 68–70, 73–74, 75
permeability, calculating, 53, 71–73
sample analysis, 70–71
vs DS PAMPA permeabilities, 53
Reagent preparation, Comet assay, 304–305
Regression analysis, acyl glucuronide degradation, 395
Relative adduct levels (RAL), calculating, 271–272, 273, 292–293
Relative total growth (RTG), calculating, 347–348
Reporter gene systems
creation of, 318
in DNA damage detection, 316–317
drug dose optimization, 319, 321–322
Reverse-phase HPLC and logP values, 10
Reversible inhibition of CYPs described, 238
RNase, 139–141, 275
RNR3-lacZ fusion gene, 317, 320–321, 322
RPMI 1640 medium in MLA, 349
Rule of Five defined, 9–10
RWJ-34130, in vitro metabolism of, 172–173
RWJ-52763, in vitro metabolism of, 174, 175, 176, 177
RWJ-68025, in vitro metabolism of, 174, 177, 178, 179, 180

S

S9 cells
in Ames testing, 325–326, 331
and drug metabolite profiling, 165–166, 167–169
obtaining, 178, 326, 332
preparation of, 179, 330–331, 332–333
Saccharolactone and glucuronidation assays, 193
Saccharomyces cervisiae in genotoxicity testing, 316
Scavengers in PAMPA, 51–52
SCGE. *See* Comet assay
Shake-flask method described, 3, 10–11, 14
Simvastatin, permeability of, 21
Single cell gel electrophoresis (SCGE). *See* Comet assay
Slide preparation, Comet assay, 304
Solubility
chlophendianol profile, 8, 9
in CYP inhibition studies, 260
described, 1, 2, 6, 7
and dimethylsulfoxide (DMSO), 13–14
LC/MS assay, 3, 6–8, 53, 57
of NCEs, 6–7, 45, 157, 160
pH and, 13
and plasma protein binding, 6
Solvents, water-soluble in PAMPA, 44

Spectroscopy methods of investigation described, 124
Stirring speed and UWL, hydrodynamic equation, 48
Stoichiometry defined, 127
Storage phosphor imaging defined, 292
Streptomycin in BMEC assays, 78–79, 80, 81
Substrates
- concentrations, CYP450 inhibition studies, 242
- CYP450 probe substrates
  - Michaelis-Menten plot (K_m, V_{max}), 234, 241
  - in vitro, 232, 242, 251
- microsome mixtures, 238
- molecule defined, 97, 100
- uncompetitive substrate inhibition equation, 194

Suicide substrates. *See* Mechanism-based inhibition
Sulfasalazine, permeability of, 21
Sulpiride, permeability of, 21
Surface plasmon resonance (SPR) described, 112, 114

T

Terfenadine and [^{3}H]Dofetilide inhibition, 359, 365
Testosterone, permeability of, 21
Thin-layer chromatography (TLC)
- in DNA adduct evaluation, 269, 284, 292, 295
- in drug metabolite profiling, 165, 167, 169, 171

Thiol conjugates
- classic fragmentations of, 378
- rCYP450 and, 374–375, 377
- in vitro detection of, 369, 373–376, 379

Time-dependent (K_{intact}) inactivation constant, determining, 258
Timolol in PAMPA, 50
Titration, 13, 60. *See also* Isothermal titration calorimetry (ITC)
Tk mutant colonies, 338, 340–341
Total concentration of drug $[D]_t$ defined, 134
Total heat content *(Q)* defined, 133–134
Toxicity
- and CYP enzymes, 280–281
- DNA damage in, 311
- evaluating, 301–302, 315–322, 337
- measuring, 344, 347

Transport
- active processes, predicting, 38
- bidirectional, studying, 104
- drug–transporter interactions, 103–110
- epithelial, 20, 104
- experiments, performing, 20, 26–27
- K_m values, estimating, 66
- measurements and ATPase assays, 101
- mechanisms, determining, 22, 30, 67
- naproxen and, 51
- rates, obtaining, 27, 29, 31
- UWL in, 47–48
- in vivo, modeling, 47

Trapping agents, effect of on CYP inhibition, 250, 258–259
Trojan horses. *See* Mechanism-based inhibition
Trypan Blue Exclusion method, 159
Trypsin and cell culture, 32
Two enzyme model equations for kinetic analysis, 194

U

UDP-glucuronosyltransferases (UGTs)
  chemical inhibition of, 190
  and drug metabolism, 185–186
  identifying, 186, 189
  isoforms, 187–188, 199
  marker activities, 190, 197
  recombinant (rUGT), activity screen with, 193, 197
  stability of, 192
UGTs. *See* UDP-glucuronosyl-transferases (UGTs)
96 well ultrafiltration methods for protein binding described, 113, 114, 116–119, 120
Uncompetitive substrate inhibition equation, 194
Unstirred water layers (UWL), 46–49
in the BBB, 47
UWL, 46–49

V

Valacyclovir
  and drug-transporter interactions, 104–110
  glycylsarcosine uptake, inhibition of, 107–108, 109
  uptake, concentration dependence of, 107–108
  uptake, time course of, 105–107
Valproic acid, product mass ion spectra, 381
Verapamil
  and permeability screening, 38
  P-gp activity and, 91, 97, 100
Vinblastine and P-gp activity, 91, 97, 100

W

Warfarin
  binding site, 128, 143, 145–146
  permeability of, 21
  sample preparation, ITC, 144
Water, deionized in CYP inhibition studies, 242

X

Xenobiotics, 279, 371–372
Xenopus laevis and membrane protein studies, 103

Y

Yasuda-Shedlovsky plot and pK_a values, 5–6, 13
Yeasts
  cell cultures, storage of, 319
  in genotoxicity testing, 315–316
  reporter strain, creation of, 318